ISGE Series

Series Editor

Andrea R. Genazzani

More information about this series at http://www.springer.com/series/11871

Charles Sultan • Andrea R. Genazzani
Editors

Frontiers in Gynecological Endocrinology

Volume 4: Pediatric and Adolescent Gynecological Endocrinology

Springer

INTERNATIONAL SCHOOL OF GYNECOLOGICAL AND REPRODUCTIVE ENDOCRINOLOGY
THE EDUCATIONAL BRANCH OF ISGE

Editors
Charles Sultan
Département Hormonologie
Hôpital Lapeyronie
CHU et Université Montpellier
Unité d'Endocrinologie et Gynécologie
Pédiatriques, Département de Pédiatrie
Hôpital Arnaud-de-Villeneuve
CHU et Université Montpellier
Montpellier
France

Andrea R. Genazzani
International Society of Gynecological
Endocrinology
Pisa
Italy

ISSN 2197-8735 ISSN 2197-8743 (electronic)
ISGE Series
ISBN 978-3-319-41431-7 ISBN 978-3-319-41433-1 (eBook)
DOI 10.1007/978-3-319-41433-1

Library of Congress Control Number: 2017932280

Printed on acid-free paper

This Springer imprint is published by Springer Nature
The registered company is Springer International Publishing AG
The registered company address is: Gewerbestrasse 11, 6330 Cham, Switzerland

Preface

We are delighted to announce the publication of another important issue in the International Society of Gynecological Endocrinology series.

This volume 4 presents important clinical and scientific data on subjects of major clinical and physiological interest, namely adolescent gynecology, presented by international opinion leaders during the ISGRE Summer School organized in Montpellier, France.

The adolescent girl is no longer a child, but not yet an adult and, for this reason, the management of adolescent endocrinology and gynecological diseases is quite specific.

Pediatric and adolescent gynecology is now a well recognized field of medicine and surgery, at the crossroads of most of the specific problems of developmental and reproductive issues. This specific area has always been of particular interest to physicians in the interface of pediatrics, gynecology, and endocrinology.

This volume presents new clinical and scientific data and includes topics of great interest, including anomalies of pubertal development, and other subjects of direct clinical relevance, such as disorders of menstrual cycles, sexuality, contraception, and pregnancy in adolescents.

This is a very well balanced edition. We are convinced that this new addition to the series will prove of great value to all pediatricians, gynecologists, endocrinologists, psychiatrics, surgeons, and public health specialists concerned with adolescent gynecology.

Montpellier, France — Charles Sultan
Pisa, Italy — Andrea R. Genazzani

Contents

Dimorphism of Human Brain: The Basis of the Gender Differences

1

Andrea R. Genazzani, Andrea Giannini, and Tommaso Simoncini

For mammals, sexual differentiation starts at conception when a fetus inherits a couple of heterologous (XY) or homologous (XX) sex chromosomes. Until the sixth week of gestation embryonal gonadal development is bi-potential, than, according to genetic sex, embryonal gonads differentiate in testes or ovaries. In presence of Y chromosome, fetus will develop testes; hormonal products of the testes, mainly testosterone, then induce the male phenotype by early permanent programming or organizational effects and later transient acute or activational effects, which disappear after withdrawal of the hormones. In the absence of Y chromosome, the fetus develops ovaries, and in the absence of male-like levels of testosterone, the female phenotype emerges. The activating effects of ovarian hormones together with endocrine and exogenous influences enhance female characteristics at puberty and beyond determining phenotyping sex [1].

Several studies affirm that gonadal determination may be controlled by various genes, such as gene Sex-determining Region Y (SRY) on short arm of Y chromosome (Yp11) involved in gonadal differentiation to testes. SRY codes for a protein containing sequence High Motility Group box (HMG) which is transient expressed in cells planned to become Sertoli cells. Moreover, gonadal determination seems to be influenced by genes, in particular, Wilm's tumor-related gene-1 (WT-1) and steroidogenic factor-1 (SF-1). Mutations of these genes in both male and female sexes are involved in the pathogenesis of agenesis and dysgenesis gonadal syndrome. It is evident that primordial gonads are inclined to an intrinsic development to female gonads and only the presence of genetic factors on Y chromosome or activated by developing testes are able to masculinize. Currently only one gene coded on X chromosome (Xp21.3), dosage-sensitive sex reversal-adrenal hypoplasia congenital on

A.R. Genazzani (✉) • A. Giannini • T. Simoncini, MD, PhD
Division of Obstetrics and Gynecology, Department of Experimental and Clinical Medicine, University of Pisa, Via Roma, 67, 56100 Pisa, Italy
e-mail: argenazzani@gmail.com; tommaso.simoncini@med.unipi.it

C. Sultan, A.R. Genazzani (eds.), *Frontiers in Gynecological Endocrinology*, ISGE Series, DOI 10.1007/978-3-319-41433-1_1

the X chromosome (DAX-1) seems to prevent possible gonadal evolution to testes in female mammals [2].

Sex chromosomes play a direct role in establishing sex differences throughout the body including the brain, thus some differences depend on chromosomal constitution and are gonadal independent. Nonetheless, increasing evidences suggest that for the large majority of neural sex differences, the modifications in gonadal hormones seem to play a dominant role. Sex differences in the central nervous system (CNS), probably may develop to direct actions of gonadal steroids which can determine neural tissue differentiation, moreover, sexual differentiation of CNS occur later than gonadal differentiation thus both processes can be independently influenced [3].

Steroid hormones synthesized by the gonads and adrenal glands easily cross the blood–brain and the blood–nerve barriers and rapidly accumulate within the nervous tissues, except for their conjugated forms such as the steroid sulfates, which cannot easily enter the brain. Neurons and glial cells possess enzymes necessary for progesterone, testosterone, dehydroepiandrosterone (DHEA), and estradiol metabolism (aromatase, 5-alpha reductase (5a-R), mainly in neurons, 3-alpha-hydroxysteroid dehydrogenase (3a-HSD), mainly in type 1 astrocytes). The activities of these steroid-metabolizing enzymes are strongly influenced by the differentiation process of the precursor stem cells into terminally differentiated CNS cells. Neurons and glial cells coordinately metabolize steroid hormones, thus forming a functional unit; as both the endocrine glands and the local metabolism contribute to the pool of steroids present in the nervous tissues and the sex and age-dependent changes in circulating levels of steroid hormones may reflect changes in brain levels. While steroid-metabolizing enzymes induce the CNS to be able to modify circulating steroids, the CNS is also able to synthesize steroids from cholesterol, at least in part, independently of peripheral steroidogenic glands secretion leading to the production of a series of potent steroidal compounds. These brain-produced steroids have been named “neurosteroids”, and have been found to exert important regulatory actions on neurons and glial cells [4] (Fig. 1.1).

The so called “neurosteroids” influence the neurobiology of sexual function acting by genomic or non-genomic effects. Genomic actions of neurosteroids are carried out directly interacting with their receptors at nuclear membrane level or indirectly throughout their effects on neuropeptides (oxytocin, beta-endorphin, etc.), neurotransmitters (dopamine, serotonin), and neurosteroids metabolites (mainly allopregnanolone). Non-genomic actions are mediated through integrate or associated membrane receptors and the activation of intracellular cascades of events determining rapid neuronal and pituitary activation via biochemical pathways of AMPc and MAP-kinases; thus resulting in a modulation of Ca2+ channels and exerting neuroprotective effects in contrast to neurotoxins and oxidative stress [5].

Estrogens have long been known to play a crucial role on coordinating many neuroendocrine events that control sexual development, sexual behavior, and reproduction. 17-β-estradiol is the primary biologically active form of estrogen in mammals which is critical for sexual differentiation of the brain, indeed it organizes neural circuits and regulates apoptosis of neurons leading to long-term differences

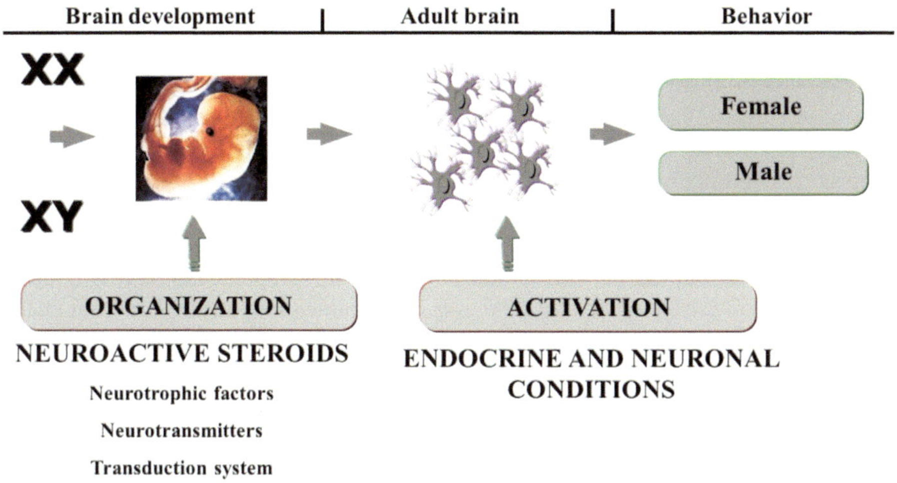

Fig. 1.1 Brain sexual differentiation is a multisignaling process presenting sex steroids as key modulators in different steps

in the male and the female brain. In addition to its role in development, estradiol prevents neuronal cell death in a variety of brain injury models, modulates learning and memory, and promotes the formation of synapses as well as cellular apoptosis. The physiological effects resulting from estradiol actions in target tissues are mediated primarily by two intracellular receptors ERα and ERβ. Both estrogen receptors together with progesterone receptors A and B (PR-A, PR-B) and androgens receptors (ARs) are observed in neurons and glia in the brain and are expressed throughout the brain with distinct patterns in different brain regions and with different levels of expression in males and females during development and in adulthood. Consequently, sexual dimorphism of human brain seems to be characterized by functional and structural differences. Functional differences are determined by hormonal and enzymatic actions or pathway modulating masculinization or feminization of different regions of CNS, while structural differences are determined by different distribution of ERs, ARs, PRs, enzymatic isoforms, and neuronal population in different cerebral areas [6].

Relating to functional differences, as previously mentioned, 17-β-estradiol is a crucial biologically active form of steroid in mammals involved in sexual differentiation of the brain, nonetheless, several experimental and pre-clinical data suggested that testosterone (T), acting on the brain, seems to regulate reproductive function, sexuality, and emotional behaviors in both sexes in a different gender-related fashion. In addition, T exerts analgesic and anxiolytic properties, affects mood and cognition, and promotes synaptic plasticity in the rat model. T also prevents neuronal death in different experimental models of neurodegeneration, and decreased T levels in plasma may represent a risk factor for the development of neurodegenerative diseases in humans. T brain effects may be directed or modulated by its metabolites, therefore, T can be aromatized to estrogen or metabolized to dihydrotestosterone (DHT) by 5a-reductase (5a-R), and DHT can be further reduced by 3-hydroxysteroid dehydrogenase (3-HSD) to 3-androstanediol (3-diol), a neurosteroid Gamma-Aminobutyric Acid-Aergic (GABA-A) agonist with anxiolytic properties. These two enzymatic pathways, aromatase and 5a-R-3HSD, are widely distributed in CNS, affecting reproductive (i.e., hypothalamus) and non-reproductive function (i.e., hippocampus, cortex) of gonadal steroids [7].

Interestingly, DHEA and its sulfate metabolite DHEA-S may act on CNS differentiation directly, by modulating several activities in different neuronal populations or as substrate for the conversion in T and DHT in such CNS target regions of androgens and estrogens. In this view, it is remarkable to highlight that brain DHEA and DHEA-S concentrations are 5–6 times higher than peripheral concentrations and several pre-clinical studies demonstrated the presence of steroidal precursors such as cholesterol and lipid derivates in mammalian brain. The effects of DHEA and DHEA-S on CNS are mediated by direct interaction with GABA-A receptors, thus blocking Cl^- channels in a dose-dependent manner and resulting in increased neuronal excitability. Experimental data also suggested putative effects of DHEA on N-methyl-D-aspartate (NMDA) and sigma (λ) receptors. DHEA administration to gonadectomized rats increased concentrations of neurosteroids not related to DHEA metabolism such as allopregnanolone (3-hydroxy-5-pregnan-20-one) (AP), in the hippocampus, in the hypothalamus, in pituitary, and in peripheral circulation and improved mnemonic ability, thus suggesting neurotrophic effects on neurons and glia cells. Moreover, gonadectomy reduced synaptic density on dendritic spines and CA1 pyramidal neurons in both male and female rats while T and DHT administrations are able to reestablish that. In this view, it has been hypothesized that the preservation of physiologic synaptic density may be an androgen-dependent process which can be elicited with different gender-specific mechanisms since that in male rats, contrary to female rats, it is not necessary synthesis of intermediate estrogens. Moreover, the ability to restore hippocampal synaptic density is not directly related to androgenic potency since that it has been demonstrated that DHEA and DHT stimulation activity on dendritic density are similar [8].

Estrogens can also increase the activity of the enzymatic pathway (5a-R)—3-hydroxysteroid-oxidoreductase, which converts progesterone into 5-dihydroprogesterone and AP, respectively. Progesterone and synthetic progestins can affect brain and peripheral content of AP divergently, both in humans and in experimental animals, suggesting distinct hormonal effects on the enzymatic pathways involved in the synthesis and release of these neurosteroids [9]. AP is a neurosteroid produced by the central nervous system, adrenals, and ovaries. AP is a 3-, 5- reduced metabolite of progesterone by the complex 5a-R-3HSD. It is a potent endogenous steroid that rapidly affects the excitability of neurons and glia cells through direct modulation of the GABA-A receptors activity. AP exerts neuropharmacological properties with hypnotic/ sedative, anxiolytic, anesthetic, analgesic, and anticonvulsive function [10]. In addition, AP exhibit neurotrophic/neuroprotective actions, reducing cell death, gliosis, and functional deficits after traumatic brain injury in rats and in experimental models of Alzheimer's disease, enhancing myelination/remyelination process. Interestingly, several experimental studies suggest that

AP positively affects all aspects of sociosexual activities, enhancing exploratory, antianxiety, social, and sexual function [11].

Genazzani and collaborators, in experimental work on male and female gonadectomized rats model, studied the effects of the administration of subcutaneous T at the dose of 10–100 μg/kg/day for female rats, and 1–5 mg/kg/day for male rats, or DHT at the doses of 1–10 and 100 μg/kg/day for females, and 0, 1–1 and 5 mg/kg/day for males, or E2V (0.05 mg/Kg/day). Ovariectomy (OVX) and orchidectomy (OCX) induced a significant decrease in AP in frontal and parietal lobe, hippocampus, hypothalamus, anterior pituitary, as well as in serum. In OVX rats, T replacement, as well as E2V, significantly increased AP content in all brain areas and in peripheral circulation, whereas in OCX, T and E2V did not actively result in influencing AP concentration in frontal and parietal lobe, while it produced a significant rise in AP levels in the hippocampus, hypothalamus, anterior pituitary, and serum. Conversely, DHT replacement had no effect on AP levels anywhere or at any administered dose, either in males or in female rats. The author concluded that gender difference and T therapy may affect brain AP synthesis/release during the reproductive aging. This effect becomes particularly evident in the brain of OVX animals, where the content of this specific neurosteroid is much more responsive than male animals to testosterone replacement. Moreover, it has been suggested that T administration should be, at least in part, dependent on a gender difference in the aromatase activity; therefore, a sexually dimorphic activity of aromatase is widely described during the fetal and postnatal life, and also, the expression and the activity of this enzyme were dimorphically affected by gonadectomy and by T replacement, supporting the hypothesis of differential enzymatic regulation also for neurosteroidogenesis [12].

The same group, focusing the attention on the homeostasis of CNS and the role of neurosteroids in the hormonal setting, investigated the gender response of endogenous opioid system to hormonal changes. The endogenous opioid system modulates responses to stress, learning and memory acquisition; it is involved in emotional regulation, pain mechanisms, and the reward system, and it is altered in various pathological states. β-endorphin (β-END) is the endogenous opiate that has received the most attention. It has been speculated that β-END may play a key role in the mechanism of sexual arousal and pleasure in both sexes and its effects seems to be inversely dose-related therefore, the administration of low physiological dose of opiate have facilitative effects and high dose exhibit inhibitory effects. Similarly, the administration of naloxone at low doses to women was able to enhance pleasure during orgasm while higher doses show contrary effects, reducing sexual arousal and orgasmic pleasure. In addition, the administration of exogenous opiates can induce an intense feeling of pleasure which has been associated to orgasm, followed by a state of relaxation and calm. Gonadal steroids are increasingly recognized as crucial factors modulating the endogenous opioid system in both sexes, suggesting the presence of additional hormone-related, neurobiological mechanisms for gender difference in brain function. The administration of above-mentioned doses of T, DHT, and E2V to male and female gonadectomized rats showed relevant results. T administration to OVX rats exerted a powerful impact on the endogenous endorphin system; therefore, it enhanced β-END concentration not only at hypothalamic level but also in several hypothalamic structures, affecting the activity of endorphinergic neurons in the hippocampus as well as in the frontal and parietal lobes. In contrast, the endorphin content of these hypothalamic structures was not affected in male rats by orchidectomy or by any steroid replacement therapy; thus suggesting that the cerebral structures receiving the endorphinergic peptide exhibit a sex-based difference in opioid system sensitivity to gonadal hormones. Since the effect of estrogen treatment was the same for both sexes, the physiological basis for this sex difference in β-END sensitivity to T therapy might depend, at least in part, on a sex difference in aromatase activity; the authors concluded that sexually dimorphic aromatase activity characterized fetal and postnatal life and this study highlighted that the expression and the activity of the enzyme were dimorphically affected by castration and T replacement [13].

As previously mentioned, structural differences are determined by different distribution of ERs, ARs, PRs, enzymatic isoforms, and neuronal population in different cerebral areas. In particular, ERα and ERβ are expressed in the amygdala, the hippocampus, in different areas of cerebral cortex, in the cerebellum, and in the hypothalamus where estrogen may determine structural and behavioral sex-specific characteristics.

Two brain regions that show robust estradiol-induced organizational changes are the preoptic area (POA) and medial basal hypothalamus (MBH), both of which are critical for sexual behavior. Estradiol-induced organizational changes are perhaps best exemplified within the POA, an area containing the medial preoptic nucleus (MPN), the sexually dimorphic nucleus of the preoptic area (SDN-POA), and the anteroventral periventricular nucleus (AVPV). The MPN is critical to the control of male sexual behavior and the SDN-POA is a sub-region within this nucleus that has been implicated in partner preference [14]. The AVPV is important for gonadotropin secretion and is believed to be the source of control of the LH surge essential for ovulation in adult females [15]. In the perinatal male brain, estradiol derived from testosterone stimulates opposing events in the SDN and AVPV, protecting neurons within the SDN-POA from apoptosis by enhancing NMDA receptor expression, while provoking expression of proapoptotic proteins such as TRIP, Bad, and Bax to induce apoptosis in the AVPV [16, 17]. In addition to modulating cell death, estradiol also mediates sex differences in synaptic patterning in the MPN by inducing synthesis of the cyclooxygenase enzymes, COX-1 and COX-2, thereby increasing the production of prostaglandin-E2 [18]. Acting via the EP2 and EP4 receptors, PGE2 activates protein kinase A and allows for glutamate-induced activation of AMPA receptors and formation of dendritic spines, the postsynaptic contact points for excitatory synapses [19]. Ultimately, the increased production of PGE2 in the male brain results in a two to three times higher density of dendritic spine synapses compared to females, and interestingly, this higher spine density positively correlates with the degree of masculinization of sexual behavior [20]. Thus, three key cellular responses, cell survival, cell death, and synaptogenesis, are all mediated by estradiol within one brain region, the preoptic area. The divergent effects of estradiol are mediated via the estrogen receptor (ER), in particular the ERα isoform. In addition to exerting organizational effects on the physiology of the POA, estradiol also induces permanent changes in synaptic connectivity in the MBH. The ventromedial nucleus of the hypothalamus (VMN) is a key region for regulating female sexual behavior. Within the VMN, male neurons have twice the number of dendritic spines and more dendritic branches than females as a result of neonatal hormone exposure. Estradiol produces sex differences in synaptic organization in this region by rapid activation of PI3-kinase which enhances glutamate release from presynaptic cells, thus provoking dendritic spine outgrowth from postsynaptic neurons. Here, too, the ERα isoform is the critical mediator of estradiol action, although the initiating steps in the signal transduction cascade appear to begin at the membrane via rapid activation of PI3 kinase, and more interestingly, the requirement for ER is restricted to the presynaptic membrane despite the induction of changes in neuronal morphology within the postsynaptic neuron. The enduring organizational changes produced by estradiol within the neonatal brain enable circulating gonadal hormones in the adult to activate sexually differentiated brain regions, such as the POA and the MBH, in a sex-specific manner. Thus, in adulthood, estrogens and progesterone act on a female brain to regulate pulsatile LH release and induce estrous cyclicity and female sexual receptivity, whereas testosterone reaches a masculinized adult brain to activate male sexual behavior [19].

As a concluding remark, some sex differences may cause differences in function, in other cases sex differences exist to ensure that function is similar in males and females. In other words, some sex differences compensate for physiological differences that if left unchecked may be maladaptive. Sex differences that perform a compensatory role may become evident when the system is perturbed. A specific example comes from looking at something as apparently basic as cell death programs in neurons. In response to hypoxia, or other conditions mimicking stroke, neurons die in both sexes of rats and mice [21].

A sex difference in a physiological process is one of nature's ways of demonstrating how that process can be modulated. Sex differences in the vulnerability to a disease may similarly reveal factors that are protective in one sex, thereby suggesting strategies to prevent or ameliorate that disease. This is especially true for many neurodevelopmental disorders, where "sex" explains more of the variance than any other known contributing factor. In humans, some treatments are known to be more effective in one sex than the other, and optimal drug doses for men and women may differ. We ignore these things at our peril and we believe that ignoring sex differences in the brain, however they arise, compromises best practices in biology and medicine, in some cases with substantiated negative health effects [22].

A deeper understanding of these mechanisms will ultimately lead to our understanding of the molecular mechanisms underlying differences in the male and female brain, and importantly, differences in how the male and female brain may be able to respond to neuronal insults encountered with injury, neurodegeneration, and normal aging.

References

1. Bao AM, Swaab DF (2011) Sexual differentiation of the human brain: relation to gender identity, sexual orientation and neuropsychiatric disorders. Front Neuroendocrinol 32(2):214–226
2. Ngun TC, Ghahramani N, Sánchez FJ et al (2011) The genetics of sex differences in brain and behavior. Front Neuroendocrinol 32(2):227–246

3. Arnold AP, Chen XQ (2009) What does the “four core genotypes” mouse model tell us about sex differences in the brain and other tissues? Front Neuroendocrinol 30(1):1–9
4. Baulieu EE (1991) Neurosteroids: a new function in the brain. Biol Cell 71:3–10
5. Frye CA (2001) The role of neurosteroids and nongenomic effects of progestins and androgens in mediating sexual receptivity of rodents. Brain Res Rev 37:201–222
6. Wright CL, Schwarz JS, Dean SL et al (2010) Cellular mechanisms of estradiol-mediated sexual differentiation of the brain. Trends Endocrinol Metab 21(9):553–561
7. Celotti F, Negri-Cesi P, Poletti A (1997) Steroid metabolism in the mammalian brain: 5alpha-reduction and aromatization. Brain Res Bull 44:365–375
8. Genazzani AR, Pluchino N, Freschi L et al (2007) Androgens and the brain. Maturitas 57(1):27–30
9. Corpechot C, Young J, Calvel M et al (1993) Neurosteroids: 3alpha-hydroxy-5 alpha-pregnan-20-one and its precursors in the brain, plasma, and steroidogenic glands of male and female rats. Endocrinology 133:1003–1009
10. Rupprecht R, Holsboer F (1999) Neuropsychopharmacological properties of neuroactive steroids. Steroids 64:83–91
11. Djebaili M, Hoffman SW, Stein DG (2004) Allopregnanolone and progesterone decrease cell death and cognitive deficits after a contusion of the rat pre-frontal cortex. Neuroscience 123:349–359
12. Pluchino N, Ninni F, Casarosa E et al (2008) Sexually dimorphic effects of testosterone administration on brain allopregnanolone in gonadectomized rats. J Sex Med 12:2780–2792
13. Pluchino N, Ninni F, Casarosa E et al (2009) Sex differences in brain and plasma beta-endorphin content following testosterone, dihydrotestosterone and estradiol administration to gonadectomized rats. Neuroendocrinology 89:411–423
14. Houtsmuller EJ, Brand T, de Jonge FH et al (1994) SDN-POA volume, sexual behavior, and partner preference of male rats affected by perinatal treatment with ATD. Physiol Behav 56:535–541
15. Dungan HM, Clifton DK, Steiner RA et al (2006) Minireview: kisspeptin neurons as central processors in the regulation of gonadotropin-releasing hormone secretion. Endocrinology 147:1154–1158
16. Krishnan S, Intlekofer KA, Aggison LK et al (2009) Central role of TRAF-interacting protein in a new model of brain sexual differentiation. Proc Natl Acad Sci U S A 106:16692–16697
17. Forger NG, Rosen GJ, Waters EM et al (2004) Deletion of Bax eliminates sex differences in the mouse forebrain. Proc Natl Acad Sci U S A 101:13666–13671
18. Amateau SK, McCarthy MM (2004) Induction of PGE2 by estradiol mediates developmental masculinization of sex behavior. Nat Neurosci 7:643–650
19. Wright CL, McCarthy MM (2009) Prostaglandin E2-induced masculinization of brain and behavior requires protein kinase A, AMPA/kainate, and metabotropic glutamate receptor signaling. J Neurosci 29:13274–13282
20. Wright CL, Burks SR, McCarthy MM (2008) Identification of prostaglandin E2 receptors mediating perinatal masculinization of adult sex behavior and neuroanatomical correlates. Dev Neurobiol 68:1406–1419
21. De Vries GJ (2004) Sex differences in adult and developing brains: compensation, compensation, compensation. Endocrinology 145:1063–1068
22. Holden C (2005) Sex and the suffering brain. Science 308:1574–1577

2 Management of Disorders of Sex Development

Charles Sultan, Laura Gaspari, Nicolas Kalfa, and Françoise Paris

Malformations of the external genitalia, formerly referred to as ambiguous genitalia, are today categorized as disorders of sex differentiation (DSD) [1]. They are secondary to the undervirilization of the 46,XY fetus or the excessive masculinization of the 46,XX fetus. These malformations are usually discovered in the neonatal period during the systematic examination of the newborn's external genital organs. However, they can also be detected during prenatal ultrasonography. These situations are extremely distressful for the families, and optimal management is therefore imperative so that the sex of rearing can be determined as quickly as possible. DSD management is thus the response to a medical emergency. It requires a multidisciplinary team that should include a pediatric endocrinologist, pediatric urological surgeon, geneticist, and psychologist. The clinical, biological, and genetic investigations, along with imaging studies and surgical and psychological management, should suggest the better choice of sex orientation or at least the less onerous one.

2.1 Diagnosis of the Disorders of Sex Differentiation (DSD)

2.1.1 Clinical Diagnosis of DSD

A scrupulous clinical examination will permit the diagnosis of a DSD (Fig. 2.1) and will also determine whether it has occurred in a context of malformation. The genital bud, genital ridges (scrotum in boys and labia majora in girls), and urogenital

C. Sultan (✉) • L. Gaspari • F. Paris
Unité d'Endocrinologie-Gynécologie Pédiatrique, Service de Pédiatrie, Hôpital Arnaud-de-Villeneuve, CHU Montpellier et Université Montpellier 1, Montpellier, France
e-mail: c-sultan@chu-montpellier.fr; f-paris@chu-montpellier.fr

N. Kalfa
Service de Chirurgie Pédiatrique, Hôpital Lapeyronie, CHU Montpellier et Université Montpellier 1, Montpellier, France

C. Sultan, A.R. Genazzani (eds.), *Frontiers in Gynecological Endocrinology*, ISGE Series, DOI 10.1007/978-3-319-41433-1_2

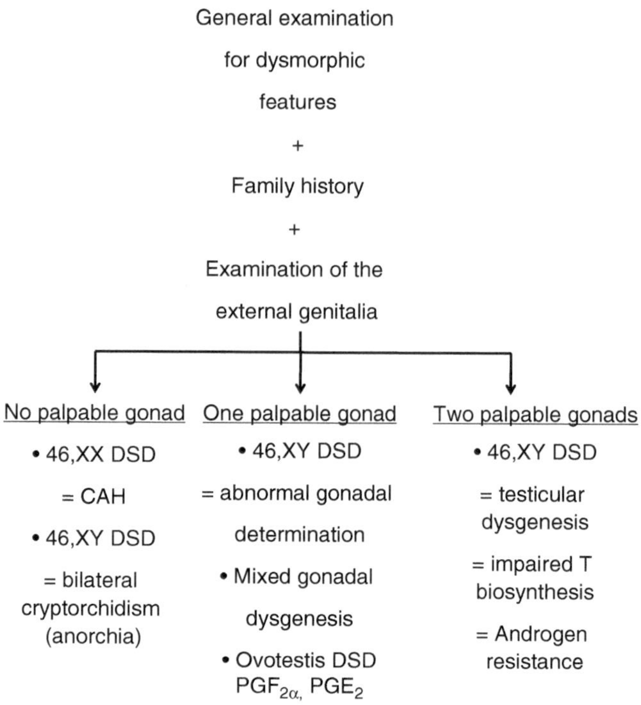

Fig. 2.1 Clinical orientation for DSD

sinus (closed in boys and open in girls) should be very carefully examined. It is important to determine whether the family has had other cases of DSD or neonatal salt-wasting.

In some cases, the external genitalia are "ambiguous" and are associated with:

A genital bud that is midway between a penis and a clitoris
Genital ridges that are incompletely fused (forked scrotum)
The urethral opening on the underside of the penis (hypospadias) or a single perineal orifice at the base of the genital bud, between the genital ridges
Gonads that are impalpable or palpable in the inguinal position

In other cases, the malformation is less clear-cut and attention should be focused on:

Bilateral cryptorchidism
Posterior hypospadias
Cryptorchidism associated with hypospadias
Micropenis (<2.5 cm)
Clitoral hypertrophy
A nonvisible vaginal orifice with posterior fusion of the genital ridges in a newborn with female phenotype

Table 2.1 The Prader scores

Stage 0	
	Normal female external genitalia
Stage 1	
	Female external genitalia with clitoromegaly
Stage 2	
	Clitoromegaly with partial labial fusion forming a funnel-shaped urogenital sinus
Stage 3	
	Increased phallic enlargement. Complete labioscrotal fusion forming a urogenital sinus with a single opening
Stage 4	
	Complete scrotal fusion with urogenital opening at the base or on the shaft of the phallus
Stage 5	
	Normal male external genitalia

Palpation of a uni- or bilateral mass in the inguinal position or in the labia majora
The degree of the DSD should be evaluated according to the Prader classification (Stage I to V) (Table 2.1).

2.1.2 Genetic Investigations

The presence of the SRY gene should be determined with PCR and the results should be ready within 24 h. This will determine whether the case is an undervirilization of a 46,XY fetus or the excessive virilization of a 46,XX fetus. It is essential to determine the karyotype, as this will enable the diagnosis of chromosomal abnormalities like 45X/46,XY mosaicism. However, this type of diagnosis will take from a couple of days to several weeks.

2.1.3 Hormonal Investigations

The hormone work-up should be performed between 6 and 36 h after birth. The following measurements are crucial: 17-hydroxyprogesterone (17-OHP), testosterone (T), and anti-Mullerian hormone (AMH). If possible, follicle-stimulating hormone (FSH), luteinizing hormone (LH), and delta4androstenedione (Δ4A) measurements should be associated.

High 17-OHP suggests congenital adrenal hyperplasia (CAH), which is usually due to a deficiency in 21-hydroxylase that results in a 46,XY DSD.

The values of T and AMH are crucial for evaluating DSD with the 46,XY karyotype. The T, FSH, and LH levels should be reevaluated during the minipuberty (days 15–90), which is the period of activation of the hypothalamic-pituitary-gonadal axis. During other periods, T and its precursors should be evaluated after the human chorionic gonadotropin (hCG) stimulation test. Most often the

Table 2.2 Comparison between the old and new DSD classification (ESPE Consensus 2006)

Previous classification	New classification
Sexual ambiguities	Disorders of Sexual Development (DSD)
MPH (Male Pseudohermaphrodisms)	46,XY DSD
FPH (Female Pseudohermaphrodisms)	46,XX DSD
True Hermaphroditism	Ovotestis, DSD
46,XX male	46,XX testicular DSD
45,X0, 46,XX Klinefelter Syndrome 47,XXY	DSD with chromosomic abnormalities

long test is used (1500 UI 1d/2 × 7). All these investigations should be able to differentiate 46,XY DSD secondary to insufficient androgen production (gonadal dysgenesis or defective androgen synthesis) from those secondary to androgen resistance associated with normal T production.

2.1.4 Imaging

Fetal ultrasonography sometimes reveals a uterus. Genitography can show evidence of Mullerian derivatives. Urogenital endoscopy under general anesthesia can be used to specify the implantation height of the Mullerian cavity when it is present.

2.2 Causes of DSD

According to the 2006 consensus statement of the european society for paediatric endocrinology (ESPE) [1] (Table 2.2), we differentiate between 46,XX DSD, 46,XY DSD, DSD with ovotestis, and DSD associated with chromosome abnormalities.

2.2.1 46,XX DSD

46,XX DSD is due to the masculinization of the 46,XX fetus because of excessive exposure to androgens during intrauterine life, whether of endogenous or exogenous origin. It may also be due to abnormal ovarian determination.

2.2.1.1 Fetal Hyperandrogenism

In the great majority of cases (75 %), the 46,XX fetus has been overexposed to fetal androgens in the context of congenital adrenal hyperplasia (CAH). The excessive adrenal androgens produced upstream of an enzymatic block are peripherally converted to T and dihydrotestosterone (DHT) and cause fetal virilization (Fig. 2.2).

DHT deficiency is the most frequent (90–95 %) of the enzymatic blocks, accounting for 1/14,000 births. Systematic screening with blotting paper is performed on the third day of life. A salt-wasting condition with hyponatremia may be associated with

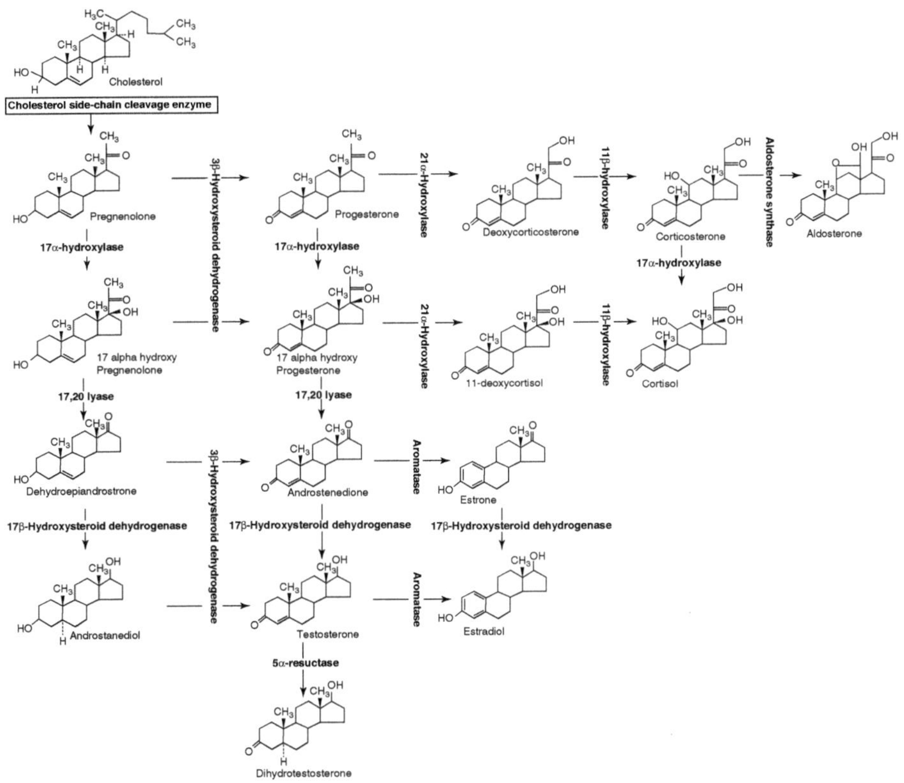

Fig. 2.2 Steroidogenesis

the virilization because of aldosterone and glucocorticoid defects downstream of the enzymatic block. The elevated plasma 17-OHP is generally >50 ng/ml. Treatment with glucocorticoids and mineralocorticoids should be undertaken as soon as possible. Molecular study of the CYP21A2 gene will confirm the diagnosis, since this disorder is recessively transmitted [2]. The sex of rearing of these newborns is almost always female; however, given the excessive androgen exposure during fetal life and the evidence of disturbed gender identification in adulthood, some authors have questioned systematic female orientation in the case of highly virilized CAH [3].

Other forms of CAH can be encountered, though these are rarer. The 11-beta-hydroxylase block is seen in 5 % of the cases. No salt-wasting occurs. The diagnosis is based on simultaneously elevated S-component and desoxycorticosterone (DOC), and a ratio of Δ4/17-OHP >1 is highly suggestive. Study of the CYP11B1 gene will confirm the diagnosis since transmission is autosomal recessive [4]. Careful substitutive therapy with glucocorticoids should be undertaken. The 3-beta-hydroxysteroid dehydrogenase block is rare (1 %). It associates salt-wasting and moderate virilization. During hormonal investigations, high 17-OH pregnenolone is evident and moderately elevated 17-OHP is also frequently noted, probably due to the effect of the hepatic 3ß HSD. An HSD3B2 gene abnormality will confirm the diagnosis, since transmission is recessive [5]. Substitutive therapy with gluco- and mineralocorticoids should be prescribed.

More rarely, the virilization of the 46,XX fetus may be caused by a lipoid adrenal hyperplasia secondary to a mutation of the StAR gene, which codes for the steroidogenic acute regulatory protein (StAR). Transmission is autosomal recessive. The StAR protein is involved in the cholesterol transport in mitochondria, which is the first step in adrenal and gonadal steroidogenesis. Lipoid adrenal hyperplasia is thus characterized by a major deficit in adrenal and gonadal steroidogenesis, evidenced by severe adrenal insufficiency and a female phenotype in both 46,XX and 46,XY fetuses. However, less severe forms – characterized by adrenal insufficiency but less pronounced undervirilization – have recently been reported [6].

The P450-oxidoreductase (POR) deficit is a possible etiology of 46,XY DSD, as well as 46,XX DSD [7]. These forms are dealt with more extensively in the chapter on 46,XY DSD.

2.2.1.2 Exogenous Hyperandrogenism

This type of fetal hyperandrogenism may be secondary to placental aromatase gene mutation, which is recessively transmitted. This abnormality is rare and is characterized by maternal virilization in the third trimester of pregnancy with spontaneous regression after delivery [8]. Another cause of exogenous androgens is one of the rare ovarian tumors, such as luteoma of pregnancy or maternal adrenal tumors [9].

2.2.1.3 Abnormalities in Gonadal Determination

Abnormalities in gonadal determination lead to 46,XX testicular DSD, and affected individuals were formerly termed XX males. These patients may present genital abnormalities during the neonatal period or a normal male phenotype. In the latter case, the diagnosis is made in adult life, frequently because of infertility. Since about 10 % of patients are SRY negative, other genes are probably involved in testis determination. It has been hypothesized that these abnormalities are secondary to either an underexpression of ovary-determining genes or an overexpression of testis-determining genes [10], and both hypotheses have been reinforced by evidence [11]. Moreover, Camerino et al. reported an RSPO1 gene mutation in the family of a 46,XX patient with male phenotype associated with palmoplantar hyperkeratosis [11].

Regarding the potential role of the testis-determining genes, the overexpression of the Sox9 gene—which has its major role during testicular development—was reported in a 46,XX man [12, 13].

2.2.2 46,XY DSD

46,XY DSD refers to the case of 46,XY newborns with undermasculinization. One or both gonads are usually palpated at birth. The hormonal levels of T, AMH, FSH, and LH, as well as the presence of Mullerian derivatives at pelvic ultrasonography, will differentiate gonadal dysgenesis (associated with insufficient gonadal secretion of T and AMH) from T production defects or T insensitivity.

2.2.2.1 Gonadal Dysgenesis

Gonadal dysgenesis is a defect in testis determination characterized by a variable alteration in Leydig and Sertoli cell function. This disorder may be secondary to mutations in any of the several genes taking part in the differentiation process of the primitive gonad to a testis.

SRY Gene Abnormalities

SRY gene abnormalities express with a clinical picture of 46,XY sex reversal with female phenotype. If gonads are not palpated at birth, it is probable that the diagnosis will be made in the pubertal period in the context of primitive amenorrhea associated with pubertal delay. However, some patients may present partial pubertal development, often caused by an association with a secreting gonadoblastoma [14]. This picture of 46,XY sex reversal is associated with a SRY gene mutation in 20 % of the cases.

Abnormalities in Other Sex Determination Genes

About 80 % of the cases of gonadal dysgenesis are not caused by a SRY gene abnormality. They may be secondary to abnormalities in the other genes that take part in testis determination, however, and they are autosomal or X-linked.

Some cases of gonadal dysgenesis have been linked to SF1 gene mutation. This gene is involved in the development of male gonads and the adrenal glands [15]. The phenotype is variable, from severe expression [16] with isolated clitoral hypertrophy to moderate expression with hypospadias or isolated micropenis [17]. Adrenal insufficiency may be associated but is not systematically observed [18].

In some patients, the gonadal dysgenesis is associated with renal dysfunction. In these cases, the diagnosis of Drash syndrome—defined as Wilms tumor associated with renal insufficiency—or Frasier syndrome—which is proteinuria secondary to focal glomerular sclerosis—may be made. Both syndromes are due to WT1 gene abnormalities that are nevertheless quite specific for each syndrome. In particular, heterozygous mutations in the open reading frame have been associated with Drash syndrome [19], while intron mutations leading to splicing abnormalities have been found in Frasier patients [20].

Sox9 gene abnormalities have been reported. Sox9 is a key gene in early male sex determination [15]. Several mutations have been identified in patients with severe skeletal malformations like campomelic dysplasia, associated in some cases with sex reversal and gonadal dysgenesis [21–23].

Homozygous or composite heterozygous mutations of the desert hedgehog (DHH) gene, which is involved in testis differentiation and perineal development, have been identified. The virilization defect is frequently severe, the phenotype is often female, and a neuropathy may be associated.

A linkage study recently identified an MAP3K1 mutation in two families with several cases of 46,XY DSD, thus indicating another player in male sex determination [24].

In addition, duplications in the short arm of the X chromosome [dosage sensitive sex reversal (DSS) locus, DAX1 gene] have been reported in several cases of gonadal dysgenesis. A DSS locus duplication was found in 46,XY DSD patients with female phenotype (46,XY complete dysgenesis). Both the DAX1 (DSS-AHC critical region on X chromosome, gene 1) and NR0B1 (nuclear receptor 0B1) genes have been identified in this locus. The NR0B1 gene belongs to the nuclear receptor family and, through its linkage with other transcription factors such as SF1, it has an "anti-testis" effect during the process of male sex determination, proportional to the gene dosage. Thus, the overexpression of the DAX gene, as in the case of duplication in a 46,XY patient, may contrast with normal testis differentiation, leading to gonadal dysgenesis [25].

Last, a chromobox homolog 2 (CBX2) gene mutation was recently identified in a newborn with complete female phenotype but a 46,XY karyotype, which had been determined in the prenatal period because of concerns about maternal age. This testis differentiation abnormality nevertheless differed from the previously presented cases of gonadal dysgenesis in that ovaries with primordial follicles were detected [26]. A mutation in the CBX2 gene, which is known for activating SF1 transcription, was identified in this patient. The CBX2 gene thus seems to actively repress ovarian development in 46,XY gonads.

2.2.2.2 Defects in Testosterone Production

Defects in T production are rare and are characterized by variable degrees of external genital undervirilization. Conversely, no Mullerian derivatives are present because AMH is normally secreted by the Sertoli cells. These defects are due to an enzymatic defect in T biosynthesis or they may be secondary to an LH receptor gene abnormality.

Defect in 3-Beta-Hydroxysteroid Dehydrogenase

This defect is associated with a variable but insufficient virilization of the 46,XY fetus, ranging from a female phenotype to minor forms of DSD, such as isolated micropenis or salt-wasting conditions. The biological and genetic investigations are the same as for 46,XX DSD.

Defect of 17-Alpha-Hydroxylase

The phenotype in cases of a 17-alpha-hydroxylase defect may also be extremely variable. In some individuals, the diagnosis is made only in the pubertal period because of pubertal delay or stagnation associated with gynecomastia. A DOC excess causes hypertension during puberty. The plasma levels of pregnenolone, progesterone, and corticosterone are elevated, which contrasts with the low values of T and D4 that are unresponsive to stimulation. The genetic abnormality concerns the CYP17 gene with recessive transmission.

Defect of 17-Beta-Hydroxysteroid Reductase

This is a rare testicular block that causes a deficit in testicular T production. The phenotype is more frequently female at birth. The diagnosis is based on a striking elevation in plasma D4 contrasting with a low T level. The mutation involves the 17ß-HSD type 3 gene, which is expressed only in testis, and its transmission is recessive. Virilization occurs at puberty associated with gynecomastia.

P450-Oxydoreductase (POR) Deficit

A POR deficit may cause 46,XY DSD as well as 46,XX DSD [7]. The cytochrome P450 oxydoreductase protein enables the electron transport from NADPH to P450 cytochromes localized in microsomes. Several cytochromes take part in cholesterol biosynthesis, while three are involved in steroid biosynthesis: P450C17 (17a-hydroxylase/17,20 lyase), P450C21 (21-hydroxylase), and P450CYP19 (aromatase). Transmission of POR gene mutations is autosomal recessive, and the study of several of these mutations has provided greater insight into DSD in association with combined deficits in 21-OH and 17-OH in cases where molecular analysis of CYP21 and CYP17 was normal. In addition to DSD, several patients present craniofacial malformations, suggestive of Antley-Bixler syndrome. The great variability in the phenotype and endocrine findings makes this diagnosis very difficult. This may be due in part to the varying degrees of the enzymatic defects and to the differences in the ability of each mutation to alter enzyme function [27].

Leydig Cell Agenesis or Hypoplasia

This is a rare form of 46,XY DSD, first identified in a patient with female phenotype associated with the 46,XY karyotype. She presented primary amenorrhea and no breast development at puberty, associated with low T at baseline and after hCG stimulation testing. The discrepancy between increased LH and normal FSH levels is generally evocative. This condition is determined by a homozygous or double heterozygous inactivating mutation of the LH receptor gene. Since the identification of these genetic abnormalities, the phenotypic expression has expanded to include conditions that range from ambiguous genitalia to partial forms such as hypospadias or isolated micropenis [28].

2.2.2.3 Androgen-Resistance Disorders

The androgen-resistance disorders are characterized by normal/high T and AMH production, in contrast to undermasculinization. These disorders are classified as 46,XY DSD, which was previously termed male pseudohermaphroditism with normal or high T.

Androgen Insensitivity (AI)

Androgen insensitivity represents more than 50 % of 46,XY DSD in our experience and is caused by a T receptor abnormality. Clinically, a gonad is palpable in the inguinal region in the majority of cases. AI is due to a recessive X-linked mutation that alters the androgen receptor (AR) gene and leads to variable degrees of undervirilization.

Regardless of the initial condition, testes are present and functional, despite cryptorchidism. They secrete T and AMH, and there are thus no Mullerian derivatives, such as uterus, Fallopian tubes or the upper part of the vagina [29]. The AI conditions are classically distinguished by two forms: complete androgen insensitivity (CAI), which is typically monomorphic, and partial androgen insensitivity (PAI), which is conversely far more heterogeneous, with phenotypes varying from Prader scores of I to V (Table 2.1).

CAI leads to the most severe phenotype of a normal female newborn. The diagnosis is often made only in the pubertal period, when primary amenorrhea associated with normal breast development and sparse axillary and pubic hair suggests this diagnosis. This adolescent also presents no acne, which is a further sign of no androgen action on target tissues.

Conversely, PAI is a quite variable condition, with phenotypes expressing all degrees of lost AR function. The range is extremely wide, with the most severe forms characterized by female external genitalia with moderate clitoral hypertrophy to the least severe forms like isolated micropenis [30] or male sterility with no external genital malformation, which is the so-called minimal androgen insensitivity syndrome (MAIS). Between these two extreme conditions, there are all degrees of undervirilization, most frequently with one or both gonads palpable. It is important to note that almost all patients develop gynecomastia in the pubertal period.

The endocrine investigations performed in neonatal PAI patients show normal or high plasma T and AMH, along with a high LH level. Conversely, in CAI patients, the T and LH levels are not always increased. In addition, the LH and T peak level observed around the sixth week of life in normal boys may be absent. The absence of Mullerian derivatives during echography or genitography is an important diagnostic element. An AR gene mutation will confirm this diagnosis. Choosing the sex of rearing at birth is relatively straightforward for CAI patients, who are always raised as females. Conversely, the choice of gender orientation for PAI patients is more difficult and needs to take into account the technical difficulties of virilizing these patients during the pubertal period. It is also important to note the absence of correlation between genotype and phenotype for several AR gene mutations, which may, moreover, express with variable phenotypes within the same family. Since most mutations are transmitted, it is important to screen all women to facilitate prenatal diagnosis.

5aR Deficiency

In the case of 5aR deficiency, T is not converted to dihydrotestosterone (DHT), which is responsible for external genital virilization. The phenotype is usually female, but it may assume all degrees of undervirilization. Clitoral hypertrophy and the association of hypospadias and micropenis were the most frequently reported findings in a recent study enrolling a large cohort of patients with a 5aR defect [31]. If the diagnosis was not made in the neonatal period, it is usually made at puberty because of amenorrhea, absence of breast development, striking virilization associated with hirsutism, clitoral hypertrophy, significant muscle development, and a masculinization in behavior. The virilization is due to the presence of an isoenzyme expressed after puberty. The hormonal investigations usually reveal an increased T/DHT ratio >10. However, 5aR defects have also been identified in patients with a normal T/DHT ratio. The diagnosis of a 5aR deficit should always be considered for a 46,XY DSD patient with increased T and AMH plasma values, regardless of the T/DHT ratio. The molecular abnormality concerns the gene coding for 5aR2. This enzyme is expressed in genital skin and prostate during fetal life and transmission is autosomal recessive; conversely, the 5aR1 enzyme expressed at puberty remains functional in skin. There is high genotype/phenotype variability, as in androgen insensitivity. In severe forms, the gender orientation is often female; conversely, this choice is more difficult in less severe cases. Sex behavior, male identity, pubertal virilization, and preserved fertility in some men with the 5aR mutation [32] provide arguments for male orientation [1].

MALD1 Gene Mutations

CXorf6 or mastermind-like domain containing 1 (MAMLD1) is a new gene discovered during a study on myotubular myopathy (MTM1 gene). This muscle disease is associated with genital malformations, since the MAMLD1 gene, which is near MTM1, is deleted. MAMLD1 is temporarily expressed in fetal gonad and may thus take part in fetal steroidogenesis. Mutations in this gene are associated with severe forms of hypospadias in a context of DSD [33]; however, this mutation has been also identified in patients with isolated hypospadias and elevated plasma T [34].

46,XY DSD and the Environment

In some cases of 46,XY DSD with elevated plasma T, no genetic abnormality is identified, leading to the diagnosis of "idiopathic" 46,XY DSD. In these cases, it is important to investigate the parental domestic and occupational exposure to environmental endocrine disrupting chemicals (EDCs) in order to identify possible fetal contamination.

Over the past 30 years, several studies have reported the undervirilization of wild animals, as well as an increasing trend in the prevalence of external genital malformations in male newborns. This trend includes isolated hypospadias [35, 36], cryptorchidism [37], and the association of two or more external genital malformations [38]. Several EDCs are known to present anti-androgenic and/or estrogenic activity, which has led to the suspicion that these chemicals may interfere with male sex differentiation during fetal life [39]. Moreover, many epidemiological studies have reinforced the EDC hypothesis by evidencing an elevated prevalence of these malformations in especially polluted areas [40, 41], and others have demonstrated an augmented concentration of EDCs in the mothers' milk of 46,XY DSD newborns [42]. In addition, animal studies have demonstrated the potentiating effect of an EDC mixture [43]. It is thus probable that the environment plays an important role in this increasing trend of external genital malformations [38–44]. We found increased estrogenic bioactivity in three 46,XY patients who were apparently exposed to EDCs during fetal life [45]. However, a geographic variation in the prevalence of these external genital malformations has also been noted, with a sharp north/south gradient in Europe, which has raised the suspicion of a genetic susceptibility to EDCs [38]. In addition to DSD, the incidence of testis cancer has increased parallel to the decline in male fertility. Based on all this evidence, Skakkebaek et al. hypothesized in 2001 that the increasing trend in external genital malformations in males, the decline in spermatogenesis, and the rise in testis cancer have a common origin: fetal exposure to EDCs, or the so-called testicular dysgenesis syndrome [46].

2.2.3 Ovotesticular DSD

True hermaphroditism is now called ovotesticular DSD, following the ESPE consensus statement of 2006 [1]. This denomination has the advantage of referring directly to the pathology, which is characterized by the coexistence of testicular and ovarian tissue. The clinical phenotype depends on the predominant tissue and may thus express any degree of DSD. It has also been reported that several virilized patients were diagnosed only in the pubertal period because of gynecomastia and growth stagnation [47]. Diagnosis is based on the histological examination of a gonadal biopsy sample, which generally shows the presence of an ovotestis or ovarian tissue on one side and testicular tissue in the contralateral side. The ovarian tissue is normal; conversely, the testicular tissue is normal in the neonatal period but becomes dysgenetic with age [48]. The karyotype is 46,XX in the majority of these patients, as the SRY gene is found in only 30 % of cases, and the 46,XY karyotype is more rarely seen. In much rarer cases, 46,XX/46,XY mosaicism is observed. Female orientation is frequently recommended because of the presence of uterus in 75 % of patients and the differentiated ovarian tissue. In addition to DSD management, surgery can preserve the gonadal tissue according to the choice of gender orientation [48].

2.2.4 DSD Caused by Chromosomal Abnormalities

Mixed gonadal dysgenesis is among the chromosomal abnormalities that cause DSD; the karyotype is 45,X0/46,XY. This genetic condition leads to DSD of variable degrees, frequently with an asymmetry characterized by one palpable gonad in the inguinal or scrotal region and the other gonad, generally a streak, in the abdominal region. The presence of Mullerian derivatives, usually on one side only, is confirmed by genitography. The choice of gender orientation may be male or female, depending on the virilization of the external and internal genitalia and the presence of Mullerian derivatives. When female gender is chosen, a gonadectomy is generally performed to eliminate the high risk of gonadoblastoma. When male gender is chosen, the gonads are surgically lowered and fixed in the scrotum to facilitate screening for gonadoblastoma.

In this classification, we find also the Klinefelter syndromes, whose karyotype is 47,XXY. The phenotype is more usually male and the diagnosis is generally made at adolescence because of pubertal delay or stagnation associated to gynecomastia and low testis volume. Much more rarely, this syndrome is associated with a mild defect of virilization such as micropenis or cryptorchidism [49].

2.3 Elements for Gender Declaration

The choice of gender orientation should always involve a multidisciplinary team and the decision must be made very carefully. Although the orientation of highly virilized 46,XX DSD is today under discussion, the choice of gender orientation for 46,XY DSD remains an extremely difficult step. The presence of testicular tissue is not an essential factor; conversely, the surgical possibilities and the potential for virilization under treatment at puberty are key factors for orientation:

In testicular dysgenesis: female orientation is standard if vaginoplasty can easily be performed.

In testicular T synthesis abnormality: female orientation is advised, since the possibility of performing a masculinizing genitoplasty is low.

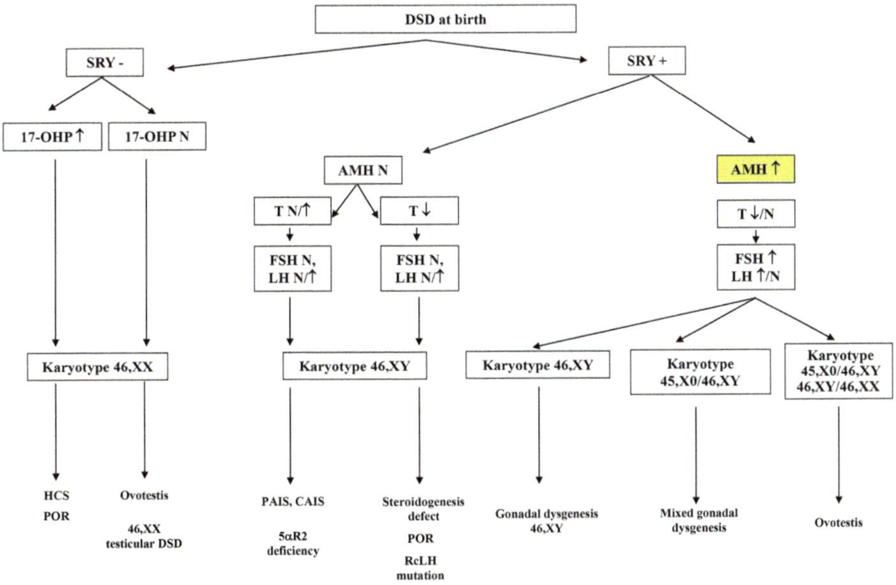

Fig. 2.3 Management of DSD

In androgen resistance: female orientation is indisputable in newborns with complete androgen resistance; conversely, in partial forms the female orientation should be considered because of the risk of insufficient virilization at puberty.

In 5α-reductase deficiency: theoretically, the orientation should be toward male gender since pubertal virilization will enable subnormal penile development, normal pubic hair, and male identity.

In the rare ovotestis DSD: female orientation is most often adopted.

Conclusions

In conclusion, scrupulous clinical examination and hormonal imaging, genetic, and molecular investigations all lead to the confirmation of DSD diagnosis (Fig. 2.3).

The families should be informed in a calm and balanced manner of the treatment options and their respective difficulties.

A multidisciplinary team should be involved in all diagnostic investigations, treatment, and follow-up.

References

1. Hughes IA, Houk C, Ahmed SF, Lee PA (2006) Consensus statement on management of intersex disorders. Arch Dis Child 91:554–563
2. Balsamo A, Baldazzi L, Menabo S, Cicognani A (2010) Impact of molecular genetics on congenital adrenal hyperplasia management. Sex Dev 4:233–248

3. Houk CP, Lee PA (2010) Approach to assigning gender in 46, XX congenital adrenal hyperplasia with male external genitalia: replacing dogmatism with pragmatism. J Clin Endocrinol Metab 95:4501–4508
4. Nimkarn S, New MI (2008) Steroid 11beta- hydroxylase deficiency congenital adrenal hyperplasia. Trends Endocrinol Metab 19:96–99
5. Krone N, Arlt W (2009) Genetics of congenital adrenal hyperplasia. Best Pract Res Clin Endocrinol Metab 23:181–192
6. Sahakitrungruang T, Soccio RE, Lang-Muritano M, Walker JM, Achermann JC, Miller WL (2010) Clinical, genetic, and functional characterization of four patients carrying partial loss-of-function mutations in the steroidogenic acute regulatory protein (StAR). J Clin Endocrinol Metab 95:3352–3359
7. Scott RR, Miller WL (2008) Genetic and clinical features of p450 oxydoreductase deficiency. Horm Res 69:266–275
8. Lin L, Ercan O, Raza J, Burren CP, Creighton SM, Auchus RJ, Dattani MT, Achermann JC (2007) Variable phenotypes associated with aromatase (CYP19) insufficiency in humans. J Clin Endocrinol Metab 92:982–990
9. Spitzer RF, Wherrett D, Chitayat D, Colgan T, Dodge JE, Salle JL, Allen L (2007) Maternal luteoma of pregnancy presenting with virilization of the female infant. J Obstet Gynaecol Can 29:835–840
10. Hughes IA (2008) Disorders of sex development: a new definition and classification. Best Pract Res Clin Endocrinol Metab 22:119–134
11. Parma P, Radi O (2010) Forgetting RSPO1. Fertil Steril 94:e39–author reply e40
12. Cox JJ, Willatt L, Homfray T, Woods CG (2011) A SOX9 duplication and familial 46, XX developmental testicular disorder. N Engl J Med 364:91–93
13. Refai O, Friedman A, Terry L, Jewett T, Pearlman A, Perle MA, Ostrer H (2010) De novo 12;17 translocation upstream of SOX9 resulting in 46, XX testicular disorder of sex development. Am J Med Genet A 152A:422–426
14. Paris F, Philibert P, Lumbroso S, Baldet P, Charvet JP, Galifer RB, Sultan C (2007) Primary amenorrhea in a 46, XY adolescent girl with partial gonadal dysgenesis: identification of a new SRY gene mutation. Fertil Steril 88(1437):e21–e25
15. Sekido R, Lovell-Badge R (2009) Sex determination and SRY: down to a wink and a nudge? Trends Genet 25:19–29
16. Lin L, Philibert P, Ferraz-de-Souza B, Kelberman D, Homfray T, Albanese A, Molini V, Sebire NJ, Einaudi S, Conway GS, Hughes IA, Jameson JL, Sultan C, Dattani MT, Achermann JC (2007) Heterozygous missense mutations in steroidogenic factor 1 (SF1/Ad4BP, NR5A1) are associated with 46, XY disorders of sex development with normal adrenal function. J Clin Endocrinol Metab 92:991–999
17. Paris F, De Ferran K, Bhangoo A, Ten S, Lahlou N, Audran F, Servant N, Poulat F, Philibert P, Sultan C (2011) Isolated "idiopathic" micropenis: hidden genetic defects? Int J Androl 34:e518–e525
18. Philibert P, Paris F, Audran F, Kalfa N, Polak M, Thibaud E, Pinto G, Houang M, Zenaty D, Leger J, Mas JC, Pienkowski C, Einaudi S, Damiani D, Ten S, Sinha S, Poulat F, Sultan C (2011) Phenotypic variation of SF1 gene mutations. Adv Exp Med Biol 707:67–72
19. Chiang PW, Aliaga S, Travers S, Spector E, Tsai AC (2008) Case report: WT1 exon 6 truncation mutation and ambiguous genitalia in a patient with Denys-Drash syndrome. Curr Opin Pediatr 20:103–106
20. Bache M, Dheu C, Doray B, Fothergill H, Soskin S, Paris F, Sultan C, Fischbach M (2010) Frasier syndrome, a potential cause of end-stage renal failure in childhood. Pediatr Nephrol 25:549–552
21. Gentilin B, Forzano F, Bedeschi MF, Rizzuti T, Faravelli F, Izzi C, Lituania M, Rodriguez-Perez C, Bondioni MP, Savoldi G, Grosso E, Botta G, Viora E, Baffico AM, Lalatta F (2010) Phenotype of five cases of prenatally diagnosed campomelic dysplasia harboring novel mutations of the SOX9 gene. Ultrasound Obstet Gynecol 36:315–323

22. Lecointre C, Pichon O, Hamel A, Heloury Y, Michel-Calemard L, Morel Y, David A, Le Caignec C (2009) Familial acampomelic form of campomelic dysplasia caused by a 960 kb deletion upstream of SOX9. Am J Med Genet A 149A:1183–1189
23. Okamoto T, Nakamura E, Nagaya K, Hayashi T, Mukai T, Fujieda K (2011) Patient reports: Two novel frameshift mutations in the SOX9 gene in two patients with campomelic dysplasia who showed long-term survival. J Pediatr Endocrinol Metab 23:1189–1193
24. Pearlman A, Loke J, Le Caignec C, White S, Chin L, Friedman A, Warr N, Willan J, Brauer D, Farmer C, Brooks E, Oddoux C, Riley B, Shajahan S, Camerino G, Homfray T, Crosby AH, Couper J, David A, Greenfield A, Sinclair A, Ostrer H (2010) Mutations in MAP3K1 cause 46, XY disorders of sex development and implicate a common signal transduction pathway in human testis determination. Am J Hum Genet 87:898–904
25. Barbaro M, Oscarson M, Schoumans J, Staaf J, Ivarsson SA, Wedell A (2007) Isolated 46,XY gonadal dysgenesis in two sisters caused by a Xp21.2 interstitial duplication containing the DAX1 gene. J Clin Endocrinol Metab 92:3305–3313
26. Biason-Lauber A, Konrad D, Meyer M, DeBeaufort C, Schoenle EJ (2009) Ovaries and female phenotype in a girl with 46, XY karyotype and mutations in the CBX2 gene. Am J Hum Genet 84:658–663
27. Miller WL, Agrawal V, Sandee D, Tee MK, Huang N, Choi JH, Morrissey K, Giacomini KM (2011) Consequences of POR mutations and polymorphisms. Mol Cell Endocrinol 10;336(1-2):174–9. https://www.ncbi.nlm.nih.gov/pubmed/?term=Miller+WL%2C+Agrawal+V%2C+Sandee+D%2C+Tee+MK%2C+Huang+N%2C+Choi+JH%2C+Morrissey+K%2C+Giacomini+KM+(2010)+Consequences+of+POR+mutations+and+polymorphisms.+Mol+Cell+Endocrinol" \o "Molecular and cellular endocrinology
28. Mendonca BB, Domenice S, Arnhold IJ, Costa EM (2009) 46, XY disorders of sex development (DSD). Clin Endocrinol (Oxf) 70:173–187
29. Werner R, Grotsch H, Hiort O (2010) 46, XY disorders of sex development--the undermasculinised male with disorders of androgen action. Best Pract Res Clin Endocrinol Metab 24: 263–277
30. Bhangoo A, Paris F, Philibert P, Audran F, Ten S, Sultan C (2010) Isolated micropenis reveals partial androgen insensitivity syndrome confirmed by molecular analysis. Asian J Androl 12:561–566
31. Maimoun L, Philibert P, Cammas B, Audran F, Bouchard P, Fenichel P, Cartigny M, Pienkowski C, Polak M, Skordis N, Mazen I, Ocal G, Berberoglu M, Reynaud R, Baumann C, Cabrol S, Simon D, Kayemba-Kay's K, De Kerdanet M, Kurtz F, Leheup B, Heinrichs C, Tenoutasse S, Van Vliet G, Gruters A, Eunice M, Ammini AC, Hafez M, Hochberg Z, Einaudi S, Al Mawlawi H, Del Valle Nunez CJ, Servant N, Lumbroso S, Paris F, Sultan C (2011) Phenotypical, biological, and molecular heterogeneity of 5{alpha}-reductase deficiency: an extensive international experience of 55 patients. J Clin Endocrinol Metab 96:296–307
32. Matsubara K, Iwamoto H, Yoshida A, Ogata T (2010) Semen analysis and successful paternity by intracytoplasmic sperm injection in a man with steroid 5alpha-reductase-2 deficiency. Fertil Steril 94(2770):e7–e10
33. Fukami M, Wada Y, Miyabayashi K, Nishino I, Hasegawa T, Nordenskjold A, Camerino G, Kretz C, Buj-Bello A, Laporte J, Yamada G, Morohashi K, Ogata T (2006) CXorf6 is a causative gene for hypospadias. Nat Genet 38:1369–1371
34. Kalfa N, Liu B, Klein O, Audran F, Wang MH, Mei C, Sultan C, Baskin LS (2008) Mutations of CXorf6 are associated with a range of severities of hypospadias. Eur J Endocrinol 159:453–458
35. Boisen KA, Chellakooty M, Schmidt IM, Kai CM, Damgaard IN, Suomi AM, Toppari J, Skakkebaek NE, Main KM (2005) Hypospadias in a cohort of 1072 Danish newborn boys: prevalence and relationship to placental weight, anthropometrical measurements at birth, and reproductive hormone levels at three months of age. J Clin Endocrinol Metab 90:4041–4046
36. Lund L, Engebjerg MC, Pedersen L, Ehrenstein V, Norgaard M, Sorensen HT (2009) Prevalence of hypospadias in Danish boys: a longitudinal study, 1977-2005. Eur Urol 55:1022–1026

37. Cortes D, Kjellberg EM, Breddam M, Thorup J (2008) The true incidence of cryptorchidism in Denmark. J Urol 179:314–318
38. Main KM, Skakkebaek NE, Virtanen HE, Toppari J (2010) Genital anomalies in boys and the environment. Best Pract Res Clin Endocrinol Metab 24:279–289
39. Stoker TE, Cooper RL, Lambright CS, Wilson VS, Furr J, Gray LE (2005) In vivo and in vitro anti-androgenic effects of DE-71, a commercial polybrominated diphenyl ether (PBDE) mixture. Toxicol Appl Pharmacol 207:78–88
40. Fernandez MF, Olmos B, Granada A, López-Espinosam MJ, Molina-Molina JM, Fernandez JM, Cruz M, Olea-Serrano F, Olea N (2007) Human exposure to endocrine-disrupting chemicals and prenatal risk factors for cryptorchidism and hypospadias: a nested case-control study. Environ Health Perspect 115:8–14
41. Gaspari L, Paris F, Jandel C, Kalfa N, Orsini M, Daurès JP, Sultan C (2011) Prenatal environmental risk factors for genital malformations in a population of 1442 French male newborns: a nested case-control study. Hum Reprod 26:3155–3162
42. Brucker-Davis F, Ducot B, Wagner-Mahler K, Tommasi C, Ferrari P, Pacini P, Boda-Buccino M, Bongain A, Azuar P, Fenichel P (2008) Environmental pollutants in maternal milk and cryptorchidism. Gynecol Obstet Fertil 36:840–847
43. Christiansen S, Scholze M, Axelstad M, Boberg J, Kortenkamp A, Hass U (2008) Combined exposure to anti-androgens causes markedly increased frequencies of hypospadias in the rat. Int J Androl 31:241–248
44. Kalfa N, Philibert P, Baskin LS, Sultan C (2011) Hypospadias: Interactions between environment and genetics. Mol Cell Endocrinol 335:89–95
45. Paris F, Jeandel C, Servant N, Sultan C (2006) Increased serum estrogenic bioactivity in three male newborns with ambiguous genitalia: a potential consequence of prenatal exposure to environmental endocrine disruptors. Environ Res 100:39–43
46. Skakkebaek NE, Rajpert-De Meyts E, Main KM (2001) Testicular dysgenesis syndrome: an increasingly common developmental disorder with environmental aspects. Hum Reprod 16:972–978
47. Alonso G, Pasqualini T, Busaniche J, Ruiz E, Chemes H (2007) True hermaphroditism in a phenotypic male without ambiguous genitalia: an unusual presentation at puberty. Horm Res 68:261–264
48. Verkauskas G, Jaubert F, Lortat-Jacob S, Malan V, Thibaud E, Nihoul-Fekete C (2007) The long-term followup of 33 cases of true hermaphroditism: a 40-year experience with conservative gonadal surgery. J Urol 177:726–731, discussion 731
49. Mazen I, El-Ruby M, El-Bassyouni HT (2010) Variable associations of Klinefelter syndrome in children. J Pediatr Endocrinol Metab 23:985–989

Central Precocious Puberty: From Diagnosis to Treatment

3

Juliane Léger and Jean-Claude Carel

3.1 Introduction

Precocious puberty (PP) is defined as the onset of clinical signs of puberty before the age of 8 years in girls and 9.5 years in boys. However, the onset of puberty may be subject to the effects of environmental (secular trends, adoption, absence of the father, and possible exposure to estrogenic endocrine-disrupting chemicals), nutritional (body mass index), and constitutional (genetics, ethnicity) factors [1–4], with implications for the definition of precocious puberty. PP may be caused by central or peripheral mechanisms [1].

Premature sexual maturation is a frequent cause for referral. Clinical evaluation is generally sufficient to reassure the patients and their families, but premature sexual maturation may reveal severe conditions and thorough evaluation is therefore required to identify its cause and potential for progression, so that appropriate treatment can be proposed. The clinical expression of precocious puberty is polymorphic. In addition to progressive central PP, with a progressive deterioration of adult height prognosis in the absence of treatment, there are very slowly progressive forms which do not modify predicted final height [5–7]. The heterogeneity of precocious puberty, in terms of its clinical presentation and definition, can be explained by the gradual nature of the transition to puberty. Indeed, the pulsatile secretion of LH begins before the onset of clinical signs of puberty, and an increase in the amplitude of the LH peaks is the key biological sign of pubertal maturation of the gonadotrophic pituitary axis. GnRH stimulation tests indirectly reveal pulsatile endogenous GnRH secretion, as this secretion determines the response

J. Léger, MD (✉) • J.-C. Carel
Department of Paediatric Endocrinology and Diabetology, INSERM UMR 1141, DHU PROTECT, Reference Center for Rare Endocrine Growth Diseases, Robert Debré Hospital, Denis Diderot Paris 7 University, 48 Bd Sérurier, F-75019 Paris, France
e-mail: juliane.leger@aphp.fr

C. Sultan, A.R. Genazzani (eds.), *Frontiers in Gynecological Endocrinology*, ISGE Series, DOI 10.1007/978-3-319-41433-1_3

to exogenous GnRH. The available data indicate that there is no clear boundary between prepubertal and pubertal status, accounting for the frequency of "marginal" forms of precocious puberty.

3.2 Etiologies and Mechanisms Underlying Premature Sexual Development

Central precocious puberty (CPP), which is much more common in girls than in boys [8], results from premature reactivation of the hypothalamo-pituitary-gonadal axis and pulsatile GnRH secretion with a hormonal pattern similar to that of normal puberty. Premature sexual development results from the action of sex steroids or compounds with sex steroid activity on target organs. CPP may be due to hypothalamic lesions, but is idiopathic in most cases, particularly in girls (Table 3.1) [1]. Recent studies have implicated the inactivation of Makorin ring finger 3 (*MKRN3*) genes in "idiopathic" CPP [9, 10]. *MKRN3* is an imprinted gene located on the long arm of chromosome 15, with a potentially inhibitory effect on GnRH secretion. *MKRN3* gene defects have been identified as a cause of paternally transmitted familial CPP, but such defects do not underlie maternally transmitted CPP and are rarely involved in sporadic forms [11].

It is also important to recognize that most cases of premature sexual maturation correspond to benign variants of normal development that can occur throughout childhood. They can mimic precocious puberty but do not lead to long term consequences and are usually benign. This is particularly true in girls below the age of 2–3 where the condition is known as premature thelarche. Similarly in older girls, at least 50 % of cases of premature sexual maturation will regress or stop progressing and no treatment is necessary [5, 6]. Although the mechanism underlying these cases of non-progressive precocious puberty is unknown, the gonadotropic axis is not activated. Premature thelarche probably represents an exaggerated form of the physiological early gonadotropin surge that is delayed in girls relative to boys.

3.3 Consequences of Precocious Puberty

Progressive premature sexual maturation can have consequences on growth and psychosocial development. Growth velocity is accelerated as compared to normal values for age and bone age is advanced in most cases. The acceleration of bone maturation can lead to premature fusion of the growth plate and short stature. Several studies have assessed adult height in individuals with a history of precocious puberty. In older published series of untreated patients, mean heights ranged from 151 to 156 cm in boys and 150 to 154 cm in girls, corresponding to a loss of about 20 cm in boys and 12 cm in girls relative to normal adult height [12]. However, these numbers correspond to historical series of patients with severe early onset precocious puberty which are not representative of the majority of patients seen in

Table 3.1 Clinical characteristics of the various forms of central precocious puberty

Cause	Symptoms and signs	Evaluation
Due to a CNS lesion		
Hypothalamic hamartoma	May be associated with gelastic (laughing attacks), focal or tonic-clonic seizures.	MRI: Mass in the floor of the third ventricle iso-intense to normal tissue without contrast enhancement.
Or other hypothalamic tumors: • Glioma involving the hypothalamus and/or the optic chiasm • Astrocytoma • Ependymoma • Pinealoma • Germ cell tumors	May include headache, visual changes, cognitive changes, symptoms/signs of anterior or posterior pituitary deficiency (e.g., decreased growth velocity, polyuria/polydipsia), fatigue, visual field defects. If CNS tumor (glioma) associated with neurofibromatosis, may have other features of neurofibromatosis (cutaneous neurofibromas, café au lait spots, Lisch nodules, etc.)	MRI: contrast-enhanced mass that may involve the optic pathways (chiasm, nerve, tract) or the hypothalamus (astrocytoma, glioma) or that may involve the hypothalamus and pituitary stalk (germ cell tumor). May have evidence of intracranial hypertension. May have signs of anterior or posterior pituitary deficiency (e.g., hypernatremia). If germ cell tumor: ßhCG detectable in blood or CSF
Cerebral malformations involving the hypothalamus: • Suprasellar arachnoid cyst • Hydrocephalus • Septo optic dysplasia • Myelomeningocele • Ectopic neurohypophysis	May have neurodevelopmental deficits, macrocrania, visual impairment, nystagmus, obesity, polyuria/polydipsia, decreased growth velocity.	May have signs of anterior or posterior pituitary deficiency (e.g., hypernatremia) or. hyperprolactinemia.
Acquired injury: • Cranial irradiation • Head trauma • Infections • Perinatal insults	Relevant history. Symptoms and signs of anterior or posterior pituitary deficiency may be present.	MRI may reveal condition-specific sequelae or may be normal.
Idiopathic – No CNS lesion	≈92 % of girls and ≈ 50 % of boys. History of familial precocious puberty or adoption may be present.	No hypothalamic abnormality on the head MRI. The anterior pituitary may be enlarged. MKRN 3 gene evaluation if paternally transmitted
Secondary to early exposure to sex steroids		
After cure of any cause of gonadotropin-independent precocious puberty.	Relevant history.	

the clinic today. Height loss due to precocious puberty is inversely correlated with the age at pubertal onset, and currently treated patients tend to have later onset of puberty than those in historical series [12].

Parents often seek treatment in girls because they fear early menarche [13]. However, there are little data to predict the age of menarche following early onset of puberty [14]. In the general population, the time from breast development to menarche is longer for children with an earlier onset of puberty, ranging from a mean of 2.8 years when breast development begins at age 9–1.4 years when breast development begins at age 12 [15].

In the general population, early puberty timing has been shown to be associated with several health outcomes in adult life with higher risks for cardiovascular disease and type 2 diabetes in both women and men [16]. However, there are no long term data on these aspects in case of precocious puberty.

Adverse psychosocial outcomes are also a concern, but the available data specific to patients with precocious puberty have serious limitations [17]. In the general population, a higher proportion of early-maturing adolescents engage in exploratory behaviors (sexual intercourse, legal and illegal substance use) and at an earlier age, than adolescents maturing within the normal age range or later [18, 19]. In addition, the risk for sexual abuse seems to be higher in girls or women with early sexual maturation [20]. However, the relevance of these findings to precocious puberty is unclear, and they should not be used to justify intervention.

3.4 Evaluation of the Child with Premature Sexual Development

The evaluation of patients with premature sexual development should address several questions: (1) Is sexual development really occurring outside the normal temporal range? (2) What is the underlying mechanism and is it associated with a risk of a serious condition, such as an intracranial lesion? (3) Is pubertal development likely to progress, and (4) Would this impair the child's normal physical and psychosocial development?

3.4.1 Clinical Diagnosis

Precocious puberty manifests as the progressive appearance of secondary sexual characteristics – breast development, pubic hair and menarche in girls, enlargement of testicular volume (testicular volume greater than 4 ml or testicular length greater than 25 mm) and the penis, and pubic hair development in boys [21, 22] – together with an acceleration of height velocity and bone maturation, which is frequently very advanced (by more than 2 years relative to chronological age). However, a single sign may remain the only sign for long periods, making diagnosis difficult, particularly in girls, in which isolated breast development may precede the appearance of pubic hair or the increase in growth velocity and bone maturation by several months. However, in some children, the increase in height velocity precedes the appearance of secondary sexual characteristics [23].

The clinical evaluation should guide the diagnosis and discussions about the most appropriate management.

The interview is used to specify the age at onset and rate of progression of pubertal signs, to investigate neonatal parameters (gestational age, birth measurements) and whether the child was adopted, together with any evidence suggesting a possible central nervous disorder, such as headache, visual disturbances or neurological signs (gelastic attacks), or pituitary deficiency, such as asthenia, polyuria-polydipsia, and the existence of a known chronic disease or history of cerebral radiotherapy. The evaluation also includes the height and pubertal age of parents and siblings, and family history of early or advanced puberty.

The physical examination assesses height, and height velocity (growth curve), weight and body mass index, pubertal stage and, in girls, the estrogenization of the vulva, skin lesions suggestive of neurofibromatosis or McCune Albright syndrome, neurological signs (large head circumference with macrocephaly, nystagmus, visual change or visual field defects, neurodevelopmental deficit), symptoms or signs of anterior or posterior pituitary deficiency (low growth velocity, polyuria/polydipsia, fatigue) and to assess the neuropsychological status of the child, which remains the major concern of the child and parents seeking help for early puberty. It is also important to recognize clinically the benign variants of precocious pubertal development, usually involving the isolated and non-progressive development of secondary sexual characteristics (breasts or pubic hair), normal growth velocity or slight increase in growth velocity, and little or no bone age advancement.

Following this assessment, watchful waiting or complementary explorations may be chosen as the most appropriate course of action. If watchful waiting is decided upon, then careful re-evaluation of progression is required 3–6 months later, to assess the rate of progression of puberty and any changes in growth.

Additional testing is generally recommended in all boys with precocious pubertal development, in girls with precocious Tanner 3 breast stage or higher and in girls with precocious B2 stage and additional criteria, such as increased growth velocity, or symptoms or signs suggestive of central nervous system dysfunction or of peripheral precocious puberty.

These tests include the assessment of bone age (which is usually advanced in patients with progressive precocious puberty), hormonal determinations, pelvic or testicular (if peripheral PP is suspected) ultrasound scans, and brain magnetic resonance imaging (MRI).

3.4.2 Biological Diagnosis

The biological diagnosis of precocious puberty is based on the evaluation of sex steroid secretion and its mechanisms. The diagnosis of central precocious puberty is based on pubertal serum gonadotrophin concentrations, with the demonstration of an activation of gonadotropin secretion [24].

Sex Steroid Determinations In boys, testosterone is a good marker of testicular maturation, provided it is assessed with a sensitive method. RIA(Radioimmunoassay) is generally used in practice. In girls, estradiol determination is uninformative, because half the girls displaying central precocious puberty have estradiol levels within the normal range of values in prepubescent girls. Very sensitive methods are required, and only RIA methods meet this requirement. The increase in estradiol concentration is also highly variable, due to the fluctuation, and sometimes intermittent secretion of this hormone. Very high estradiol levels are generally indicative of ovarian disease (peripheral PP due to cysts or tumors). Estrogenic impregnation is best assessed by pelvic ultrasound scans, on which the estrogenization of the uterus and ovaries may be visible [25].

Gonadotrophin Determinations Basal gonadotropin levels are informative, and are generally significantly higher in children with PP than in prepubertal children [26]. However, basal serum LH concentration is much more sensitive than basal FSH concentration and is the key to diagnosis. Ultrasensitive assays should be used to determine serum LH concentration. Prepubertal LH concentrations are <0.1 IU/L, so LH assays should have a detection limit close to 0.1 IU/L [27–29].

The response to GnRH stimulation is considered the gold standard for the diagnosis of central precocious puberty. Stimulation tests involving a single injection of LHRH analogs can also be used [30, 31]. The major problem is defining the decision threshold. In both sexes, a central cause of precocious puberty is demonstrated an increase in pituitary gonadotropin levels. Indeed, the underlying mechanism of early central puberty is linked to premature activation of the hypothalamic-pituitary-gonadal axis, with the onset of pulsatile LH secretion and an increase in the secretion of pituitary gonadotropins both in basal conditions and after stimulation with LHRH. Before the onset of puberty, the FSH peak is greater than the LH surge. During and after puberty, the LH surge predominates. In cases of central precocious puberty, basal serum LH concentration usually is ≥0.3 IU/L and serum LH concentration after stimulation is ≥5 IU/L [1, 32]. FSH is less informative than LH, because FSH levels vary little during pubertal development. However, the stimulated LH/FSH ratio may make it easier to distinguish between progressive precocious puberty (with an LH/FSH ratio >0.66) and non-progressive variants not requiring GnRHa therapy.

3.4.3 Place of Imaging in the Evaluation of Precocious Puberty

Pelvic ultrasound scans can be used to assess the degree of estrogenic impregnation of the internal genitalia in girls, through measurements of size and morphological criteria. A uterine length ≥35 mm is the first sign of estrogen exposure. Morphological features are also important, as the prepubertal state is marked by a tubular uterus, which becomes more pearl-like in shape during the course of puberty, with a bulging fundus. Measurements of uterine volume increase the reliability of the examination (prepubertal ≤2 ml). Endometrial thickening on an endometrial ultrasound scan

Table 3.2 Differentiation between true precocious puberty and slowly progressive forms

		Progressive precocious puberty	Slowly progressive precocious puberty
Clinical	*Pubertal stage*	Passage from one stage to another in 3–6 months	Spontaneous regression or stabilization of pubertal signs
	Growth velocity	Accelerated: > 6 cm/year	Normal for age
	Bone age	Typically advanced, variable, at least 2 years	Variable, but usually within 1 year of chronological age
	Predicted adult height	Below-target height or decreasing on serial determinations	Within target height range
Pelvic ultrasound scan	*Uterus*	Length > 34 mm or volume > 2 ml	Length ≤ 34 mm or volume ≤ 2 ml
		Pearl-shaped uterus	Prepubertal, tubular uterus
		Endometrial thickening (endometrial ultrasound scan)	
	Ovaries	Not very informative	Not very informative
Hormonal evaluation	*Estradiol (RIA ++)*	Not very informative, usually measurable	Not detectable or close to the detection limit
	LH peak after stimulation with GnRH	In the pubertal zone ≥ 5 IU/L	In the prepubertal range
	Basal LH determination	Useful if value is high (≥3 IU/L) and frankly in the pubertal range	No definitive value

provides a second line of evidence. Ovary size and the number of follicles are not criteria for the assessment of pubertal development [25, 31, 33]. Testicular ultrasound should be performed if the testicles differ in volume or if peripheral precocious puberty is suspected, to facilitate the detection of Leydig cell tumors, which are generally not palpable.

Neuroimaging is essential in the etiological evaluation in progressive central precocious puberty. Magnetic resonance imaging (MRI) is the examination of choice in the study of the brain and of the hypothalamic-pituitary region, for the detection of hypothalamic lesions. The prevalence of such lesions is higher in boys (30–80 % of cases) than in girls (8–33 %) and is much lower when puberty starts after the age of 6 years in girls, this population accounting for the majority of cases. It has been suggested that an algorithm based on age and estradiol levels could replace MRI, but such an approach has not been clearly validated [34–36].

At the end of this analysis, the diagnostic approach should help to determine the progressive or non-progressive nature of pubertal precocity (Table 3.2) and to differentiate between the etiologies of central or peripheral precocious puberty.

Indeed, many girls with idiopathic precocious puberty display very slow progressive puberty, or even regressive puberty, with little change to predicted adult height and a normal final height close to their parental target height [5, 6]. Therapeutic abstention is the most appropriate approach in most of these cases, because puberty progresses slowly, with menarche occurring, on average, 5.5 years after the onset of clinical signs of puberty, and patient reaching a normal final height relative to parental target height. However, in some cases (about one third of subjects), predicted adult stature may decrease during the progression of puberty, in parallel with the emergence of evident biological signs of estrogenization and a highly progressive form of central PP. Thus, children for whom no treatment is justified at the initial assessment should undergo systematic clinical assessment, at least until the age of 9 years, to facilitate the identification of girls subsequently requiring treatment to block central precocious puberty.

3.4.4 The Normal Variants of Puberty

The distinction between early puberty and normal puberty is not clear-cut. There are several variants of normal puberty, which may pose problems for differential diagnosis, particularly as they have a high prevalence [37–39].

Premature thelarche is isolated breast development before the age of 8 years. There are two peaks in the frequency of premature thelarche: the neonatal period, which is marked by gonadotropin activation, this peak potentially lasting for 2–3 years, and the prepubertal period [33]. Premature thelarche differs from early puberty in the absence of any other aspect of sexual development, usually with a lack of scalability of breast development and no acceleration of height velocity or significant advance in bone maturation (≥2 years). Uterine ultrasound scans provide a simple means of checking that there is no change in the uterus. No further exploration or treatment is required and the outcome is the persistence of moderate breast development (in two thirds of cases) or regression. However, isolated premature breast development may precede the onset of central precocious puberty, which should not be ignored if patients develop other pubertal signs and an acceleration of height velocity.

Premature pubarche is the appearance of pubic hair before the age of 8 years in girls and 9 years in boys. It may be accompanied by clinical signs of hyperandrogenism: acne, axillary hair, accelerated growth rate. It corresponds to adrenal maturation (adrenarche) and is not a differential diagnosis for central precocious puberty. Possible differential diagnoses to be systematically excluded include adrenal tumors and congenital adrenal hyperplasia [40, 41].

Slowly Progressive Forms of Precocious Puberty Such forms present clinically as early puberty with the development of secondary sexual characteristics and a moderate advance in bone age. On ultrasound scans, the uterus may show very early estrogen impregnation. However, the response to GnRH is of the prepubertal type. The mechanism underlying these cases of non-progressive precocious puberty is unknown, but the gonadotropic axis is not activated. Studies monitoring these benign variants of precocious puberty have shown that treatment with GnRH agonists is not appropriate because there tends to be either a total regression of pubertal signs or a slow progression towards puberty [5, 6]. Table 3.2 provides elements guiding differentiation between slowly progressive and progressive forms of central precocious puberty.

3.4.5 Psychosocial Aspects

Psychosocial aspects of early puberty are the major concern of patients and families seeking help for early puberty, whereas doctors generally focus on etiological aspects and height prognosis. Psychological assessment usually reveals a normal IQ. Patients tend to be rather solitary, with high scores for isolation, and a tendency to become depressed. They are mostly concerned about their appearance, whereas parents are generally worried about the onset of periods. Little is known about the long-term psychosocial consequences of early puberty or about the psychosocial integration of patients treated for precocious puberty [13, 42].

3.5 Management of Central Precocious Puberty

3.5.1 GnRH Agonists

GnRH agonists are generally indicated in progressive central precocious puberty, with the aim to restore genetic growth potential and to stabilize or regress pubertal symptoms. GnRH agonists continuously stimulate the pituitary gonadotrophs, leading to desensitization and decreases in LH release and, to a lesser extent, FSH release [43]. Several GnRH agonists are available in various depot forms and the approval for use of the various formulations varies with countries. Despite nearly 30 years of use of GnRH agonists in precocious puberty, there are still ongoing questions on their optimal use and an international consensus statement has summarized the available information and the areas of uncertainty as of 2007 [17].

GnRH agonist treatments should be followed by experienced clinicians and result in the regression or stabilization of pubertal symptoms, decrease of growth velocity, and bone age advancement [17]. GnRHa-injection dates should be recorded and adherence with the dosing interval monitored. A suppressed LH response to the stimulation by GnRH, GnRH agonist, or after an injection of the depot preparation (which contains a fraction of free GnRH agonist) is indicative of biochemical efficacy of the treatment but is not recommended routinely. Progression of breast or testicular development usually indicates poor compliance, treatment failure, or incorrect diagnosis and requires further evaluation.

There are no randomized controlled trials assessing *long term outcomes* of the treatment of central precocious puberty with GnRH agonists and height outcome have been mostly evaluated. Among approximately 400 girls treated until a mean age of 11 years, the mean adult height was about 160 cm and mean gains over predicted height varied from 3 to 10 cm [12]. Individual height gains were very variable, but were calculated using predicted height, which is itself poorly reliable. Factors affecting height outcome include initial patient characteristics (lower height if bone age is markedly advanced and shorter predicted height at initiation of treatment) and, in some series, duration of treatment (higher height gains in patients starting treatment at a younger age and with longer durations of treatment). No height gain benefit has been shown in girls treated after the age of 9 years.

Other outcomes to consider include bone mineral density, risk of obesity and metabolic disorders, and psychosocial outcomes. Bone mineral density may decrease during GnRH agonist therapy. However, subsequent bone mass accrual is preserved, and peak bone mass does not seem to be negatively affected by treatment [17]. There has been concern that GnRH agonists use may affect BMI. However, childhood obesity is associated with earlier pubertal development in girls, and early sexual maturation is associated with increased prevalence of overweight and obesity. Altogether, the available data indicate that long-term GnRH agonist treatment does not seem to cause or aggravate obesity or have repercussions for body composition, bone mineral density, fertility, and metabolic or cancer comorbidities. General health status is not different as compared to women with normal puberty [44–46]. The development of polycystic ovarian syndrome remains controversial [47–50] and further studies are still required to assess the potential risk of premature ovarian dysfunction. Data concerning psychosocial outcomes are scarce and there is little evidence to show whether treatment with GnRH agonists are associated with improved psychological outcome [13, 46]. Studies of this aspect are required.

Although *tolerance* to GnRH agonist treatment is generally considered good, it may be associated with headaches and menopausal symptoms such as hot flushes. Local complications (3–13 %) such as sterile abscesses may result in a loss of efficacy and anaphylaxis has been described [51].

The *optimal time to stop treatment* has not been established and factors that could influence the decision to stop GnRH agonists include aiming at maximizing height, synchronizing puberty with peers, ameliorating psychological distress, or facilitating care of the developmentally delayed child. However, data only permit analysis of factors that affect adult height. Several variables can be used to decide on when to stop treatment including chronological age, duration of therapy, bone age, height, target height, growth velocity. However these variables are closely interrelated and cannot be considered independently. In addition, retrospective analyses suggest that continuing treatment beyond the age of 11 years is associated with no further gains [52]. Therefore, it is reasonable to consider these parameters and informed parent and patient preferences, with the goal of menarche occurring near the population norms [17]. Pubertal manifestations generally reappear within months of GnRH agonist treatment being stopped, with a mean time to menarche of 16 months [53]. Long-term fertility has not been fully evaluated, but preliminary observations are reassuring [46, 53].

The addition of growth hormone [54] or oxandrolone [55] when growth velocity decreases or if height prognosis appears to be unsatisfactory has been proposed, but data are limited on the efficacy and safety of these drugs in children with precocious puberty.

3.5.2 Management of Causal Lesions

When precocious puberty is caused by a hypothalamic lesion (e.g., mass or malformation), management of the causal lesion generally has no effect on the course of pubertal development. Hypothalamic hamartomas should not be treated by surgery for the management of precocious puberty. Precocious puberty associated with the presence of a hypothalamic lesion may progress to gonadotropin deficiency.

Conclusion

Knowledge of the different clinical forms of precocious puberty is essential to determine whether there is a tumor (intracranial) or other disease, and the indications for treatment or an abstention from treatment.

References

1. Carel JC, Leger J (2008) Clinical practice. Precocious puberty. N Engl J Med 358(22): 2366–2377
2. Kaplowitz PB, Slora EJ, Wasserman RC, Pedlow SE, Herman-Giddens ME (2001) Earlier onset of puberty in girls: relation to increased body mass index and race. Pediatrics 108(2): 347–353
3. Biro FM, Galvez MP, Greenspan LC, Succop PA, Vangeepuram N, Pinney SM et al (2010) Pubertal assessment method and baseline characteristics in a mixed longitudinal study of girls. Pediatrics 126(3):e583–e590
4. Sorensen K, Mouritsen A, Aksglaede L, Hagen CP, Mogensen SS, Juul A (2012) Recent secular trends in pubertal timing: implications for evaluation and diagnosis of precocious puberty. Horm Res Paediatr 77(3):137–145
5. Palmert MR, Malin HV, Boepple PA (1999) Unsustained or slowly progressive puberty in young girls: initial presentation and long-term follow-up of 20 untreated patients. J Clin Endocrinol Metab 84(2):415–423
6. Leger J, Reynaud R, Czernichow P (2000) Do all girls with apparent idiopathic precocious puberty require gonadotropin-releasing hormone agonist treatment? J Pediatr 137(6): 819–825
7. Prete G, Couto-Silva AC, Trivin C, Brauner R (2008) Idiopathic central precocious puberty in girls: presentation factors. BMC Pediatr 8:27
8. Teilmann G, Pedersen CB, Jensen TK, Skakkebaek NE, Juul A (2005) Prevalence and incidence of precocious pubertal development in Denmark: an epidemiologic study based on national registries. Pediatrics 116(6):1323–1328
9. Abreu AP, Dauber A, Macedo DB, Noel SD, Brito VN, Gill JC et al (2013) Central precocious puberty caused by mutations in the imprinted gene MKRN3. N Engl J Med 368(26):2467–2475
10. Bulcao Macedo D, Nahime Brito V, Latronico AC (2014) New causes of central precocious puberty: the role of genetic factors. Neuroendocrinology 100(1):1–8
11. Macedo DB, Abreu AP, Reis AC, Montenegro LR, Dauber A, Beneduzzi D et al (2014) Central precocious puberty that appears to be sporadic caused by paternally inherited mutations in the imprinted gene makorin ring finger 3. J Clin Endocrinol Metab 99(6):E1097–E1103
12. Carel JC, Lahlou N, Roger M, Chaussain JL (2004) Precocious puberty and statural growth. Hum Reprod Update 10(2):135–147

13. Xhrouet-Heinrichs D, Lagrou K, Heinrichs C, Craen M, Dooms L, Malvaux P et al (1997) Longitudinal study of behavioral and affective patterns in girls with central precocious puberty during long-acting triptorelin therapy. Acta Paediatr 86(8):808–815
14. Giabicani E, Lemaire P, Brauner R (2015) Models for predicting the adult height and age at first menstruation of girls with idiopathic central precocious puberty. PLoS One 10(3):e0120588
15. Marti-Henneberg C, Vizmanos B (1997) The duration of puberty in girls is related to the timing of its onset. J Pediatr 131(4):618–621
16. Day FR, Elks CE, Murray A, Ong KK, Perry JR (2015) Puberty timing associated with diabetes, cardiovascular disease and also diverse health outcomes in men and women: the UK Biobank study. Sci Rep 5:11208
17. Carel JC, Eugster EA, Rogol A, Ghizzoni L, Palmert MR, Antoniazzi F et al (2009) Consensus statement on the use of gonadotropin-releasing hormone analogs in children. Pediatrics 123(4):e752–e762
18. Michaud PA, Suris JC, Deppen A (2006) Gender-related psychological and behavioural correlates of pubertal timing in a national sample of Swiss adolescents. Mol Cell Endocrinol 254–255:172–178
19. Schoelwer MJ, Donahue KL, Bryk K, Didrick P, Berenbaum SA, Eugster EA (2015) Psychological assessment of mothers and their daughters at the time of diagnosis of precocious puberty. Int J Pediatr Endocrinol 2015(1):5
20. Wise LA, Palmer JR, Rothman EF, Rosenberg L (2009) Childhood abuse and early menarche: findings from the black women's health study. Am J Public Health 99(Suppl 2):S460–S466
21. Marshall WA, Tanner JM (1969) Variations in pattern of pubertal changes in girls. Arch Dis Child 44(235):291–303
22. Marshall WA, Tanner JM (1970) Variations in the pattern of pubertal changes in boys. Arch Dis Child 45(239):13–23
23. Papadimitriou A, Beri D, Tsialla A, Fretzayas A, Psychou F, Nicolaidou P (2006) Early growth acceleration in girls with idiopathic precocious puberty. J Pediatr 149(1):43–46
24. Nathan BM, Palmert MR (2005) Regulation and disorders of pubertal timing. Endocrinol Metab Clin North Am 34(3):617–641, ix
25. de Vries L, Horev G, Schwartz M, Phillip M (2006) Ultrasonographic and clinical parameters for early differentiation between precocious puberty and premature thelarche. Eur J Endocrinol 154(6):891–898
26. Resende EA, Lara BH, Reis JD, Ferreira BP, Pereira GA, Borges MF (2007) Assessment of basal and gonadotropin-releasing hormone-stimulated gonadotropins by immunochemiluminometric and immunofluorometric assays in normal children. J Clin Endocrinol Metab 92(4):1424–1429
27. Neely EK, Wilson DM, Lee PA, Stene M, Hintz RL (1995) Spontaneous serum gonadotropin concentrations in the evaluation of precocious puberty. J Pediatr 127(1):47–52
28. Pasternak Y, Friger M, Loewenthal N, Haim A, Hershkovitz E (2012) The utility of basal serum LH in prediction of central precocious puberty in girls. Eur J Endocrinol 166(2): 295–299
29. Houk CP, Kunselman AR, Lee PA (2009) Adequacy of a single unstimulated luteinizing hormone level to diagnose central precocious puberty in girls. Pediatrics 123(6):e1059–e1063
30. Yazdani P, Lin Y, Raman V, Haymond M (2012) A single sample GnRHa stimulation test in the diagnosis of precocious puberty. Int J Pediatr Endocrinol 2012(1):23
31. Sathasivam A, Rosenberg HK, Shapiro S, Wang H, Rapaport R (2011) Pelvic ultrasonography in the evaluation of central precocious puberty: comparison with leuprolide stimulation test. J Pediatr 159(3):490–495
32. Fuqua JS (2013) Treatment and outcomes of precocious puberty: an update. J Clin Endocrinol Metab 98(6):2198–2207
33. de Vries L, Guz-Mark A, Lazar L, Reches A, Phillip M (2010) Premature thelarche: age at presentation affects clinical course but not clinical characteristics or risk to progress to precocious puberty. J Pediatr 156(3):466–471

34. Chalumeau M, Hadjiathanasiou CG, Ng SM, Cassio A, Mul D, Cisternino M et al (2003) Selecting girls with precocious puberty for brain imaging: validation of European evidence-based diagnosis rule. J Pediatr 143(4):445–450
35. Stanhope R (2003) Gonadotrophin-dependent [correction of dependant] precocious puberty and occult intracranial tumors: which girls should have neuro-imaging? J Pediatr 143(4):426–427
36. Pedicelli S, Alessio P, Scire G, Cappa M, Cianfarani S (2014) Routine screening by brain magnetic resonance imaging is not indicated in every girl with onset of puberty between the ages of 6 and 8 years. J Clin Endocrinol Metab 99(12):4455–4461
37. Atay Z, Turan S, Guran T, Furman A, Bereket A (2012) The prevalence and risk factors of premature thelarche and pubarche in 4- to 8-year-old girls. Acta Paediatr 101(2):e71–e75
38. Mogensen SS, Aksglaede L, Mouritsen A, Sorensen K, Main KM, Gideon P et al (2011) Diagnostic work-up of 449 consecutive girls who were referred to be evaluated for precocious puberty. J Clin Endocrinol Metab 96(5):1393–1401
39. Kaplowitz P (2004) Clinical characteristics of 104 children referred for evaluation of precocious puberty. J Clin Endocrinol Metab 89(8):3644–3650
40. Oberfield SE, Sopher AB, Gerken AT (2011) Approach to the girl with early onset of pubic hair. J Clin Endocrinol Metab 96(6):1610–1622
41. Ghizzoni L, Gasco V (2010) Premature pubarche. Horm Res Paediatr 73(5):420–422
42. Baumann DA, Landolt MA, Wetterwald R, Dubuis JM, Sizonenko PC, Werder EA (2001) Psychological evaluation of young women after medical treatment for central precocious puberty. Horm Res 56(1–2):45–50
43. Lahlou N, Carel JC, Chaussain JL, Roger M (2000) Pharmacokinetics and pharmacodynamics of GnRH agonists: clinical implications in pediatrics. J Pediatr Endocrinol Metab 13(Suppl 1):723–737
44. Thornton P, Silverman LA, Geffner ME, Neely EK, Gould E, Danoff TM (2014) Review of outcomes after cessation of gonadotropin-releasing hormone agonist treatment of girls with precocious puberty. Pediatr Endocrinol Rev 11(3):306–317
45. Lazar L, Meyerovitch J, de Vries L, Phillip M, Lebenthal Y (2014) Treated and untreated women with idiopathic precocious puberty: long-term follow-up and reproductive outcome between the third and fifth decades. Clin Endocrinol (Oxf) 80(4):570–576
46. Lazar L, Lebenthal Y, Yackobovitch-Gavan M, Shalitin S, de Vries L, Phillip M et al (2015) Treated and untreated women with idiopathic precocious puberty: BMI evolution, metabolic outcome, and general health between third and fifth decades. J Clin Endocrinol Metab 100(4):1445–1451
47. Heger S, Partsch CJ, Sippell WG (1999) Long-term outcome after depot gonadotropin-releasing hormone agonist treatment of central precocious puberty: final height, body proportions, body composition, bone mineral density, and reproductive function. J Clin Endocrinol Metab 84(12):4583–4590
48. Franceschi R, Gaudino R, Marcolongo A, Gallo MC, Rossi L, Antoniazzi F et al (2010) Prevalence of polycystic ovary syndrome in young women who had idiopathic central precocious puberty. Fertil Steril 93(4):1185–1191
49. Magiakou MA, Manousaki D, Papadaki M, Hadjidakis D, Levidou G, Vakaki M et al (2010) The efficacy and safety of gonadotropin-releasing hormone analog treatment in childhood and adolescence: a single center, long-term follow-up study. J Clin Endocrinol Metab 95(1): 109–117
50. Chiavaroli V, Liberati M, D'Antonio F, Masuccio F, Capanna R, Verrotti A et al (2010) GNRH analog therapy in girls with early puberty is associated with the achievement of predicted final height but also with increased risk of polycystic ovary syndrome. Eur J Endocrinol 163(1):55–62
51. Carel JC, Lahlou N, Jaramillo O, Montauban V, Teinturier C, Colle M et al (2002) Treatment of central precocious puberty by subcutaneous injections of leuprorelin 3-month depot (11.25 mg). J Clin Endocrinol Metab 87(9):4111–4116

52. Carel JC, Roger M, Ispas S, Tondu F, Lahlou N, Blumberg J et al (1999) Final height after long-term treatment with triptorelin slow-release for central precocious puberty: importance of statural growth after interruption of treatment. J Clin Endocrinol Metab 84:1973–1978
53. Heger S, Muller M, Ranke M, Schwarz HP, Waldhauser F, Partsch CJ et al (2006) Long-term GnRH agonist treatment for female central precocious puberty does not impair reproductive function. Mol Cell Endocrinol 254–255:217–220
54. Pasquino AM, Pucarelli I, Segni M, Matrunola M, Cerroni F, Cerrone F (1999) Adult height in girls with central precocious puberty treated with gonadotropin-releasing hormone analogues and growth hormone. J Clin Endocrinol Metab 84(2):449–452
55. Vottero A, Pedori S, Verna M, Pagano B, Cappa M, Loche S et al (2006) Final height in girls with central idiopathic precocious puberty treated with gonadotropin-releasing hormone analog and oxandrolone. J Clin Endocrinol Metab 91(4):1284–1287

Management of Peripheral Precocious Puberty in Girls

4

Charles Sultan, Laura Gaspari, Nicolas Kalfa, and Françoise Paris

The premature appearance of secondary sexual characteristics like breast development and pubic hair is upsetting and prompts many families to consult endocrinologists. Yet the management of precocious puberty is not always straightforward [1], especially given the unusually wide range of clinical expression: most presentations of precocious puberty are peripheral precocious puberty (PPP).

- Ten to twenty percent of all cases are instances of central precocious puberty (CPP). The course of its development needs to be carefully assessed and a central tumor must be eliminated. In its typical form, CPP progresses rapidly and the accelerated bone maturation leads to early fusion of the bone plates, thus compromising final adult height. Other clinical presentations have been identified and will be discussed further on.
- In 50–60 % of the cases, only one secondary sexual characteristic shows premature development and the diagnosis is premature thelarche (breast development), premature pubarche (appearance of pubic hair). In these cases, the etiology should be sought, and clinical, biological, and radiographic management is devoted to preventing the precocious onset of puberty.

C. Sultan (✉) • L. Gaspari • F. Paris
Unité d'Endocrinologie-Gynécologie Pédiatriques, Departement de Pédiatrie, Hôpital Arnaud de Villeneuve, CHU Montpellier et Université Montpellier 1, Montpellier, France

Service d'Hormonologie (Développement et Reproduction), Hôpital Lapeyronie, CHU Montpellier et Université Montpellier 1, Montpellier, France
e-mail: c-sultan@chu-montpellier.fr

N. Kalfa
Service de Chirurgie Pédiatrique, Hôpital Lapeyronie, CHU Montpellier, Montpellier, France

Service d'Hormonologie (Développement et Reproduction), Hôpital Lapeyronie, CHU Montpellier et Université Montpellier 1, Montpellier, France

C. Sultan, A.R. Genazzani (eds.), *Frontiers in Gynecological Endocrinology*, ISGE Series, DOI 10.1007/978-3-319-41433-1_4

- The development of secondary sexual characteristics has an ovarian cause, with an autonomous hyperproduction of estrogens causing precocious pseudopuberty independently of gonadotropin activation. In more and more cases, it has become evident that the hyperestrogenism may have an exogenous origin such as environmental chemical pollutants in the air, water, and food chain. These xenoestrogens have a chemical structure that mimics the actions of natural estrogens by stimulating the activity of target tissues.

In all cases, the initial step is to evaluate the level of estrogen secretion, in terms of both its impact on target organs (breasts, growth rate, bone maturation, etc.) and its course over time. A good understanding of the various ways that precocious puberty clinically presents in girls is vital for the decision on therapeutic management, as the optimal treatment is often not evident during the initial evaluation.

4.1 Evaluation of the Pubertal Stage

One of the first steps in diagnosis is the estimation of pubertal stage. The Tanner stages have been the reference for many years, as they are very well codified (Table 4.1). In routine clinical practice, this relatively precise staging is complemented by examination of the sesamoid bone of the hand. This marker of bone maturation appears towards 11 years and signals the start of puberty.

The Tanner stages have been the reference for generations of pediatric endocrinologists. In an American study of a very large cohort of girls examined between the ages of 3 and 11 years, most of the girls appeared to enter puberty at a younger age (9.9 years for B2 and 10.5 years for P2). This drop in the age of puberty onset was most evident in black girls. The authors attributed their findings to the impact of environmental factors (chemical pollution). The findings that most of the girls entering puberty at the youngest ages (between 6 and 8 years) do not present with short adult height and that the duration of puberty (tempo) is inversely linked to the age of onset (timing) should be considered as relevant to clinical practice, especially to any decision about therapeutic management.

These works as a whole have done much to elucidate the development of secondary sexual characteristics and the normal course of puberty in girls.

Table 4.1 Mean ages for normal pubertal development stages in girls, based on Tanner stages for breast development (B) and pubic hair (P)

Pubertal stage	Age (years)
Breast buds (B2)	10.1
Sparse pubic hair growth (P2)	11.2
Darker, coarser pubic hair growth (P3)	12.2
Growth spurt	12.2
Menarche	12.7
Adult pubic hair in type and quantity (P5)	14
Mature breast (B5)	14

The activation of the gonadotropic axis is marked by a peak in LH above 5 μUI/ml and an LH/FSH ratio above 1 during LHRH testing. Conversely, to the assertions of other groups, we do not accept the basal values of LH (whatever the standard used) as a marker of pubertal onset.

The measurement of plasma estradiol by radioimmunology is not a reliable method to evaluate the onset of puberty because of its low specificity and high fluctuations. Only the analysis of the biological activity of estrogens using ultrasensitive methods is able to provide useful information on pubertal onset [2].

Last, pelvic ultrasonography with measurement of the uterus should be systematically performed: onset of puberty shows an increase in ovarian volume (>1.5 cm^3) and uterine size with length exceeding 3.5 cm. The finding of an increased diameter of the uterine fundus and a uterine vacuity line reflects significant estrogenization.

Clinical, biological, anthropometric, and radiographic evaluations are all helpful in distinguishing normal puberty from precocious puberty, which may have important clinical, psychological, and therapeutic implications.

4.2 Clinical Expression of Peripheral Precocious Puberty

Precocious puberty is eight times more frequent in girls than in boys [3]. Premature breast development, pubic hair, and growth acceleration should prompt several questions (Table 4.2), the answers to which will provide clues as to the best adapted treatment strategy.

1. Did puberty clinically begin before 8 years?
2. What has been the progression of the clinical symptoms?
3. Are there biological or radiographic signs of exaggerated maturation?
4. How is predicted adult height affected?
5. What are the psychological consequences?
6. Is the hormonal secretion gonadotropin-dependent or -independent?
7. In the case of central gonadotropin activation, is it due to a tumor or is it idiopathic?

Premature thelarche is the most common clinical expression of PPP. Premature thelarche refers to isolated breast development in girls between 2 and 7 years, which differs from the genital crisis of the newborn whose breast development (associated with strong estrogenization and even milk production) may last for the first 18

Table 4.2 Clinical forms of peripheral precocious puberty

Peripheral precocious puberty: precocious pseudopuberty
Ovarian autonomy
McCune-Albright syndrome, ovarian cyst
Granulosa cell tumor
Adrenal tumor (feminizing)
Environmental pollution (pesticides)

months of life. This premature breast development is bilateral in half the cases, unilateral, or, less frequently, asymmetric. Volume varies: 60 % at B2, 30 % at B3, and 10 % at B4. The breast is often tender and palpation is sometimes painful. There is no discharge.

In persistent or marked forms of thelarche, the hormonal work-up should be limited to the LHRH test to confirm a predominant FSH response [4]. Bone maturation is rarely accelerated. The progression is characterized by fluctuations over time: spontaneous remission, persistence, and aggravation of breast volume, which should evoke the possibility of puberty onset. In this case, pelvic ultrasound can provide useful information.

When estrogen secretion is patent (simultaneous increase in uterine volume), contamination by products with estrogen-like activity should be considered and sought (soy-rich foods, environmental pesticides, etc.). In its usual form, premature thelarche requires no treatment.

Peripheral precocious or precocious pseudopuberty is not characterized by the premature activation of the gonadotropic axis: it is caused by an abnormally high production of estrogens and, more rarely, androgens because of a "tumor" on the ovary or adrenal glands. It is iso- or heterosexual depending on the whether the excess steroid hormone strengthens or transforms the child's phenotype.

4.2.1 Peripheral Precocious Puberty Caused by Ovarian Autonomy

The considerable progress in determining the molecular mechanisms of hormone transduction signals has greatly contributed to our understanding of the physiopathology and clinical expression of peripheral precocious puberty caused by ovarian autonomy. This progress may one day culminate in a specific treatment for this rare but incapacitating disorder. Heterosexual precocious pseudopuberty secondary to a virilizing adrenal or ovarian tumor is much rarer.

4.2.1.1 McCune-Albright Syndrome

McCune-Albright syndrome (MAS) is a sporadic disorder characterized by the classic triad of precocious puberty, fibrous bone dysplasia, and *café-au-lait* spots [5]. Diverse endocrine abnormalities can also be associated: somatotrophic pituitary adenomas, hypothyroid goiter, and adrenal hyperplasia.

Precocious Puberty

MAS affects girls almost exclusively and is characterized by its extreme precociousness and the gravity of the immediate clinical picture: isolated menstruation as early as the first months or first years of life. The full clinical picture will develop later, with breast enlargement and pubic hair. The often voluminous ovarian cysts discovered by ultrasound are cyclic and are difficult to treat: cystectomy or ovariectomy is often necessary when all other treatments fail. The acceleration of growth velocity is considerable (+2, +3 SD) and constant, on the order of 9–10 cm per year.

Bone maturation is also accelerated and will thus compromise the prognosis for final adult height.

The biological work-up will show very high plasma estradiol associated with dramatically low plasma gonadotropins and no response to GnRH stimulation. This indicates LH/FSH-independent precocious puberty and situates this type of precocious puberty within the context of the ovarian-autonomous syndromes.

Café-au-lait Spots

The *café-au-lait* spots of MAS are hyperpigmented, typically light brown or brown, with irregular borders ("coast of Maine") that distinguish them from the smooth-bordered spots observed in neurofibromatosis. The spots are usually unilaterally distributed, on the same side as the bone lesions. When associated with precocious puberty, they are an essential diagnostic element.

Fibrous Bone Dysplasia

Fibrous bone dysplasia is the third element in the classic triad. This bone abnormality may remain silent for many years, only to be revealed by a spontaneous fracture or on the occasion of a slight injury. X-rays reveal pseudocysts of the bone cortex that rapidly invade the entire skeleton.

Other Endocrine Pathologies

Other endocrine pathologies are seen to varying degrees: hyperthyroidism, acromegaly, gigantism, hypercorticism, hyperprolactinemia, and hyperparathyroidism. These types of endocrine hyperfunctioning are also caused by autonomous hormonal hyperproduction.

Molecular Bases of McCune-Albright Syndrome

The specific location of the skin lesions and the sporadic character of MAS (no documented cases of hereditary transmission) suggest that this disorder is due to a somatic mutation that occurs early in development. The result is a mosaic distribution of abnormal cells. The appearance and the severity of the bone, skin, and endocrine abnormalities thus depends on the number of cells carrying the mutation.

Moreover, the diverse endocrine hyperfunctioning syndromes observed in the course of MAS have in common the presence and activation of cells that respond to extracellular signaling by activation of the adenyl cyclase system. The hypothesis of local hyperproduction of cyclic adenosine monophosphate (AMPc) was confirmed several years ago: MAS is caused by a genetic abnormality that causes a constitutive activation of adenyl cyclase. The evidence of activating $G\alpha_s$ mutations in various tissues of MAS patients further supports this mechanism.

4.2.1.2 Granulosa Cell Tumors

Although rare (10% of the ovarian tumors in children), granulosa tumors are expressed in early childhood by strong estrogen secretion that results in marked breast development, accelerated growth velocity, and by menstruation. These ovarian tumors are discovered in a wide variety of circumstances:

- Endocrine disturbances
  - The hormonal activity of the tumor explains why 80–90 % of the girls under 8 years present isosexual precocious pseudopuberty. This pubertal advance induced by the estrogen secretion of the tumor cells is independent of the low levels of GnRH and prepubertal gonadotropins. On clinical examination, breast development is frequently noted but this is variable; metrorrhagia, accelerated growth velocity, and sometimes advanced bone age are also noted. The preoperative plasma estrogen concentration is almost always elevated. Virilization with precocious pubarche, acnea, hirsutism, and rarely clitoromegaly is related to aromatase deficiency inside the tumor.
  - Endocrine symptoms may also be present in cases of ovarian granulose cells in the post pubertal period. Symptoms are more difficult to detect, such menometrorragia and hyperandrogenism.
  - Precocity of diagnosis and an early recognition of endocrine signs from ovarian granulosa cell tumors significantly improve its prognosis with a lower risk of peritoneal extension.

In most patients, the levels of inhibin and AMH are elevated and return to normal post-surgery. The level of inhibin is correlated with tumor extension and eventual relapse. If the estradiol level is initially high, this too can be useful for follow-up. However, its interest is limited because [1] 30 % of granulosa tumors are nonsecreting [2], its level depends on the surrounding theca cells and is thus variable, and [3] physiological puberty can interfere with measurement.

- During emergency surgery (10 % of the cases) for acute abdominal pain and vomiting that are mistakenly diagnosed as acute appendicitis. These symptoms are due to torsion of the ovary or more rarely tumor rupture..
- An abdominal-pelvic mass that may be quite voluminous. This mass is frequently asymptomatic and it is discovered by the parents. It may also cause compression of the urinary tract (lumbar pain, colic nephritic, urinary infection) or the intestine (constipation, incomplete occlusion syndrome).
- As a fortuitous discovery during surgical intervention for other reasons, such are inguinal hernia repair, or as calcifications or ossifications of abdominal X-rays.
- By discovery of an ovarian cyst during prenatal diagnosis, which is an exceptional situation.

Surgery is the treatment of choice for a granulosa cell tumor. A careful preoperative evaluation is necessary to preserve fertility and future hormonal functioning. Staging includes peritoneal cytology and exploration of the abdominal cavity. Limited tumors can be treated by salpingo ovariectomy, as the rate of relapse is minimal. For bilateral tumor, a conservative treatment of the contralateral ovary should be discussed. In stages with extraovarian extension, chemotherapy is recommended. Follow up includes careful clinical, hormonal, and ultrasonographic evaluation.

Due to its excellent prognosis and the often complete recovery after initial surgery, juvenile ovarian granulosa cell tumors (OGCT) has usually been considered as benign condition. Survival of the patients with stage Ia tumors is around 90 %, the overall survival in the whole group approximating 85 %. However, the minority of the tumors that have spread within the abdomen or recurred after initial therapy have a much poorer prognosis and OGCT should be considered an ovarian cancer of good prognosis rather than a benign condition. It is still not possible to identify those patients who will relapse in the future, and the mechanism of this relapse remains to be elucidated. Nevertheless, molecular biology has identified two markers of prognosis:

- Mutations of the Gs alpha protein – a protein included in the transduction of the FSH signal – have been found in hot spot position 201 in 30 % of patients' DNAs [6]. The oncologic stages were significantly different according to the gsp oncogene status. Patients with a hyperactivated Gαs exhibited a significantly more advanced tumor ($P < 0.05$). Gsp oncogene is indeed implicated in cell proliferation level and cell invasion capacity.
- Another prognostic factor of OGCT could be the level of the differentiation of the tumoral cell. One of the earliest differentiating genes of granulosa cell in the fetus is FOXL2. FOXL2, a forkhead transcription factor, is a regulatory element of the organogenesis of the mammalian ovary. The patients with no or reduced expression of FOXL2 in their tumor exhibit significantly more advanced oncologic staging. All patients requiring complementary treatment (chemotherapy or complementary surgery) showed reduced FOXL2 expression in the tumor [7]. The extinction of this gene implicated in granulosa cell differentiation is compatible with an uncontrolled proliferation of these cells.

4.2.1.3 Ovarian Cysts

Functional nonneoplastic ovarian cysts and masses are frequent in peripubertal girls and are generally follicular or luteal in origin [8].

Ovarian cysts are mostly unilateral, unilocular, and simple with the size varying between 2 and 5 cm in diameter.

Rapid prepubertal breast development is usual followed by metrorrhagia in some cases. Pelvic US is mandatory.

If the cyst is anechogenic, the patient should be monitored for a period of 3–6 months. If there is any clinical or sonographic change, surgery can be discussed.

4.2.2 Feminizing Tumors of the Adrenal Gland

Feminizing tumors of the adrenal gland are relatively rare causes of precocious pseudopuberty.

4.2.3 Precocious Pseudopuberty and Environmental Pollution

Increasing attention should be given to precocious pseudopuberty secondary to environmental contamination by chemical products such as pesticides, herbicides, and fungicides. Endocrine disruptors with the capacity to mimic estrogens are able to generate estrogen secretion, resulting in simple thelarche to true central PP.

A decline in the age of pubertal onset and a rise in the prevalence of precocious puberty in girls (PP) (pubertal development before 8 years in girls) have been widely documented throughout the world [9, 10]. A better understanding of the "endocrine disrupting" activities of many environmental pollutants, particularly estrogen-mimetic compounds, has prompted the medical and research communities to consider their role in the increased prevalence of PP.

Environmental endocrine disruptors (EEDs) are able to disrupt the endocrine system at various levels, affecting, for example, the hypothalamic-pituitary axis, steroidogenesis, and the binding of steroid nuclear receptors; they therefore theoretically have the ability to interfere with the course of physiological puberty. Most notably, EEDs can mimic estrogen activity, which is why they are called "xenoestrogens" [11]. The acceleration in the incidence of PP cases and greater knowledge of the "endocrine disrupting" activities of EEDs have prompted the scientific community to hypothesize their role in the increased prevalence of pubertal precocity [12, 13].

Endocrine disruptors may be natural or synthetic and are listed below.

Phyto and mycoestrogens
Pesticides
Plastics
Synthetic Estrogens (OCP)
Cosmetics
Dioxin

Over the last 20 years, we have developed an ultrasensitive assay for EED in patient blood.

We have been able to demonstrate the role of EED contamination in a 4-month-old girl with precocious puberty seen in our pediatric endocrinology clinic, as we found very high concentrations of lindane and DDT in the child, her mother, and soil samples taken from their home to confirm our results [14]. In addition, we recently observed that premature thelarche can sometimes be associated with prenatal or postnatal exposure to EEDs, in a study we conducted in a group of young girls in whom we identified an abnormally high ultrasensitive estrogenic activity [15].

Over the last years, we have clearly observed an advance in the age of pubertal onset and it is ongoing. In addition, a rise in the incidence of PP has been reported in France as well as in many countries. Studies conducted in animals and humans support the role of EEDs in peripheral precocious puberty. It is however evident that a central action of EED cannot be excluded. This interaction of EED with the Kiss neurons may also contribute to the increase prevalence of central PP in girls. Beyond their impact on pubertal development, the relationships among the duration of estrogen exposure, the pervasiveness of EEDs, and the rising incidence of breast cancer appear to be generally acknowledged, which underlines—if need be—the importance of this issue for public health.

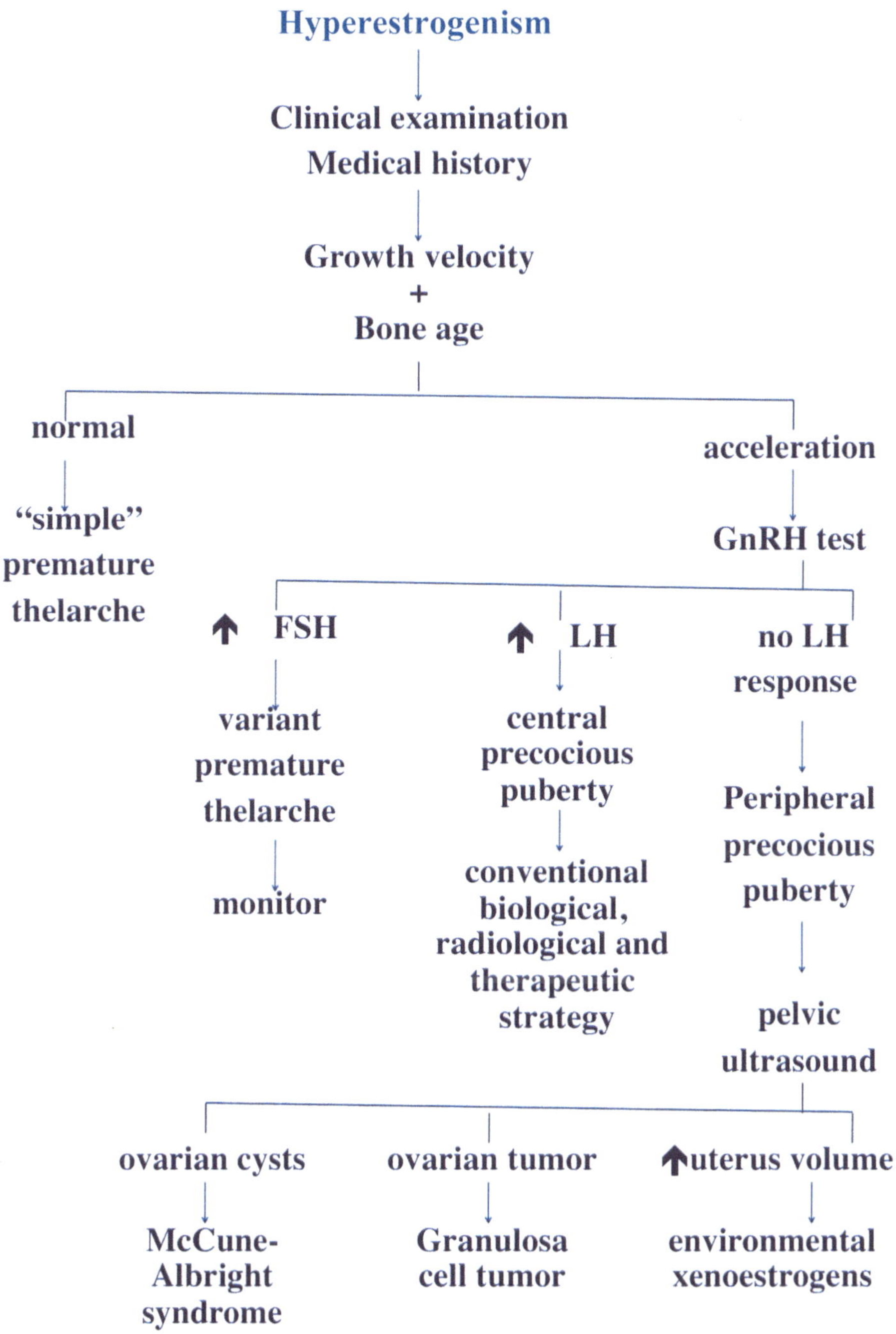

Fig. 4.1 Decision tree for peripheral precocious puberty

Conclusion

In girls, the prevalence of precocious puberty is rapidly increasing all over the world. PPP may be due to ovarian autonomous hyperactivity that should be identified and specifically treated (Fig 4.1). However, the role of EED seems predominant and raises a key question of a health and economic problem.

References

1. Fuqua JS (2013) Treatment and outcomes of precocious puberty: an update. J Clin Endocrinol Metab 98:2198–2207
2. Paris F, Servant N, Terouanne B, Balaguer P, Nicolas JC, Sultan C (2002) A new recombinant cell bioassay for ultrasensitive determination of serum estrogenic bioactivity in children. J Clin Endocrinol Metab 87:791–797
3. Sultan C, Gaspari L, Kalfa N, Paris F (2012) Clinical expression of precocious puberty in girls. Endocr Dev 22:84–100
4. Traggiai C, Stanhope R (2003) Disorders of pubertal development. Best Pract Res Clin Obstet Gynaecol 17:41–56
5. Lumbroso S, Paris F, Sultan C (2004) Activating Gsalpha mutations: analysis of 113 patients with signs of McCune-Albright syndrome--a European Collaborative Study. J Clin Endocrinol Metab 89:2107–2113
6. Kalfa N, Ecochard A, Patte C, Duvillard P, Audran F, Pienkowski C, Thibaud E, Brauner R, Lecointre C, Plantaz D, Guedj AM, Paris F, Baldet P, Lumbroso S, Sultan C (2006) Activating mutations of the stimulatory g protein in juvenile ovarian granulosa cell tumors: a new prognostic factor? J Clin Endocrinol Metab 91:1842–1847
7. Benayoun BA, Kalfa N, Sultan C, Veitia RA (2010) The forkhead factor FOXL2: a novel tumor suppressor? Biochim Biophys Acta 1805:1–5
8. Pienkowski C, Baunin C, Gayrard M, Lemasson F, Vaysse P, Tauber M (2004) Ovarian cysts in prepubertal girls. Endocr Dev 7:66–76
9. Aksglaede L, Sorensen K, Petersen JH, Skakkebaek NE, Juul A (2009) Recent decline in age at breast development: the Copenhagen Puberty Study. Pediatrics 123:e932–e939
10. Biro FM, Greenspan LC, Galvez MP, Pinney SM, Teitelbaum S, Windham GC, Deardorff J, Herrick RL, Succop PA, Hiatt RA, Kushi LH, Wolff MS (2013) Onset of breast development in a longitudinal cohort. Pediatrics 132:1019–1027
11. Paris F, Balaguer P, Terouanne B, Servant N, Lacoste C, Cravedi JP, Nicolas JC, Sultan C (2002) Phenylphenols, biphenols, bisphenol-A and 4-tert-octylphenol exhibit alpha and beta estrogen activities and antiandrogen activity in reporter cell lines. Mol Cell Endocrinol 193:43–49
12. Buck Louis GM, Gray LE Jr, Marcus M, Ojeda SR, Pescovitz OH, Witchel SF, Sippell W, Abbott DH, Soto A, Tyl RW, Bourguignon JP, Skakkebaek NE, Swan SH, Golub MS, Wabitsch M, Toppari J, Euling SY (2008) Environmental factors and puberty timing: expert panel research needs. Pediatrics 121(Suppl 3):S192–S207
13. Ozen S, Darcan S (2011) Effects of environmental endocrine disruptors on pubertal development. J Clin Res Pediatr Endocrinol 3:1–6
14. Gaspari L, Paris FO, Jeandel C, Sultan C (2011) Peripheral precocious puberty in a 4-month-old girl: role of pesticides? Gynecol Endocrinol 27:721–724
15. Paris F, Gaspari L, Servant N, Philibert P, Sultan C (2013) Increased serum estrogenic bioactivity in girls with premature thelarche: a marker of environmental pollutant exposure? Gynecol Endocrinol 29:788–792

Premature Pubarche

5

Charles Sultan, Laura Gaspari, Nicolas Kalfa,
and Françoise Paris

Pubertal maturation involves two associated processes: adrenarche due to adrenal androgen production and gonadarche linked to the reactivation of the hypothalamus-pituitary-gonadal axis.

5.1 Definition

Premature pubarche (PP) is characterized by the presence of pubic hair developing in girls younger than 8 years [1].

It is referred to as premature or exaggerated adrenarche and is considered a benign condition of normal development, occurring in 4–10 % of prepubertal girls. However, other causes of androgen excess should be considered and ruled out:

- Precocious puberty
- Enzymatic defects of adrenal steroidogenesis (late onset of 21-hydroxylase deficiency)
- Adrenal tumors

C. Sultan (✉) • L. Gaspari • F. Paris
Unité d'Endocrinologie-Gynécologie Pédiatriques, Departement de Pédiatrie, Hôpital Arnaud-de-Villeneuve, CHU Montpellier et Université Montpellier 1, Montpellier, France
e-mail: c-sultan@chu-montpellier.fr

N. Kalfa
Service de Chirurgie Pédiatrique, Hôpital Lapeyronie, CHU Montpellier et Université de Montpellier, Montpellier, France

C. Sultan, A.R. Genazzani (eds.), *Frontiers in Gynecological Endocrinology*, ISGE Series, DOI 10.1007/978-3-319-41433-1_5

5.2 Adrenarche

Adrenarche is the maturation of the adrenal zona reticularis, a physiological process unique to higher primates. In humans it occurs before pubertal onset at a mean age of 6 years, and the result is an increase in adrenal androgens: Dehydroepiandrosterone (DHEA) and dehydroepiandrosterone sulfate (DHEAS) (Fig. 5.1). Unconjugated DHEA can be converted directly to androgens (to Δ4-androstenedione → testosterone), whereas the conversion of DHEAS to androgens first requires cleavage of the sulfate group [2].

The mechanism of adrenarche onset remains unknown, although the implication of leptin, IGF1, and ACTH has been conjectured. In addition, MC-2 receptor, CYP19, IGF1, and AR gene polymorphisms have been reported to be associated with PP in some cases.

The physiological role of adrenarche in the pubertal maturational process has never been elucidated.

5.3 Clinical Features

The consequences of exposure to androgen excess in prepubertal girls are:

- Development of pubic hair
- Development of axillary hair
- Acne
- Oily skin/hair

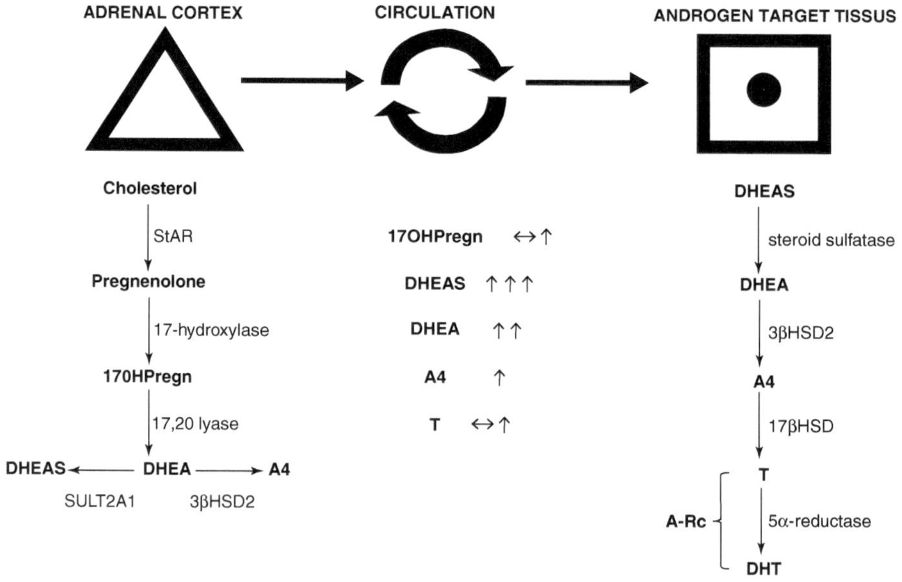

Fig. 5.1 Adrenal steroid biosynthesis

- Adult body odor
- Mood swings and/or behavioral changes

In a recent work, R. Voutilanen reported that 63 girls with PP presented the following characteristics: 89 % adult-type body odor, 70 % oily hair, 56 % acne, 48 % pubic hair, 38 % axillary hair, and 12 % acanthosis nigricans. In 20–50 % of these girls, higher than normal childhood weight was observed. Moreover, a bone age advance of 1–2 years was noted. Although some of these girls presented earlier menarche, normal adult target height was reached [3].

5.4 Evaluation of Girls with PP

The diagnosis of PP is based on the exclusion of other causes of pubertal hyperandrogenism. The focus should be on the age at the onset of signs, the tempo of their changes, and recent acceleration of growth. Examination of the girl should include pubertal staging, a search for other signs of hyperandrogenism, and the evaluation of BMI. Laboratory assessment is limited to the measurement of basal serum 17-OH progesterone, DHEAS, Δ4-androstenedione, and testosterone. An adrenocorticotropic hormone (ACTH) stimulation test must be performed if the basal 17-OH progesterone level is found to be above 2 ng/dL. A bone age evaluation is systematically carried out: in most cases, a 1–2 year advance in bone age is found.

Abdominal MRI should be considered when an adrenal androgen-secreting tumor is suspected.

A definitive algorithm for the evaluation of PP cannot be recommended. We nevertheless propose the following decision tree (REF. *Sultan PAG*), which has usually been helpful in our clinical experience (Fig. 5.1).

5.5 Differential Diagnosis

PP must be distinguished from a number of pathological conditions:

- Precocious puberty
- Non-classical congenital adrenal hyperplasia (NC-CAH), due to 21-OH gene mutation
- Virilizing adrenal tumors
- Exogenous androgen exposure

5.5.1 Precocious Puberty

PP may be a marker for the early onset of puberty: idiopathic central precocious puberty may present with pubic and/or axillary hair [4]. Bone age and growth velocity are accelerated and plasma androgens are abnormally elevated for age (Fig. 5.2d).

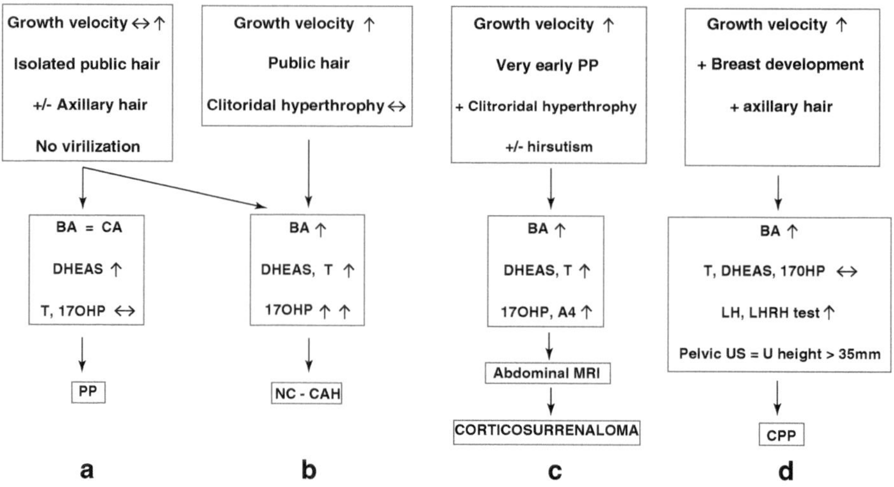

Fig. 5.2 Clinical presentation of pre pubertal hyperandrogenism

5.5.2 Non-classical Congenital Adrenal Hyperplasia (NC-CAH)

NC-CAH is usually related to 21-OH deficiency [5]. In this condition, NC-CAH has an extremely variable presentation. In prepubertal girls, the presenting signs include: PP, cystic acne, accelerated growth, and advanced bone age (Fig. 5.2b).

NC-CAH has been found in 1–30 % of girls with PP. This wide range is likely related to ethnic differences. The biological diagnosis of NC-CAH is suspected when early morning basal 17-OH progesterone is above 200 ng/dL and when an increase in 17-OH progesterone above 1200 ng/dL is found after the ACTH stimulation test [6].

In our experience [7] with a cohort of 40 girls with PP, 24 % of them presented a molecular defect within the 21-OH gene.

5.5.3 Virilizing Adrenal Tumors

Virilizing tumors are rare but not exceptional (Fig. 5.2c): we recently had the opportunity to manage two very young girls referred to our clinic for PP without exaggerated symptoms of virilization. MRI was performed because abdominal palpation revealed an abdominal mass [8]. In both cases, an adrenocortical carcinoma was diagnosed and surgically removed.

5.5.4 Exogenous Androgen Exposure

Exogenous androgen exposure occurs exceptionally through creams or gels containing testosterone.

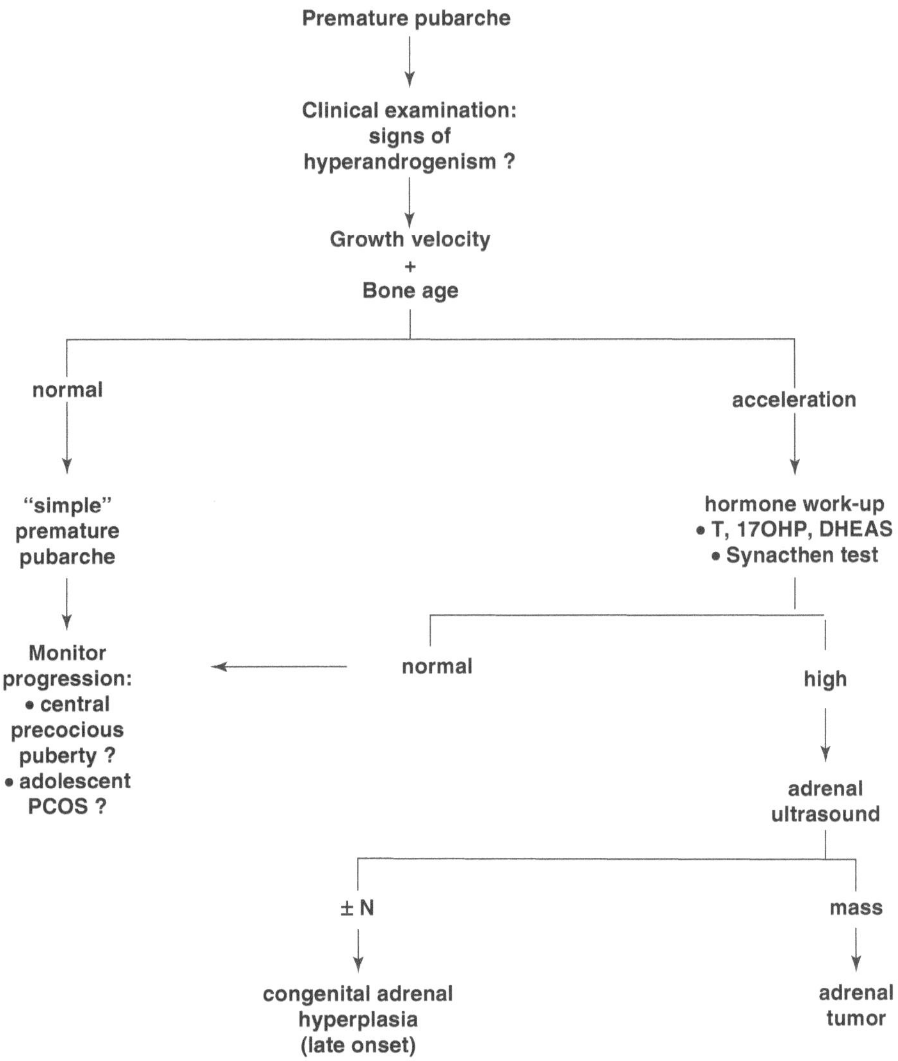

Fig. 5.3 Decision tree for premature pubarche

5.6 Management

There are few recommendations for the management of PP [9] (Fig. 5.3):

- If there is unusual weight gain, fasting measures of glycemic and insulin levels are recommended.
- If rapid pubertal progress occurs, laboratory and imaging assessment must be performed.

- In the majority of cases, when clinical and laboratory findings are consistent with idiopathic PP, these girls may be followed at 6-month intervals till menarche.
- The girls should be followed at least yearly after menarche, since they are considered to be at high risk for further adolescent polycystic ovary syndrome (PCOS) essentially for those who had a low birth weight and a prepubertal weight gain [10].

Table 5.1 Grading of hypothalamic amenorrhea on the basis of the progestogen, clomiphene, and Gn-RH tests, respectively

1	Clomiphene positive with bleeding following
1a	Normal luteal phase
1b	Insufficient luteal phase
1c	Anovulatory cycle
2	Progestogen positive
	Clomiphene negative
3	Progestogen negative with pituitary response to 100 μg of Gn-RH i.v.
3a	"Adult response"
3b	"Prepubertal response"
3c	No response

From Leyendecker, G., Wildt, L. and Plotz, E.J. et al. [11].

Conclusions

- PP is a frequent condition in girls, particularly in the Mediterranean area.
- The prevalence of PP is increasing, likely due to the recent higher incidence of obesity among prepubertal girls.
- Clinical and laboratory investigations are useful for distinguishing early adrenal maturation from the first signs of persistent hyperandrogenism.
- Extended longitudinal studies are necessary to confirm the link between early onset of androgen excess, insulin resistance, and PCOS.
- PP is not always a benign condition.

References

1. Voutilainen R, Jaaskelainen J (2015) Premature adrenarche: etiology, clinical findings, and consequences. J Steroid Biochem Mol Biol 145:226–236
2. Miller WL (2009) Androgen synthesis in adrenarche. Rev Endocr Metab Disord 10:3–17
3. Utriainen P, Voutilainen R, Jaaskelainen J (2009) Continuum of phenotypes and sympathoadrenal function in premature adrenarche. Eur J Endocrinol / Eur Fed Endocr Soc 160:657–665
4. Biro FM, Huang B, Daniels SR, Lucky AW (2008) Pubarche as well as thelarche may be a marker for the onset of puberty. J Pediatr Adolesc Gynecol 21:323–328

5. Turcu AF, Auchus RJ (2015) Adrenal steroidogenesis and congenital adrenal hyperplasia. Endocrinol Metab Clin North Am 44:275–296
6. Armengaud JB, Charkaluk ML, Trivin C, Tardy V, Breart G, Brauner R, Chalumeau M (2009) Precocious pubarche: distinguishing late-onset congenital adrenal hyperplasia from premature adrenarche. J Clin Endocrinol Metab 94:2835–2840
7. Paris F, Tardy V, Chalancon A, Picot MC, Morel Y, Sultan C (2010) Premature pubarche in Mediterranean girls: high prevalence of heterozygous CYP21 mutation carriers. Gynecol Endocrinol 26:319–324
8. Paris F, Kalfa N, Philibert P, Jeandel C, Gaspari L, Sultan C (2012) Very premature pubarche in girls is not a pubertal variant. Hormones (Athens) 11:356–360
9. Oberfield SE, Sopher AB, Gerken AT (2011) Approach to the girl with early onset of pubic hair. J Clin Endocrinol Metab 96:1610–1622
10. Neville KA, Walker JL (2005) Precocious pubarche is associated with SGA, prematurity, weight gain, and obesity. Arch Dis Child 90:258–261
11. Leyendecker, G., Wildt, L. and Plotz, E.J. *Gynäkologe* 1982;14:84

6 Maturation of the Hypothalamic-Pituitary-Ovarian Axis and the Onset of Puberty

Françoise Paris, Laura Gaspari, and Charles Sultan

6.1 Introduction

Puberty is an essential life event, the period in which somatic and sexual maturation and reproductive capacity are achieved [36]. Far from being a punctual event, it is the culmination of a complex series of maturational events that start in utero, are reactivated in the neonatal period, and progress throughout the entire span of childhood [34]. Although the age of puberty onset is in great part genetically determined [17], the downward trends reported by several authors have led to the hypothesis of an interaction between genes and the environment [3, 22, 36]. Puberty has indeed come to be regarded as a biological sensor, and the changes in its timing, which have been detected in recent years in several wildlife species and human populations, suggest that it may serve as a potential biomarker for negative environmental influences on reproduction. Yet this issue is still contested by some, and an evaluation of worldwide epidemiological data is therefore needed to either confirm or invalidate this reported trend. In this short review, we focus on the major neuroendocrine factors involved in puberty onset, as well as its modulation by metabolic signals or epigenetic mechanisms (Fig. 6.1).

F. Paris (✉) • C. Sultan
Unité d'Endocrino et Gynéco Pédiatriques, Département de Pédiatrie, Hôpital Arnaud-de-Villeneuve, CHU et Université Montpellier, Montpellier, France

Département Hormonologie, Hôpital Lapeyronie, CHU et Université Montpellier, Montpellier, France
e-mail: f-paris@chu-montpellier.fr

L. Gaspari
Unité d'Endocrino et Gynéco Pédiatriques, Département de Pédiatrie, Hôpital Arnaud-de-Villeneuve, CHU et Université Montpellier, Montpellier, France

C. Sultan, A.R. Genazzani (eds.), *Frontiers in Gynecological Endocrinology*, ISGE Series, DOI 10.1007/978-3-319-41433-1_6

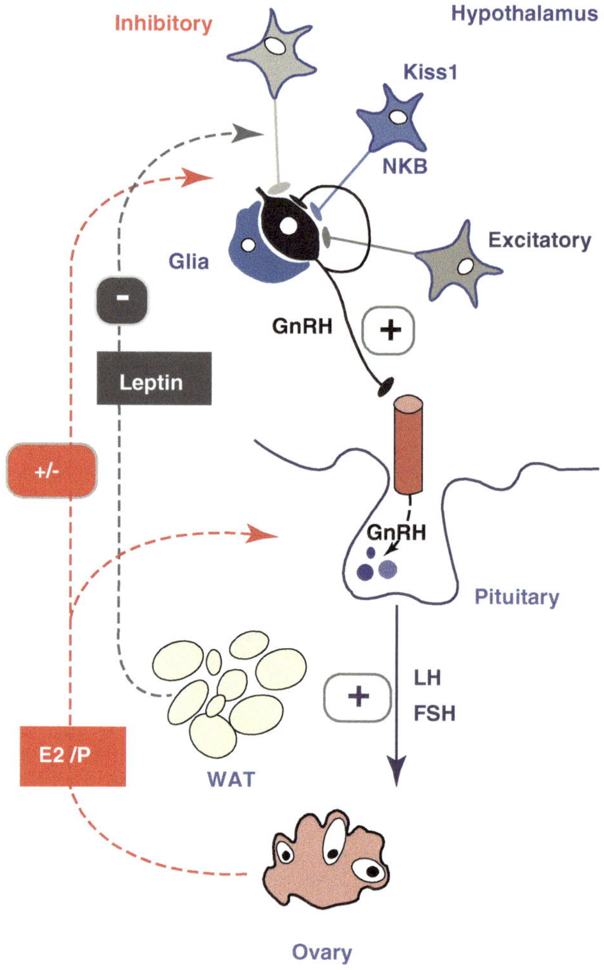

Fig. 6.1 Hypothalamic-pituitary-gonadal (HPG) axis and puberty according to [49]. Hypothalamic GnRH neurons receive trans-synaptic inhibitory and excitatory inputs that modulate the pulsatile release of GnRH. This neuropeptide drives the secretion of FSH and LH from the anterior pituitary, which in turn stimulates the secretion of gonadal sex steroids. These steroids have both negative and positive feedback effects for estradiol (E2) or only negative one for testosterone (T). Leptin produced by the white adipose tissue (WAT) is involved in the metabolic regulation of HPG

6.2 Neuronal Control of Puberty: Essential Roles of GnRH and Kisspeptin (KP) Neurons

During puberty onset, GnRH pulsatility increases in both amplitude and frequency and stimulates the gonadotroph cells of the anterior pituitary gland. This increases the secretion of FSH and LH, which in turn stimulates the secretion of sex steroids:

testosterone by the Leydig cells of the testis and androstenedione by the thecal cells of the ovarian follicles, which is then converted into estrogen by the aromatase enzyme in granulosa cells [4]. The increase in sex steroids stimulates the somatotroph axis, causing growth acceleration, progressive growth plate maturation, and the development of secondary sexual characteristics, all of which lead to the clinical expression of pubertal development. This key role of GnRH neurons has been clearly demonstrated by the clinical model of Kallmann's hypogonadotropic hypogonadism due to a migration defect of GnRH neurons [43]. Nevertheless, pubertal changes in pulsatile GnRH secretion are induced by modifications in the axodentritic inputs to the GnRH neuronal network [24, 35]. Puberty may thus be the end point in the hierarchical activation/inactivation of excitatory and inhibitory GnRH regulators [35].

Among the neuropeptide regulators of GnRH neurons, kisspeptin (KP) has been recognized as essential for the control of puberty onset [48]. KP is encoded by the Kiss1 gene and operates through the kisspeptin receptor (KissR), a G protein-coupled receptor also called Gpr54 . In rodents, two prominent populations of KP neurons have been reported in the arcuate nucleus (ARC) and the rostral periventricular area of the third ventricle (RP3V) of the hypothalamus, whereas in other mammals including primates, KP neurons are significantly expressed in the ARC/infundibular region [38]. In recent years, genetic endocrine disorders have proved useful for gaining a better understanding of physiological processes. With regard to puberty, inactive mutations of the Kiss1 gene or Gpr54 gene result in hypogonadotropic hypogonadism [12, 44]. Conversely, activating mutations of either of these genes lead to precocious puberty [46, 47].

Experimental data have also pointed to the key role of KP neurons in puberty onset. First, a rise in hypothalamic expression of the Kiss1 and Gpr54 genes has been reported during pubertal transition in rats [30]. Second, KP in mice elicits a better LH response in adults than in prepubertal mice, giving evidence of an increase in the sensitivity to the stimulatory effects of KP on GnRH/LH secretion [21]. The increase in the depolarizing KP action on GnRH neurons from juvenile to adult age reinforces the better Gpr54 signaling efficiency during the pubertal period [21]. Last, an elevation in the number of KP-positive neurons and their projections toward GnRH neurons has been also demonstrated at the time of puberty [11]. This mechanism is more marked in female than in male mice, leading to the hypothesis of a sexual dimorphism in Kiss1 gene expression.

6.3 Roles of KP Partners in Pubertal Onset

In addition to the crucial role of KP in the control of puberty onset, other endocrine signals have been reported to modulate GnRH neuron activity by several groups.

Anatomical analyses have demonstrated that a high percentage of KP neurons co-expresses neurokinin B (NKB) and its receptor (NK3R) in the ARC [20, 32, 49]. Since most of these neurons also express dynorphin-A (Dyn), they have been termed KNDy neurons [25]. As for KP, pubertal disorders underline the role of NKB and its receptor in pubertal regulation. For example, Topoglu reported four human pedigrees with severe congenital gonadotrophin deficiency and pubertal failure that were homozygous for loss-of-function mutation in TAC3 (encoding NKB) or TACR3 (encoding NK3R) [50]. These data, as well as the demonstration of an increase in TAC3 and TACR3 expression during puberty in mice [19], suggest that NKB is a central regulator of human gonadotropic function. Moreover, numerous experimental studies have reported a potent stimulatory action of the

NKB agonist senktide on LH secretion [18]. This stimulatory effect is nevertheless absent in Gpr54 null mice, suggesting that KP signaling may be a link between NKB and GnRH neurons [18]. In support of this hypothesis, experimental data demonstrate the stimulatory action of the NKB agonist senktide on KP neurons, but not directly on GnRH neurons [31]. In parallel, it was demonstrated that KNDy neurons express TACR3 gene, whereas GnRH do not [31]. All these data confirm that NKB activates GnRH neurons indirectly through kisspeptin [32].

Sex steroid levels are also involved in the regulation of pubertal onset. It is well known that sex steroids have both negative and positive feedback effects [4]. This has been corroborated by several clinical reports of central precocious puberty occurring during peripheral pubertal progression [37]. Recent works have underlined that the ARC hypothalamic area may be involved in the negative feedback of estrogens (E), whereas the rostral periventricular region of the hypothalamus (AVPV) is involved in its positive feedback [24]. Comparisons of wild type and ERα knock-out mice revealed that both negative and positive estrogen feedback are mediated by ERα [10]. Nevertheless, ERβ, but not ERα, is expressed in GnRH neurons, raising a question about the link between E and GnRH neurons [23]. A good candidate for this interaction would again be the KNDy neurons. First, increased Kiss1 gene expression was reported in postmenopausal women and ovariectomized monkeys [41]. Conversely, estrogen replacement in the monkeys markedly reduced Kiss-1 gene expression [41]. Second, the ablation of KNDy neurons prevents the rise of LH in ovariectomized mice [29]. Nevertheless, the positive feedback of E2 on the preovulatory LH surge is not fully understood, although it may involve estrogen-receptive histamine-containing neurons [16, 24].

6.4 Metabolic Control of Puberty

A substantial quantity of data points to the essential role of metabolic factors in the control of puberty. First, the concept of a critical fat mass – that is, the necessity of a minimal weight for normal puberty – emphasizes the role of leptin produced by adipose tissue [8]. In addition, leptin and leptin receptor deficiency in humans are known to be responsible for hypogonadotropic hypogonadism [14, 15], while overweight and obese prepubertal girls present earlier puberty onset [2]. These data underline the important role of leptin in puberty. However, the normalization of mean leptin concentrations in the condition of negative energy balance failed to restore normal gonadotropin levels in female rats [51]. Moreover, pharmacological studies in humans and rodents with leptin deficiency have clearly demonstrated that leptin alone cannot trigger early puberty [9]. All these data suggest that rather than being a trigger, leptin plays a permissive role in puberty onset [40]. Other impacts of leptin at other levels of the hypothalamic-pituitary-gonadal (HPG) axis have also been considered. This principal central leptin action seems indirectly mediated since leptin receptor (LepR) mRNA was not found in GnRH neurons [39, 42]. It is currently unknown where leptin conducts its reproductive actions. Negative energy balance was reported to induce suppression of Kiss1 mRNA in pubertal rat hypothalamus, whereas administration of KP increased both serum LH levels and hypothalamic Kiss1 mRNA levels [6]. On the other hand, premature onset overweight in female rats increased Kiss1 gene expression [7]. Although these data stress the important role of leptin in GnRH pubertal activation via the KP neurons, one issue remains unresolved: does leptin have a direct or indirect action on the KP neurons? The above-cited works have demonstrated that leptin exerts both a direct and an indirect action on KP neurons. The detection of LepR mRNA in KP neurons of the ARC strengthens the assumption of direct leptin action on these neurons [5]. Nevertheless, not only congenital selective ablation of these LepR from KP neurons is compatible with preserved puberty and fertility [13], but LepR is also expressed in various hypothalamic area [28] underlying an indirect action of leptin via pathways that have yet to be identified.

6.5 Novel Mechanism in the Control of Puberty

As described above, substantial efforts have been made in the past decade to identify the factors involved in the initiation of puberty. This body of work has not only shown the major role of the KP/GPR54 system in pubertal development, but has also indicated that the initiation of puberty requires the involvement of many other genes such as TAC, TACR3, Lep, and LepR. A new concept of pubertal initiation is related to upstream mechanisms involving gene silencing (Fig. 6.2). These upstream mechanisms can also include epigenetic regulation [33]. Kiss1 gene was thus found to be repressed in the ARC before puberty by the polycomb group transcriptional silencing complex (EED and CBX7) [26]. DNA methylation of two key members of this complex lifted this repression at the initiation of puberty, which coincided with an increase in the expression of the Kiss1 gene. Further insight into pubertal regulation was recently provided by several cases of familial central precocious puberty due to MKRN3 mutations [1, 45]. MKRN3 is a maternally expressed gene that encodes the protein MKRN3, whose transcription decreases in mice during peripuberty. These humans as well as experimental data strongly suggest that MKRN3 represses the initiation of puberty during the juvenile pause [1].

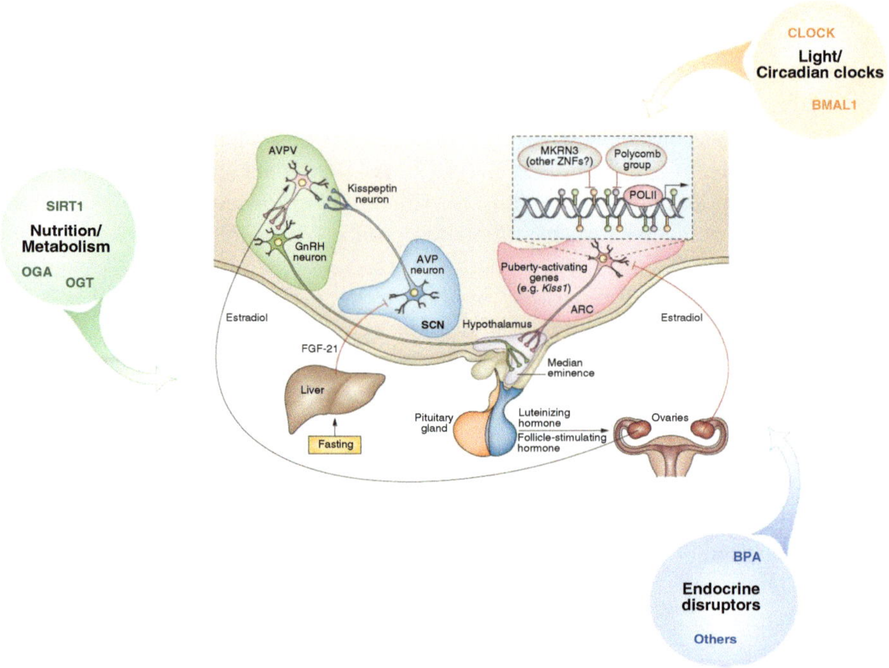

Fig. 6.2 The repressive control of puberty according to [27, 33]. The polycomb group complex and the MKRN3 are the two gene-silencing systems expressed in the ARC. The loss of transcriptional repression identified as a main mechanism underlying the onset of puberty. Different external and internal environmental stimuli (nutrition/metabolism, light/circadian clocks, endocrine disruptors) also modulate the timing and progression of puberty. Abbreviation: *SCN* suprachiasmatic nucleus, *ARC* arcuate nucleus, *AVPV* anteroventral periventricular nucleus, *AVP* vasopressin, *MKRN3* markorin

Conclusion

Puberty is not a punctual phenomenon. It is the culmination of a general maturation process that starts in fetal life, is reactivated in the neonatal period, and is finally expressed in adolescence. Pubertal timing is shaped by the dynamic interplay between gene load and the environment. Puberty has thus been regarded as a biological sensor, and downward trends in the timing of puberty, as have been detected in recent years in wildlife species and human populations, are considered as potential biomarkers for the suspected deterioration of the hypothalamic-pituitary-gonadal axis due to environmental influences. Our understanding of pubertal regulation has progressed greatly over the past decade, especially with the identification of novel neuropeptide pathways (Kiss, NKB, etc.) and molecular mechanisms (epigenetics, mRNA) involved in its regulation.

References

1. Abreu AP, Dauber A, Macedo DB, Noel SD, Brito VN, Gill JC, Cukier P, Thompson IR, Navarro VM, Gagliardi PC, Rodrigues T, Kochi C, Longui CA, Beckers D, de Zegher F, Montenegro LR, Mendonca BB, Carroll RS, Hirschhorn JN, Latronico AC, Kaiser UB (2013) Central precocious puberty caused by mutations in the imprinted gene MKRN3. N Engl J Med 368:2467–2475
2. Ahmed ML, Ong KK, Dunger DB (2009) Childhood obesity and the timing of puberty. Trends Endocrinol Metab: TEM 20:237–242
3. Aksglaede L, Sorensen K, Petersen JH, Skakkebaek NE, Juul A (2009) Recent decline in age at breast development: the Copenhagen Puberty Study. Pediatrics 123:e932–e939
4. Alonso LC, Rosenfield RL (2002) Oestrogens and puberty. Best Pract Res Clin Endocrinol Metab 16:13–30
5. Backholer K, Smith JT, Rao A, Pereira A, Iqbal J, Ogawa S, Li Q, Clarke IJ (2010) Kisspeptin cells in the ewe brain respond to leptin and communicate with neuropeptide Y and proopiomelanocortin cells. Endocrinology 151:2233–2243
6. Castellano JM, Bentsen AH, Mikkelsen JD, Tena-Sempere M (2010) Kisspeptins: bridging energy homeostasis and reproduction. Brain Res 1364:129–138
7. Castellano JM, Bentsen AH, Sanchez-Garrido MA, Ruiz-Pino F, Romero M, Garcia-Galiano D, Aguilar E, Pinilla L, Dieguez C, Mikkelsen JD, Tena-Sempere M (2011) Early metabolic programming of puberty onset: impact of changes in postnatal feeding and rearing conditions on the timing of puberty and development of the hypothalamic kisspeptin system. Endocrinology 152:3396–3408
8. Cheung CC, Thornton JE, Kuijper JL, Weigle DS, Clifton DK, Steiner RA (1997) Leptin is a metabolic gate for the onset of puberty in the female rat. Endocrinology 138:855–858
9. Cheung CC, Thornton JE, Nurani SD, Clifton DK, Steiner RA (2001) A reassessment of leptin's role in triggering the onset of puberty in the rat and mouse. Neuroendocrinology 74:12–21
10. Christian CA, Glidewell-Kenney C, Jameson JL, Moenter SM (2008) Classical estrogen receptor alpha signaling mediates negative and positive feedback on gonadotropin-releasing hormone neuron firing. Endocrinology 149:5328–5334
11. Clarkson J, Herbison AE (2006) Postnatal development of kisspeptin neurons in mouse hypothalamus; sexual dimorphism and projections to gonadotropin-releasing hormone neurons. Endocrinology 147:5817–5825
12. de Roux N, Genin E, Carel JC, Matsuda F, Chaussain JL, Milgrom E (2003) Hypogonadotropic hypogonadism due to loss of function of the KiSS1-derived peptide receptor GPR54. Proc Natl Acad Sci U S A 100:10972–10976
13. Donato J Jr, Cravo RM, Frazao R, Gautron L, Scott MM, Lachey J, Castro IA, Margatho LO, Lee S, Lee C, Richardson JA, Friedman J, Chua S Jr, Coppari R, Zigman JM, Elmquist JK, Elias CF (2011) Leptin's effect on puberty in mice is relayed by the ventral premammillary nucleus and does not require signaling in Kiss1 neurons. J Clin Invest 121:355–368
14. Dubern B, Clement K (2012) Leptin and leptin receptor-related monogenic obesity. Biochimie 94:2111–2115
15. Farooqi IS, Wangensteen T, Collins S, Kimber W, Matarese G, Keogh JM, Lank E, Bottomley B, Lopez-Fernandez J, Ferraz-Amaro I, Dattani MT, Ercan O, Myhre AG, Retterstol L, Stanhope R, Edge JA, McKenzie S, Lessan N, Ghodsi M, De Rosa V, Perna F, Fontana S, Barroso I, Undlien DE, O'Rahilly S (2007) Clinical and molecular genetic spectrum of congenital deficiency of the leptin receptor. N Engl J Med 356:237–247
16. Fekete CS, Strutton PH, Cagampang FR, Hrabovszky E, Kallo I, Shughrue PJ, Dobo E, Mihaly E, Baranyi L, Okada H, Panula P, Merchenthaler I, Coen CW, Liposits ZS (1999) Estrogen receptor immunoreactivity is present in the majority of central histaminergic

neurons: evidence for a new neuroendocrine pathway associated with luteinizing hormone-releasing hormone-synthesizing neurons in rats and humans. Endocrinology 140:4335–4341
17. Gajdos ZK, Henderson KD, Hirschhorn JN, Palmert MR (2010) Genetic determinants of pubertal timing in the general population. Mol Cell Endocrinol 324:21–29
18. Garcia-Galiano D, van Ingen SD, Leon S, Krajnc-Franken MA, Manfredi-Lozano M, Romero-Ruiz A, Navarro VM, Gaytan F, van Noort PI, Pinilla L, Blomenrohr M, Tena-Sempere M (2012) Kisspeptin signaling is indispensable for neurokinin B, but not glutamate, stimulation of gonadotropin secretion in mice. Endocrinology 153:316–328
19. Gill JC, Navarro VM, Kwong C, Noel SD, Martin C, Xu S, Clifton DK, Carroll RS, Steiner RA, Kaiser UB (2012) Increased neurokinin B (Tac2) expression in the mouse arcuate nucleus is an early marker of pubertal onset with differential sensitivity to sex steroid-negative feedback than Kiss1. Endocrinology 153:4883–4893
20. Goodman RL, Lehman MN, Smith JT, Coolen LM, de Oliveira CV, Jafarzadehshirazi MR, Pereira A, Iqbal J, Caraty A, Ciofi P, Clarke IJ (2007) Kisspeptin neurons in the arcuate nucleus of the ewe express both dynorphin A and neurokinin B. Endocrinology 148:5752–5760
21. Han SK, Gottsch ML, Lee KJ, Popa SM, Smith JT, Jakawich SK, Clifton DK, Steiner RA, Herbison AE (2005) Activation of gonadotropin-releasing hormone neurons by kisspeptin as a neuroendocrine switch for the onset of puberty. J Neurosci: Off J Soc Neurosci 25:11349–11356
22. Herman-Giddens ME (2013) The enigmatic pursuit of puberty in girls. Pediatrics 132:1125–1126
23. Hrabovszky E, Kallo I, Szlavik N, Keller E, Merchenthaler I, Liposits Z (2007) Gonadotropin-releasing hormone neurons express estrogen receptor-beta. J Clin Endocrinol Metab 92:2827–2830
24. Hrabovszky E, Liposits Z (2013) Afferent neuronal control of type-I gonadotropin releasing hormone neurons in the human. Front Endocrinol 4:130
25. Lehman MN, Coolen LM, Goodman RL (2010) Minireview: kisspeptin/neurokinin B/dynorphin (KNDy) cells of the arcuate nucleus: a central node in the control of gonadotropin-releasing hormone secretion. Endocrinology 151:3479–3489
26. Lomniczi A, Loche A, Castellano JM, Ronnekleiv OK, Bosch M, Kaidar G, Knoll JG, Wright H, Pfeifer GP, Ojeda SR (2013) Epigenetic control of female puberty. Nat Neurosci 16:281–289
27. Lomniczi A, Wright H, Ojeda SR (2015) Epigenetic regulation of female puberty. Front Neuroendocrinol 36:90–107
28. Louis GW, Greenwald-Yarnell M, Phillips R, Coolen LM, Lehman MN, Myers MG Jr (2011) Molecular mapping of the neural pathways linking leptin to the neuroendocrine reproductive axis. Endocrinology 152:2302–2310
29. Mittelman-Smith MA, Williams H, Krajewski-Hall SJ, Lai J, Ciofi P, McMullen NT, Rance NE (2012) Arcuate kisspeptin/neurokinin B/dynorphin (KNDy) neurons mediate the estrogen suppression of gonadotropin secretion and body weight. Endocrinology 153:2800–2812
30. Navarro VM, Castellano JM, Fernandez-Fernandez R, Barreiro ML, Roa J, Sanchez-Criado JE, Aguilar E, Dieguez C, Pinilla L, Tena-Sempere M (2004) Developmental and hormonally regulated messenger ribonucleic acid expression of KiSS-1 and its putative receptor, GPR54, in rat hypothalamus and potent luteinizing hormone-releasing activity of KiSS-1 peptide. Endocrinology 145:4565–4574
31. Navarro VM, Gottsch ML, Wu M, Garcia-Galiano D, Hobbs SJ, Bosch MA, Pinilla L, Clifton DK, Dearth A, Ronnekleiv OK, Braun RE, Palmiter RD, Tena-Sempere M, Alreja M, Steiner RA (2011) Regulation of NKB pathways and their roles in the control of Kiss1 neurons in the arcuate nucleus of the male mouse. Endocrinology 152:4265–4275
32. Navarro VM, Tena-Sempere M (2012) Neuroendocrine control by kisspeptins: role in metabolic regulation of fertility. Nat Rev Endocrinol 8:40–53

33. Ojeda SR, Lomniczi A (2014) Puberty in 2013: unravelling the mystery of puberty. Nat Rev Endocrinol 10:67–69
34. Ojeda SR, Lomniczi A, Sandau U, Matagne V (2010) New concepts on the control of the onset of puberty. Endocr Dev 17:44–51
35. Ojeda SR, Roth C, Mungenast A, Heger S, Mastronardi C, Parent AS, Lomniczi A, Jung H (2006) Neuroendocrine mechanisms controlling female puberty: new approaches, new concepts. Int J Androl 29:256–263; discussion 286–290
36. Parent AS, Teilmann G, Juul A, Skakkebaek NE, Toppari J, Bourguignon JP (2003) The timing of normal puberty and the age limits of sexual precocity: variations around the world, secular trends, and changes after migration. Endocr Rev 24:668–693
37. Partsch CJ, Heger S, Sippell WG (2002) Management and outcome of central precocious puberty. Clin Endocrinol (Oxf) 56:129–148
38. Pinilla L, Aguilar E, Dieguez C, Millar RP, Tena-Sempere M (2012) Kisspeptins and reproduction: physiological roles and regulatory mechanisms. Physiol Rev 92:1235–1316
39. Quennell JH, Mulligan AC, Tups A, Liu X, Phipps SJ, Kemp CJ, Herbison AE, Grattan DR, Anderson GM (2009) Leptin indirectly regulates gonadotropin-releasing hormone neuronal function. Endocrinology 150:2805–2812
40. Roa J, Navarro VM, Tena-Sempere M (2011) Kisspeptins in reproductive biology: consensus knowledge and recent developments. Biol Reprod 85:650–660
41. Rometo AM, Krajewski SJ, Voytko ML, Rance NE (2007) Hypertrophy and increased kisspeptin gene expression in the hypothalamic infundibular nucleus of postmenopausal women and ovariectomized monkeys. J Clin Endocrinol Metab 92:2744–2750
42. Sanchez-Garrido MA, Tena-Sempere M (2013) Metabolic control of puberty: roles of leptin and kisspeptins. Horm Behav 64:187–194
43. Schwanzel-Fukuda M, Bick D, Pfaff DW (1989) Luteinizing hormone-releasing hormone (LHRH)-expressing cells do not migrate normally in an inherited hypogonadal (Kallmann) syndrome. Brain Res Mol Brain Res 6:311–326
44. Seminara SB, Messager S, Chatzidaki EE, Thresher RR, Acierno JS Jr, Shagoury JK, Bo-Abbas Y, Kuohung W, Schwinof KM, Hendrick AG, Zahn D, Dixon J, Kaiser UB, Slaugenhaupt SA, Gusella JF, O'Rahilly S, Carlton MB, Crowley WF Jr, Aparicio SA, Colledge WH (2003) The GPR54 gene as a regulator of puberty. N Engl J Med 349:1614–1627
45. Settas N, Dacou-Voutetakis C, Karantza M, Kanaka-Gantenbein C, Chrousos GP, Voutetakis A (2014) Central precocious puberty in a girl and early puberty in her brother caused by a novel mutation in the MKRN3 gene. J Clin Endocrinol Metab 99:E647–E651
46. Silveira LG, Noel SD, Silveira-Neto AP, Abreu AP, Brito VN, Santos MG, Bianco SD, Kuohung W, Xu S, Gryngarten M, Escobar ME, Arnhold IJ, Mendonca BB, Kaiser UB, Latronico AC (2010) Mutations of the KISS1 gene in disorders of puberty. J Clin Endocrinol Metab 95:2276–2280
47. Teles MG, Bianco SD, Brito VN, Trarbach EB, Kuohung W, Xu S, Seminara SB, Mendonca BB, Kaiser UB, Latronico AC (2008) A GPR54-activating mutation in a patient with central precocious puberty. N Engl J Med 358:709–715
48. Tena-Sempere M (2008) Timeline: the role of kisspeptins in reproductive biology. Nat Med 14:1196
49. Tena-Sempere M (2013) Keeping puberty on time: novel signals and mechanisms involved. Curr Top Dev Biol 105:299–329
50. Topaloglu AK, Reimann F, Guclu M, Yalin AS, Kotan LD, Porter KM, Serin A, Mungan NO, Cook JR, Ozbek MN, Imamoglu S, Akalin NS, Yuksel B, O'Rahilly S, Semple RK (2009) TAC3 and TACR3 mutations in familial hypogonadotropic hypogonadism reveal a key role for Neurokinin B in the central control of reproduction. Nat Genet 41:354–358
51. True C, Kirigiti MA, Kievit P, Grove KL, Smith MS (2011) Leptin is not the critical signal for kisspeptin or luteinising hormone restoration during exit from negative energy balance. J Neuroendocrinol 23:1099–1112

7 From Primary Hypergonadotropic Amenorrhea to "POI": Aetiology and Therapy

Vincenzina Bruni, Sandra Bucciantini, and Simona Ambroggio

Ovarian function can cease precociously before menarche (primary hypergonadotropic amenorrhea) or can occur after a period of regular ovarian function, leading to the condition defined as "primary ovarian insufficiency." Various terms have been used to define this deviation from healthy ovarian function including "premature ovarian failure" (POF); "premature ovarian dysfunction" and "occult or incipient ovarian failure" describe lesser forms of partial ovarian failure with raised serum FSH concentration but more or less regular menstrual cycles. The term "primary ovarian insufficiency" (POI), proposed by Albright in 1942 [1] describes a continuum of impaired ovarian function rather than a dichotomous state based on the hypothesis that ovarian follicular activity might resume intermittently, even years after diagnosis, leading to pregnancy in some women. Thus, this term could be considered more appropriate than those used previously [2]. The term "early menopause" is used commonly to refer to ovarian damage in 40–45 year-old women.

The common denominator of POI is amenorrhea lasting 4 or more months accompanied by serum FSH increase to menopausal level (usually over 30–40 IU, minimum three measurements done at least a month apart) and estradiol levels under 50 pg mL. It is estimated to affect approximately 1 % of women under 40 years of age, 0.1 % of women under 30 years of age, and 0.01 % of women under 20 years of age [3] but actually the prevalence is less certain [4]. Progress and improvements in diagnosis and oncological treatments will certainly lead to an increase in the future of the number of recognized cases of POI [5].

V. Bruni (✉)
University of Florence, Florence, Italy
e-mail: vbruni@unifi.it

S. Bucciantini
Pediatric and Adolescent Gynecology Unit, AOUC Careggi, Florence, Italy

S. Ambroggio
CIDIMU Centro italiano di Diagnostica Medica Ultrasonica, Turin, Italy

C. Sultan, A.R. Genazzani (eds.), *Frontiers in Gynecological Endocrinology*, ISGE Series, DOI 10.1007/978-3-319-41433-1_7

7.1 POI Pathophysiology

Although the cause of primary ovarian insufficiency is undefined in most cases, the disorder generally arises from dysfunction or depletion of ovarian follicles [6, 7]. In rare cases of follicular dysfunction, sufficient ovarian follicles are present but they do not function properly. For example, primary ovarian insufficiency can be caused by mutations in *FSHR*, which encodes the FSH receptor [8, 9]. Alternatively, destruction of primordial follicles by toxic agents, autoimmune response, activation of proapoptotic pathways, or accelerated follicular recruitment might result in premature depletion of the pool of primordial follicles.

7.2 POI Aetiology

Most cases of POF are idiopathic, with no identifiable etiology. However, diverse etiologies have been associated with POF, in particular genetic aberrations, autoimmune ovarian damage, iatrogenic factors, infectious agents, toxins, and environmental factors [10].

7.2.1 Genetic Disorders

The various genetic mechanisms implicated in the pathogenesis of POF include reduced gene dosage and non-specific chromosome effects that impair meiosis. These can lead to premature ovarian failure by causing a decrease in the pool of primordial follicles, increased atresia of the ovarian follicles due to apoptosis, or lack of follicle maturation [10, 11].

Chromosomal abnormalities have been recognized as a cause of POF, but percentages vary widely among reported series. The numerous different karyotype anomalies responsible for precocious ovarian deficiency can be classified as follows.

7.2.2 X Chromosome Numerical Defects

The X chromosome has been known to play an essential role in the maintenance of ovarian development and function; therefore, females lacking an X chromosome or those showing an extra X chromosome are predisposed to develop POF [4]. The most frequent X chromosome anomaly is Turner's Syndrome, with X monosomy (45,X) in 50% of cases. In the remaining 50% of cases, the karyotype presents either a two-long-armed X chromosome (isochromosome) or a ring shaped X chromosome or mosaicism (45,X/46,XX). POF in these patients is due to accelerated follicular loss [12]. X monosomy without mosaicism is more typically found in primary amenorrhea, while mosaicism and other forms of association are also associated with POF. Either haploinsufficiency of pivotal genes on the X chromosome or non-specific meiotic impairment could explain the accelerated atresia of oocytes [4]. 47,XXX: the presence of three X chromosomes can lead to meiotic disturbance and ovarian failure, but the mechanism remains to be defined [13]. Patients presented different symptoms, such as genitourinary tract abnormalities, tall stature, epicanthus, and high incidence of autoimmune diseases [14].

7.2.3 X Chromosome Structural Abnormalities and X–Autosome Translocations

Women with structural abnormalities of the X chromosome have primary ovarian insufficiency. The most important of the numerous genes implicated in the mechanisms of POF and located on the X chromosome is FMR1, involved in X fragile syndrome, a pleiotropic Mendelian disorder (when POF is part of the phenotypic spectrum). This dominant, hereditary disease with incomplete penetration is the most frequent cause of hereditary mental retardation with a prevalence of 1:8000 women. The gene is located on Xq27.3 and it has an expandable region composed of repeats of CGG nucleotide in 5'UTR position. A normal subject possesses fewer than 55 repetitions of the CGG triplet. The syndrome depends on amplification of the site of repetition and involves the presence of more than 200 triplets; the clinical features include mental retardation, characteristic facial features with large ears and prominent jaw, joint laxity, and behavioral abnormalities. Pre-mutation is characterized by the presence of an intermediate number of triplets, 55–200, with a 15–20 % risk of POF when there are between 80 and 100 triplets. In adult females pre-mutation may be associated with the neurological condition fragile X associated tremor/Ataxia Syndrome (FXTAS) which requires genetic consultation [4, 12, 14–16].

The FMR2 gene is located at Xq28, and the mechanisms generating disease (fragile X and mental retardation syndrome) are similar to those of FMR1. Furthermore, deletions in FMR2 have been described in women with POF [15].

A critical region on the X chromosome is specifically related to ovarian development and function. This region extends from Xq13.3 to Xq27: deletion of the short or long arm of the X chromosome results in either early primary or secondary amenorrhea. Moreover, the site of deletion or translocation can influence POF typology with primary amenorrhea when the Xq13 region is involved or when the Xq25 or Xq26 is involved [4, 14].

Multiple genes on the X chromosome have been identified by X-autosomal translocations, including DIAPH (Xq22), XPNPEP2 (Xq25), DACH2 (Xq21.3), POF1B (Xq21.1), CHM (Xq21.1), PGRMCI (Xq24), COL4A6 (Xq22.3), NXF5 (Xq22.1) [4]. Studies on X-autosome translocation have been significant in evidencing gene influence on autosomes and X-chromosome in the development of POF. The position of the X-autosome translocation is a feasible pathogenetic explanation. In fact, genes transferred to the highly heterochromatic region of the X chromosome tolerate epigenetic effects after a rearrangement which changes their chromatin structure: the result is lesser expression of genes associated with normal ovarian function and fertility [14, 17].

7.2.4 Autosomal Rearrangements

Robertsonian and reciprocal autosomal translocation have been observed in sporadic cases of POF, but no specific autosomal regions are preferentially associated with ovarian deficit. It has been suggested that functional changes and interruptions in certain genes critical for ovarian function on acrocentric chromosome due to translocation could be possible causes of POF [14].

7.2.5 Single Genes Responsible for Non-syndromic POF

Many genes have emerged as POF candidates, but in non-syndromic POI only a minority have been proven unequivocally causative, with notable differences in frequency among different populations [4].

Single genes associated with POF may be expressed on the X chromosome or autosomal genes. The genes expressed on chromosome X that are most frequently associated with POF are: BMP15 (Xp11.2), AR (Xq12), and FOXO4 (Xq13.1), as well as PGRMCI (Xq22-q24), POF1B (Xq21.2), DACH2 (Xq21.3), and FMRI (Xq27.3). Mutations in various autosomal genes have been associated with POF. However, genetic-linkage studies are difficult to do; the role of many mutations is unknown and they are not a common cause of primary ovarian insufficiency [18].

7.2.6 Chromosomes with Autosomal Genes that Are Strong Candidates as a Cause of POF

Chromosome 1: FIGLA (1p13.3), a germ-cell specific transcription factor that plays a crucial role in the formation of the primordial follicle and coordinates expression of zona pellucida genes; TGFBR3 (1p33-p32); GPR3 (1p36-p35); WNT4 (1p36.23-P35.1); MSH4 (1p31)

Chromosome 2: FSHR (2p21-p16); LHR (2p21); Inhibin alpha-INHA (2q35); Inhibin beta B–INHBB (2cen-q13)

Chromosome 5: GDF9 (5q31.1), expressed in oocytes

Chromosome 6: POU5FI (6p21.31); MSH5 (6p21.3); FOXO3 (6q21); CITED2 (6q23.3), gene essential for early embryonic development; ESR1 (6q25.1), coding Estrogen Receptor alpha

Chromosome 7: NOBOX (7q35), an oocyte-specific homeobox gene that plays a critical role in early folliculogenesis; Inhibin beta A-INHBA (7p15-p13)

Chromosome 9: NR5AI (9q33), SF-I (9q33); SOLHLHI (9q34.3)

Chromosome 10: NANOSI (10q26.11); PTEN (10q23.3)

Chromosome 12: Anti-Mullerian hormone receptor type II-AMHR2 (12q13); CDKNIB (12p13.1-p12); KITLG (12q22)

Chromosome 13: SOLHLH2 (13q13.3); FOXOI (13q14.1), an important gene for granulosa cell function and follicle maturation

Chromosome 14: ESR2 (14q23.3), coding Estrogen Receptor 2 (ER beta)

Chromosome 19: NANOS2 (19q13.32); NANOS3 (19p13.13)
Chromosome 20: SALL4 (20q13.2); SPOII (20q13.31)
Chromosome 22: DMCI (22q13.1) [4]

Protein and enzyme deficits implicated in steroid genesis are also responsible for deficiencies in estrogen production, notwithstanding the stimulation of FSH on granulosa cells. The steroidogenic acute regulatory protein (Star) regulates intramitochondrial transport of cholesterol. Mutation of this protein causes congenital adrenal hyperplasia. Mutations of certain enzymes such as aromatase, 17–20 desmolase, and 17alpha hydroxylase desmolase cholesterol cause POF [19].

7.2.7 Pleiotropic Single Gene Disorders in POF

The fragile X syndrome described above is the most frequent.

Other pathological syndromes associated with POF are:

- Galactosemia (GALT gene, at 9p13): Ovarian failure is a common long-term complication in girls with this disease. Pathogenesis involves excess galactose toxicity that impairs folliculogenesis, induces resistance to gonadotropins and accelerates follicular atresia. These patients present poor growth, poor intellectual function, and neurological deficit (predominant ataxia) [4, 20].
- Blepharophimosis-ptosis-epicanthus syndrome (BPES) type I (FOXL2 gene, at 3q23): BPES is associated with a characteristic facies (drooping upper eyelids with narrow horizontal eyelid openings, a fold of skin that runs upward and inward from the lower eyelids, and lateral displacement of the inner canthi) and premature ovarian failure. This is a pleiotropic autosomal dominant syndrome with an estimated de novo mutation rate of over 50 % [12].
- Polyendocrinopathy-candidiasis-ectodermal dystrophy (AIRE gene, at 21q22.3): The AIRE gene can lead to various multi-system abnormalities such as alopecia, vitiligo, keratopathy, malabsorption, hepatitis, mucocutaneous candidiasis, Addison's disease, hypoparathyroidism, DM1, chronic atrophic gastritis, pernicious anemia, and autoimmune thyroid disorders. POF is common with onset usually in the third decade [4].
- Ovarian leukodystrophy (EIF2B2 gene, at 14q24.3; EIF2B4 gene, at 2p23.3; EIF2B5 gene, at 3q27.1): Ovarian failure may be associated with this genetic disease that is characterized by variable but progressive neurological degeneration [4].
- Carbohydrate-deficient glycoprotein syndrome type I (PMM2 gene, at 16p13): This genetic disorder may include also neurological abnormalities and ovarian failure [4].
- Perrault syndrome (HSD17B4 gene, at 5q21): An extremely rare pleiotropic autosomal recessive disorder characterized by progressive sensorineural deafness, ovarian failure, and sometimes neurological manifestations [4, 12].
- Proximal symphalangism and multiple synostose syndrome (NOG gene, at 17q22): Ankylosis of the proximal interphalangeal joints and POF.

- Bloom syndrome (BLM gene, on 15q26.1): In addition to POF, this disorder is characterized by early aging, short stature, and elevated rates of cancer
- Ataxia telangiectasia (ATM gene, at 11q22–q23): Progressive cerebellar degeneration with telangiectasia, immunodeficiency, recurrent infections, insulin-resistant diabetes, premature aging, high risk for epithelial cancer, radiosensitivity, and POF are characteristic features.
- Werner syndrome (WRN gene, at 8p12): Involves premature aging of the skin, bones, and vasculature with elevated rates of certain cancers (sarcoma) and POF.
- Rothumnd-Thomson syndrome (RECQL4 gene, at 8q24.3): Involves small stature, skeletal/dental anomalies, cutaneous rash, cataracts, premature aging, increased risk for cancer, and POF.
- Nijmegen breakage syndrome (NBN/NBS1 gene, at 8q21): Autosomal recessive disorder characterized by microcephaly, facial dysmorphia, growth retardation, immune deficiency, and predisposition to develop cancer [12].

A complete list of syndromes associated with POF is available on line at http://links.lww.com/COOG/A25. [21]. However, since these conditions account for only about 1 % of cases, genetic investigation is not routine in the absence of anamnestic and clinical findings indicative of POF.

7.2.8 Mitochondrial Genes Causing POF

Since the mature oocyte has the greatest number of mitochondria of any human cell perturbations of mitochondrial genes or nuclear gene affecting mitochondria are candidates for POF. Dysregulation of mitochondrial dynamics contributes to excessive oxidative stress and initiation of apoptosis, accelerating follicle depletion. Perturbation of mitochondrial genes is known to be present in various syndromes involving POF, in particular:

- Progressive external ophthalmoplegia (POLG gene, at 15q25) with additional clinical features of proximal myopathy (progressive weakness of the motor muscles of the eyeballs and upper lids), sensory ataxia, and Parkinsonism.
- Perrault syndrome (HARS 2 gene, at 5q31.3; LARS 2 gene, at 3p21.3; CLPP gene, at 19p13.3; C10orf2 gene, at 10q24): ovarian failure is one of the characteristic features of Perrault syndrome in females (as specified above in the paragraph on *pleiotropic single gene disorders in POI*), but the genes specified encode mitochondrial tRNA synthetase.

7.2.9 Other Genetic Syndromes

Primary or secondary ovarian failure is associated also with other genetic syndromes, but the causative genes have not been individuated. It is important to remember that only a minority of genes have been proven to be unequivocally, via functional validation, the cause of non-syndromic POF. The list includes BPMI5, PGRMCI, and FMR1 permutation on the X chromosome, GDF9, FIGLA, FSHR, NOBOX, NR5AI, NANOS3, and the recently discovered STAG3, SYCEI, MCM8, MCM9, HFMI on autosome genes. Note that only 1.5 % of the genome is protein-coding, and non-coding variants must be investigated more thoroughly. Perturbations could affect non-coding RNA (microRNA, long non-coding RNA), disruption or creation of alternative splicing or transcription factor-binding sites, and epigenetic modifications (DNA methylation, chromatin modification) [4] .

7.2.10 Autoimmunologic Causes

Abnormal self-recognition of the immune system may account for 4–30 % of cases of POF due to the exaggerated autoimmune reaction involved in atretic acceleration, oocyte wastage, and impaired folliculogenesis. The autoimmune attack can be general or partial; it may be reversible and even responsible for the fluctuating course of POI [22]. The presence of lymphocytic oophoritis, demonstration of ovarian or other organ-specific autoantibodies, and associated autoimmune disorders are evidence of autoimmune etiology in a context of general autoimmune dysregulation [10].

There appear to be three different types of autoimmune POI:

- Related to adrenal immunity where the closest association is with autoimmune polyendocrine syndrome autoimmune polyglandular syndromes (APS) type 1 (candidiasis, hypoparathyroidism, hypoadrenalism, and possible comorbidities) and type 2 (hypoadrenalism and hypothyroidism with possible comorbidities)
- Associated with non-adrenal autoimmunity (related to thyroid disease, hypoparathyroidism, hypophysitis, DM1, rheumatoid arthritis, vitiligo, alopecia areata, celiac disease, Sjoegren's syndrome, pernicious anemia, myasthenia gravis, SLE, immune thrombocytopenic purpura, glomerulonephritis)
- Isolated idiopathic [23].

The closest association is with adrenal immunity in Autoimmune Polylgandular Syndromes (APS).

Type 1 APS is a rare autosomal recessive disorder characterized by multiple organ-specific autoimmunity secondary to a variety of autoantibodies directed against key intracellular enzymes; it includes oophoritis in 60 % of cases.

Type 2 APS is an autosomal dominant disorder that is associated with gonadal failure in 4 % of patients. Addison's disease is present in both types of APS [10].

Adrenocortical and steroidogenic cell autoantibodies (SCA) are recognized as the best markers of autoimmune POF, but they are also commonly found in POI associated with autoimmune Addison's disease [11, 23]. In fact, more than 60 % of cases of POI associated with APS have positive SCA directed against steroidogenic cells or enzymes found in adrenal cortex, placenta, ovaries, and testicles, such as StC Ab, anti- CYP21 Ab, P450SccAb, CYP17A1Ab; the same autoantibodies are found in fewer than 10 % of cases of POF that do not present adrenal autoimmunity as well as in idiopathic POF. About 15–20 % of POI subjects present anti-TPO antibody, 3β-hydroxysteroid dehydrogenase autoantibodies, gonadotropin receptor autoantibodies, zona pellucida autoantibodies, and/or anti-oocyte cytoplasm antibodies without SCA [11, 22, 23]. Circulating 21-hydroxylase antibodies may be immune markers of autoimmune adrenal insufficiency [24].

There have been several reports of antiovarian antibodies in POF, but their specificity and pathognomonic roles are questionable. Clinical or subclinical hypothyroidism is the disorder most commonly associated with POI, with TPO antibodies in 25–60 % of patients [22].

Abnormalities in T-lymphocytes, macrophages, and dendritic cells play an important role in autoimmune reactions, and, of specific interest to our topic, in the development of autoimmune lesions in POI, where they support the mechanism of the disease [25]. Autoimmune oophoritis is characterized by mononuclear inflammatory cell infiltrate in the teca cells of growing follicles; early stage follicles do not present lymphocytic inflammation. The infiltrate includes plasma and B and T cells and may also be found in perivascular and perineural regions [26]. Ovarian biopsy might be useful for detection of autoimmune oophoritis, but it is generally not recommended because it is an invasive procedure of uncertain clinical value [11]. Commercially available antiovarian antibody tests give unsatisfactory findings. Certain non-ovarian autoantibodies, in particular autoantibodies to steroid producing cells, may mediate autoimmune damage in POF, but the prognostic value is uncertain and few laboratories carry out the necessary tests [27]. It has been suggested that a significant increase in CD8 density on T cells might be a reliable indicator of immune system involvement in POI [28].

7.2.11 Iatrogenic Causes

Even when bilateral ovariectomy is not performed, pelvic surgery can cause early menopause, presumably due to damage to ovarian blood vessels or post surgical local inflammation. However, the risks of pelvic surgery are difficult to quantify and they are generally considered minimal except in subjects with endometriosis, especially in the presence of bilateral endometrial ovarian cysts [12, 29].

Chemotherapy can cause damage by impairing follicle maturation or primordial follicle depletion or both. The effects of chemotherapy on ovarian reserve depend on various factors, in particular patient age, substances used, and duration of treatment [18, 27, 30]. Regarding age, the younger the patient is at the time of chemotherapy, the lower the risk of ovarian failure.

Anthracyclines, alkylating agents, cisplatin and derivatives, and antimetabolites are the most frequently used agents. Anthracyclines (i.e., doxorubicin) are cytotoxic antibiotics whose antineoplastic action is due to interaction with DNA. The mechanism of ovarian damage caused by anthracycline appears to be follicular depletion by apoptosis associated with serious vascular toxicity [30].

Table 7.1 Risk of POI related to intake of gonadotoxic drugs

POI risk level	Gonadotoxic drugs
High	Busulfan, chlorambucil, chlormethine, cyclophosphamide, ifosfamide, melphalan, procarbazine
Medium	Adriamycin, carboplatin, cisplatin, docetaxel, doxorubicin, paclitaxel
Low	Bleomycin, dactinomycin, 5-Fluoruracil, mercaptopurine, methotrexate, vinblastine, vincristine

Cisplatin and its derivatives cause massive apoptosis of early follicles causing in turn ovarian dysfunction. Alkylating agents (e.g., cyclophosphamide) are the chemotherapeutic agents most frequently associated with gonadal damage (up to 40 % of patients risk ovarian failure at childbearing age) because they destroy resting oocytes and possibly also the pregranulosa cells of primordial follicles. Cyclophosphamide triggers follicular atresia with vessel occlusion, focal corticoid fibrosis, and the disappearance of primordial follicles from fibrotic areas [30].

Antimetabolites instead cause less ovarian damage because they act on dividing cells.

Three risk categories have been established for certain chemotherapeutic agents based on their gonadotoxicity: various alkylating agents are classified as high risk; platinum agents, certain anthracycline antibiotics, and taxoids are medium-risk; and vinca plant alkaloids, some anthracycline antibiotics, and antimetabolites are low-risk [18] (Table 7.1).

Oocytes are very sensitive to radiation, and women exposed to total body and/or pelvic/abdominal irradiation are especially likely to suffer irreversible damage to the ovaries. The degree of risk depends on patients' age at the time of exposure, dose, and site of treatment [12, 18, 30].

Ionizing radiation can cause direct DNA damage to ovarian follicles resulting in follicular atrophy and decreased ovarian follicular reserve. Oocyte radiosensivity presumably varies during the growth phase, and primordial follicles seem more radioresistant than maturing follicles [31]. One mathematical model used suggested that less than 2 Gy would destroy 50 % of immature oocytes. Another model used to predict estimated surviving follicles in relation to dose of ionizing radiation showed that the effective sterilizing dose is inversely related to age at time of treatment. Ovarian damage occurs immediately after treatment in 97.5 % of cases with the following sterilizing doses or doses of fractionated radiotherapy: 20.3 Gy at birth, 18.4 Gy at 10 years, 16.5 Gy at 20 years, 14.3 Gy at 30 years, and 1 Gy at 50 years [32].

7.2.12 Infectious Causes

Oophoritis due to mumps can cause POF, but in the majority of cases, ovarian function returns to normal following recovery [10, 27]. There have been various anecdotal reports of POF following other viral and microbic infections, such as tuberculosis, varicella, cytomegalovirus, malaria, and shigella [10, 12, 33]. HIV and/or even related antiretroviral therapy may have negative effects on ovarian function and fertility leading to POF [27, 34].

7.2.13 Environmental Toxins

People of all ages worldwide, but especially in developing countries, are exposed to increasing amounts of environmental chemicals that can influence fertility. Animal studies and human observations have individuated certain chemical substances that target ovarian cells:

- Phthalates – practically ubiquitous diesters, commonly used as plasticizers in flexible PVC products. They cause large follicle destruction.
- Methoxychlor – a pesticide, widely used against insects that attack fruit and vegetables. Methoxychlor can be metabolized and a variety of its metabolites cause follicle atresia and lack of corpus luteum.
- Dioxin – a product of waste incineration, forest fires, and volcanic eruptions. It has a direct toxic influence on ovarian function.
- Bisphenol-A – a chemical widely used in the production of polycarbonate plastics and epoxy resins. It inhibits follicular growth and induces follicular atresia.
- Polycyclic aromatic hydrocarbons (PAH) – a class of several hundred compounds ubiquitous in the environment as a result of various combustion processes including automobile exhaust and cigarette smoking. Many PAHs and their metabolites are present in ground, surface, and waste water. They are highly lipophilic and extremely bioavailable and thus have easy entry into the food chain. They are toxic for the ovaries causing oxidative stress and reduction in the number of primordial follicles.
- Occupational chemicals, such as butadiene diepoxide, vinylcyclohexane, and bromopropane, are products of various industrial processes. They have been shown to have toxic influence on the ovaries and are able to damage and even destroy primordial and primary follicles, accelerating atretic processes.

The stage of development at which the oocyte-containing follicle is destroyed determines the outcome of xenobiotic damage within the ovary. Temporary infertility can be the result of selective influence of an environmental factor on the ovarian follicle population. The infertility may be reversible after exposure to the negative environmental factor ceases, but when the primordial follicles have been targeted, the stem cell population of germ cells may be destroyed, resulting in irreversible ovarian failure [30, 35].

7.2.14 Other Causes of POF

Smoking is the most widely studied toxin responsible for ovarian function. Cigarette smoking has been shown to comport increased risk of idiopathic POF. Tobacco toxins can have a negative influence on ovarian reserve by increasing apoptosis in primordial germ cells, leading to accelerated follicular atrophy and atresia [10, 27]. Women with epilepsy have been reported to have increased risk of developing POF [10, 36].

Personal and Family History There is no specific menstrual history that is characteristic of the development of spontaneous 46,XX primary ovarian insufficiency. In most cases, the condition develops after a normal puberty and established regular menses (secondary amenorrhea), although primary amenorrhea may be present in about 10% of cases [6, 37]. Occasionally, menses stop abruptly. In some women, menses fail to resume after a pregnancy or after they have stopped taking hormonal contraceptives. Most commonly there is a prodrome of oligomenorrhea, polymenorrhea, or dysfunctional uterine bleeding, usually prior to final cessation of menstruation. Also, we must point out that for young subjects it is inappropriate to attribute amenorrhea to stress without further evaluation. Symptoms of estrogen deficiency (hot flashes and night sweats, sleep disturbance, and dyspareunia related to vaginal dryness) develop in many, but not all, patients. Furthermore, not all patients have profound estrogen deficiency, and vaginal examination often reveals signs suggesting normal estrogen levels.

Physical examination may reveal stigmata indicative of Turner's syndrome such as short stature, webbed neck, and high, arched palate or evidence of an associated disorder such as hyperpigmentation or vitiligo (which is associated with autoimmune adrenal insufficiency), thyroid enlargement, galactorrhea, and/or signs of androgen excess.

Endocrine evaluation must be done, specifically serum FSH, LH, prolactin, TSH, and estradiol, at the very least and after pregnancy has been ruled out. Similar to the situation in natural menopause, POI is characterized by elevated FSH levels and reduced estrogen production. FSH evaluation should be repeated after 1 month, together with serum estradiol, if the first test shows levels in menopausal range. To date, there is no agreement on the minimum FSH increase necessary to establish a diagnosis of POI [5]. Inhibin A and inhibin B levels are reduced due to the decreased number of follicles and follicle development [2, 38]. Specifically, a decrease in inhibin B production appears to be the first sign of incipient ovarian insufficiency in Turner's syndrome [39]. However, normal levels of inhibin A and inhibin B have been demonstrated in the first stage of autoimmune POI, in agreement with the hypothesis of selective theca cell destruction in auto-immune oophoritis, with initial preservation of granulose cells [40].

Antimullerian hormone (AMH) is currently considered the best hormonal marker to estimate ovarian follicle pool. AMH is a dimeric glycoprotein member of the TGF-β super family produced in women only by the ovaries. AMH expression is absent in primordial follicles and appears in granulose cells of primary follicles. The strongest staining of AMH is observed in preantral and small antral follicles, and AMH is present in growing follicles until dominance [41]. The main physiological role of AMH is to inhibit the early stages of follicular development and control recruitment from the primordial pool of follicles [42]. AMH levels have been found to be normal in women with hypogonadotropic amenorrhea, whereas they are very low or undetectable in women with physiological menopause and premature or primary ovarian insufficiency. The data in the literature confirm that knowledge of serum AMH levels improves menopause prediction and the monitoring of ovarian damage caused by spontaneous events and medical and surgical treatments in young women and adolescents [43]. AMH is considered a biomarker in menopause staging because it declines before FSH levels increase [44]. Recently, AMH was demonstrated to be more sensitive than FSH (80 % vs. 28.57 %), but the two presented almost equal specificity (78.89 % vs. 78.65 %) [45]. Caution is required when interpreting a single AMH measurement because biological fluctuations, surgical procedures, medications, and different laboratory methodologies frequently lead to dramatic changes in AMH levels [43].

Pelvic ultrasonography helps establish good morphological evaluation and provides some information regarding functioning of the lower genital tract. Antral follicle count (AFC) via trans-vaginal sonography done in the early follicular phase (second to fifth day) is a method for evaluating follicle residue (thus, ovarian reserve) that is more sensitive than FSH levels in normal subjects. There should be 3–8 antral follicles measuring 2–10 mm in each ovary in conditions of normal ovarian function. Some studies consider such counts valid also for young subjects with POI. Serum AMH levels show a strong correlation with antral follicle count [46], but they are more consistently correlated with the clinical degree of follicle pool depletion than inhibin B and AFC in young women with elevated FSH levels [47].

Genetic investigations center on specific chromosomal and genetic studies (karyotype, FMR1 gene mutation if there is family history of premature ovarian failure, fragile X syndrome, or mental retardation). When there is no dysmorphism and the family anamnesis is negative for particular pathological conditions, the starting point of genetic workup for women with POF is investigation of FMR1 gene status and karyotype analysis [21]. Specialized centers extend diagnostic testing to include FSHR, BMP15, GDF9, NR5A1, and NOBOX genes.

Immunological Investigations When there are symptoms suggestive of adrenal insufficiency (asthenia, apathy, hypoglycemia, vitiligo), it may be necessary to test for adrenocortical and/or steroidogenic antibodies, that are, however, quite rare in idiopathic POI. 17α-OH antibodies, P450scc antibodies, and 3β-hydroxysteroid dehydrogenase (3β-HSD) antibodies are considered the main serologic markers for ovarian failure in POF patients with autoimmune Addison's disease, but testing for these antibodies have limited application in routine clinical practice [23, 48]. On the other hand, the presence of 21-OH antibodies in women with idiopathic POF might be an important marker for identifying patients at risk of developing autoimmune adrenal insufficiency [48]. One must always look for thyroid peroxidase antibodies in cases of POF without adrenal autoimmune involvement because thyroiditis is the most prevalent autoimmune endocrine abnormality in POF patients. The search for antiovarian autoantibodies, a possible independent marker of autoimmune ovarian disease, is not done routinely given their questionable specificity in POF [22, 23]. Finally, in cases with positive anamnesis for other autoimmune conditions (vitiligo, hypothyroidism) or patients who present sideropenic anemia, it is useful to screen for celiac disease and look for anti-gastric parietal cell antibodies to evidence eventual polyendocrine disorders associated with autoimmune atrophic gastritis [49].

Bone mineral density measurement is particularly important in establishing bone growth in Turner's syndrome subjects. Over the last decade various methods have been used, in particular:

- X-ray (standard)
- DXA single or dual photon absorptiometry
  - Dual-energy X-ray absorptiometry
  - Three-dimensional volumetric (vBMD) (cm$^{3)}$
- QUS (quantitative ultrasonography)
- pQCT (peripheral quantitative computed tomography)
- HR-pQCT (high resolution peripheral quantitative computed tomography

Studies using these different methods are commented on under the heading *Bone mineral density* in the THERAPY section 7. 3.10.

Associated medical condition evaluation is often a useful complement to diagnosis and can be important in establishing appropriate therapy, in particular substitute therapies in specific syndromes and for high cardiovascular risk patients [50].

7.3 Hormonal Replacement Therapy (HRT) in POI

7.3.1 Choice of Therapy

What substitute hormonal therapy to choose depends on:

- Patient's age at the time of ovarian damage (e.g., before full puberal development, including maturation of the genital tract and achievement of peak bone mass, or after years of menstruation)
- Cause of the ovarian damage (genetic, immunologic or neoplastic; hormonal or non-hormonal; etc.)
- Individual congenital and/or acquired risk factors

7.3.2 Therapeutic Targets

- In younger subjects therapy aims to correct one or more specific problems, such as restoring an appropriate endocrine milieu for normal growth, enhancing bone mass accrual, promoting uterine growth and maturation, stimulating development of secondary sexual characteristics and/or sexuality, improving cognitive, behavioral, and psychosocial functions, providing cardiovascular protection.
- In subjects who have experienced a period of normal ovarian function the aim is to restore normal hormone milieu.

7.3.2.1 Estrogen Replacement Therapy for Puberty Induction in Gonadal Dysgenesis

We note that approximately one third of these patients experience spontaneous puberty, most commonly girls with XX mosaicism. Pubarche is the first feature in most patients and about 20 % present pubarche only after estrogen therapy [51]. Growth failure and altered ovarian function are present in virtually all individuals with Turner's syndrome, and the average adult stature of untreated individuals is about 20 cm shorter than that of their peers. This problem generally begins in utero, continues into infancy and childhood, and is accentuated by the absence of pubertal growth spurt. Growth hormone therapy is now standard care for 90 % of girls with Turner's syndrome [52]. Induction of puberty requires drugs, dosages, times and methods of administration that stimulate normal puberal patterns and facilitate growth processes. Thus, since the ovaries of prepuberal girls secrete measurable, albeit modest, quantities of estradiol, the current trend is to initiate estrogen therapy in childhood, at very low dose, to achieve E2 levels typical for normal girls at onset of puberty and to add cyclic progesterone therapy 2–4 years after initiation of estrogen therapy or when break-through bleeding occurs. The same protocols are followed for subjects who have suffered irreversible ovarian damage due to other causes.

7.3.3 Estrogens Used in HRT

Specific treatment schedules have been established using:

- 17β-Estradiol – transdermal or transcutaneous administration
- Depot 17β-estradiol (as estradiol cypionate), which consists of 67 % estradiol, administered by single monthly intramuscular injection
- 17β-Estradiol – oral administration
- Ethinyl-estradiol (synthetic estrogen) – oral administration

7.3.4 Puberty Induction with Transdermal 17β-Estradiol

There are sound theoretical reasons for favoring transdermal administration. Transdermal E2 produces close to normal concentrations of E2, E1, and bioestrogen, and even low doses produce greater reduction in LH/FSH levels than normal doses administered by other methods [53, 54]. The most favorable findings regarding use of transdermal E2 are seen with substitute hormone therapy in normal age menopause subjects, in whom transdermal E2 exerted favorable or neutral effects on serum lipids and hs-CRP, including decrease in serum triglyceride and Lp(a) levels and increase of HDL-2 cholesterol concentration [55]; the risk of venous thromboembolism (VTE) was not increased [56–58]. Physiological transdermal estrogen-based regimens may lead to lower systemic blood pressure and minor activation of the renin-angiotensin system than oral synthetic estrogen-based therapies in POI subjects under 40 years old [59]. No reduction in IGF1 levels was demonstrated in subjects with hyper- and hypo-hypogonadism [60, 61].

As early as 2001, a group of Swedish investigators recommended increasing the dosages of transdermal 17β-estradiol, adding nocturnal applications to attain levels of estradiol similar to those seen at the onset of spontaneous puberty in normal girls. The starting dose was 0.05–0.07 μg/kg body weight administered via transdermal matrix patch (25 μg/24 h) cut into pieces corresponding to 3.1, 4.2, or 6.2 μg/24 h. Dosages were doubled after 4–14 months depending on serum E2 profile. The patch was applied at bedtime and removed the next morning. Progestogen was also administered, beginning within 2 years of the onset of treatment [62]. Subsequently, in 2014, lower starting doses were proposed, except for older girls for whom, when breast development was of high priority, the starting dose ranged from 0.08 to 0.12 μg/kg body weight [63] (Table 7.2).

The Turner's syndrome Consensus Study Group also proposed a protocol for induction of puberty:

Age (years)	
10–11	Monitor for spontaneous puberty based on Tanner staging and FSH level
12–13	If no spontaneous development and FSH elevated, begin low dose E2 therapy
12.5–15	Gradually increase E2 dose over about 2 years (e.g., 14, 25, 37, 50, 75, 100, 200 g daily via patch) to adult dose
14–16	Begin cyclic progesterone treatment after 2 years of estrogen or when breakthrough bleeding occurs
16–30	Continue full doses at least until age 30 (normally estrogen levels are highest between age 15 and 30 years)

Bondy [52]

Davenport [64] proposed a similar protocol, with scaled doses using portioned patches applied in the evening and removed the following morning, aimed at achieving specific E2 levels:

E2 target level	Patch portion	Dosage equivalent
3–4 pg/ml	Usually 1/6 or 1/8 of 25 μg patch	0.1 μg/kg for 6 months
6–8 pg/ml		0.2 μg/kg for 12 months
↔12 pg/ml	½ patch	12.5 μg/kg for 18 months
↔ 25 pg/ml	1 patch	25 μg/kg for 24 months
↔ 37 pg/ml	1 patch	37.5 μg/kg for 30 months
↔ 50 pg/ml	1 patch	50 μg/kg for 36 months (opportune time to start Progesterone or Progestin therapy, which should be started earlier if breakthrough bleeding occurs)
↔ 75 pg/ml	1 patch	75 μg/kg for 42 months
↔ 50–150 pg/ml	1 patch	100 μg/kg for 48 months (normal adult dose)

Table 7.2 Ankarberg-Lindgren et al. protocols for treatment of subjects with hyper- and hypo-hypogonadism

	Age	N° cases	Pathology	Dose	End points
Ankarberg-Lindgren et al. [62]	12.3–18.1	15	Hyper- or hypogonadotropic hypogonadism 8 Turner's syndrome 1 craniopharyngioma 1 hypopituitarism 1 medulloblastoma; PNET 1 ovarian insufficiency 1 androgen insensitivity 1 Mb Glaucher	17β-estradiol 0.08–0.12 μg/kg/day in transdermal matrix patch (TD 25 mg/24 h) cut into pieces corresponding to 3.1, 4.2, or 6.2 μg/24 h Dose doubled after 4–14 months, depending on serum E2 profile. Application of patch at bedtime and removal the next morning Addition of Progestogen within 2 years of the start of treatment	Achieve spontaneous levels as well as diurnal pattern of serum 17β-estradiol in early puberty
Ankarberg-Lindgren et al. [63]		54 (88 observa-tions)	Hyper- or hypogonadotropic hypogonadism 31 Turner's syndrome 7 hypopituitarism 3 androgen resistance (gonadectomized) 7 primary ovarian failure 6 ovarian failure (chemotherapy)	17β-estradiol 0.05–0.07 μg/kg/day as puberty induction starting dose in 29 girls (age range 10.5–16.9 years) 17β-estradiol 0.08–0.12 μg/kg in 42 girls (age range 9.9–18 years) 17β-estradiol 0.13–0.15 μg/kg in 17 girls (age range 11.7–17 years) Application of patch at bedtime and removal the next morning For older girls, when breast development was high priority, the starting dose was 0.08–0.12 μg/kg.	Establishment of *Guidelines* for the induction of puberty via transdermal E2 patch in a large out-patient setting

7.3.5 Puberty Induction with Percutaneous 17β-Estradiol in Hydroalcoholic Gel

Twenty-three girls ranging in age from 10.7 to 17.7 years (median age 13.6 years) with Turner's syndrome (17,XO/45,X karyotypes and six mosaics) and hypogonadism were enrolled in an uncontrolled, open, multicenter study, carried out between 1992 and 1999. Bone age at onset of treatment was > 9 years. Single-dose sachets containing 0.1 mg estradiol were prepared specifically for the study. The starting dose was 0.1 mg (22.2 pmol/L serum E2 concentrations) in the1st year, increased to 0.2 mg the 2nd year, 0.5 mg the 3rd year, 1 mg the 4th year, and 1.5 mg (corresponding to 162.2 pmol/L serum E2 concentrations) the 5th year. The starting dose of 0.1 mg of E2 is equal to 0.13 mg of E2V or 0.04 mg of conjugated equine estrogen.

All girls reached at least stage B4P4, and there were no significant differences between GH users and nonusers with regard to height SD score, weight SD score, bone age acceleration, or adult height. The treatment was safe and well accepted [65].

7.3.6 Puberty Induction with Depot 17β-Estradiol Cypionate

Preliminary reports have demonstrated that low doses of estrogen (monthly estradiol cypionate at doses of 1.0–1.5 mg) stimulate statural growth in hypogonadal girls. The association between GH therapy (very low dose) and a monthly intramuscular dose of depot 17β-estradiol cypionate, beginning with 0.2 mg, and increasing at 6-month intervals to 0.4, 0.6, and, in 7 of the girls, 0.8 mg achieved better results regarding increased final height. The data support the hypothesis that early (age 12–12.9 years) administration of 17β-E2 preserves height without interfering with the effect of GH on the enhancement of height potential. We note that this preparation is not available in Europe [66–68].

7.3.7 Puberty Induction with Oral Estrogens

17β-Estradiol, ethinyl-estradiol, and conjugated estrogens have been used to induce puberty in subjects with hyper- and hypo-gonadotropic hypogonadism. The metabolic action of these estrogens varies depending on the method of administration. Oral estrogens have a first pass hepatic effect with supra-physiological exposure, reduced production of IGF1, and increases in its binding protein (IGF BP-1); GH production is increased, but its activity is reduced; lipolysis and postprandial oxidation of fatty acids are reduced; triglyceride storage increases (experimental data on rats [69, 70], and postmenopausal women [71]); fat mass increases with tendency to central deposition of fat, and lean mass is reduced due to the reduction in the anabolic action of IGF1 [72]). These effects are, theoretically at least, more remarkable with ethinyl-estradiol, which exercises a stronger influence than natural estradiol on estrogen-dependent markers such as liver proteins (estrogen-dependent clotting factors, angiotensinogen, VLDL, SHBG, HDL-C) [73]. The doses administered and the individual patient characteristics (including age) condition the clinical effects of the treatment.

Comparison of transdermal E2 (50 μg) and oral E2 (2 mg) therapy in young subjects with hypopituitarism evidences that oral administration achieves a more significant reduction in IGF1 levels and increase in IGFBP1 levels without modifying IGFBP3 levels. However, high-density lipoprotein cholesterol levels increased after 3 months of treatment with oral E2. No differences were found between the two treatments regarding anthropometric measurements; blood pressure; heart rate; glucose, insulin, and C-peptide levels; or the homeostasis model assessment index [61] (Table 7.3).

7.3.7.1 Puberty Induction with 17β-Estradiol (E2)

Oral 17β-estradiol is widely used to induce puberty in girls with Turner's syndrome. The drug is composed of metabolized estrone (E1), estriol (E3), and estrone sulfate (E1S), but the pronounced reconversion of these metabolites to estradiol contributes to the maintenance of elevated estradiol levels for up to 12 h after intake [74]. The impact of estradiol on estrogen-dependent markers, such as liver proteins (estrogen-dependent clotting factors, angiotensinogen, VLDL, SHBG, HDL-C), is low with oral E2 and totally absent with E2 transdermal patch. The normally very short half-life of natural oral estradiol is prolonged in micronized formulations (Table 7.4).

There are no substantial negative data that discourage use of oral E2. Neither rates of protein turnover, lipolysis, lipid oxidation rates, nor IGF-levels are adversely affected by either oral (E2) or transdermal estrogen [80]. More recent data confirm that the different routes of 17-E2 delivery do not have different effects on body composition, lipid oxidation, and lipid concentrations in hypogonadal girls with Turner's syndrome [81].

7.3.7.2 Puberty Induction with Ethinyl Estradiol (EE2)

This estrogen has a remarkably strong metabolic impact on adult women, and the route of delivery, whether oral, vaginal, or transdermal, does not affect the impact. EE2 is characterized by long half-life, slow metabolism, and long tissue retention, and it is 200–20,000 times more potent than E2. Ample studies show good results for EE2 administration in young subjects. One study in particular (a

Table 7.3 E2 plasma levels with 25, 50, 100 μg patches in different phases of menstrual cycle

E2 plasma levels with matrix patch		E2 plasma levels during ovulatory menstrual cycle	
Patch delivery	Peak E2 levels	Cycle phase	Normal values (Pg/mL)
25 mcg	30–45 pg/ml	Follicular	10–98
50 mcg	40–80 pg/ml	Ovulatory	170–770
100 mcg	90–140 pg/ml	Luteal	190–340
		Post-menopause	10–38

Table 7.4 Oral E2 combined with GH therapy in puberty induction

Authors	Age (years)	N°cases	Oral E2 dose	Endpoints
Naeraa et al. [75]	16.3 ± 0.7 (12.8–20.0) BA13.8	10	E2 6–11 μg/kg/day (total dose 600 μg/day)	Morning vs. evening E2 administration; metabolism
Gravholt et al. [76]	16 ± 2	8	Placebo+placebo Placebo+GH Placebo+GH+E2 [0.39±0.12 mg/day (0.25–0.6)]	Body composition; metabolism
Bannink et al. [77]	11.8–15	56	5 μg/kg/day × 2 years 7.5 μg/kg/day 3rd year 10 μg/kg/day >3rd year	Breast and uterus development
Cleemann et al. [78]	22–65 (mean 37)	54 (TS)	E2 2 mg (1–22 day) + NETA 1 mg (13–22)+ Calcium and Vit D	Bone density
Cleemann et al. [79]	12.2–24.9 (16.7 ± 3.3)	41	Mean starting dose: 0.23 ± 012 mg (0.10–0.50 mg) Maintenance dose: E2 2 mg (1–22 day) +NETA 1 mg (13–22) + E2 1 mg (23–28)	Uterus and ovary evaluation

randomized, double-blind, placebo-controlled clinical trial on GH and low-dose ethinyl estradiol administered to girls 5–12 years old) showed significantly earlier thelarche (median 11.6 years vs. 12.6 years, *P* 0.001) and slower tempo of puberty (median, 3.3 years vs. 2.2 years, *P* 0.003) in the EE2 treated girls than controls [82] (Table 7.5).

7.3.7.3 Puberty Induction with Conjugated Equine Estrogens (CEE)

One study focused on establishing the impact of age on the effects of estrogen replacement to influence final height in Turner's syndrome patients receiving GH therapy. Subjects received a daily dose of 0.3 mg conjugated estrogens for 6 months, after which the dose was increased to 0.625 mg daily. After 1 year of this treatment the patients also received 10 mg of MAP for 10 days each month to induce regular menstrual cycles [91]. Another study on the induction of puberty in Turner's syndrome girls compared the results of oral administration of CEE and transdermal E2 patch. Twelve (12) girls with Turner's syndrome naive to estrogen and on GH therapy for at least 6 months were randomly assigned to receive conjugated oral estrogen at a dose of 0.3 mg daily for the first 6 months followed by 0.3 mg or 0.625 mg, on alternating days for the next 6 months, or transdermal E2 0.025-mg patch twice a week for 6 months followed by a 0.0375 mg patch twice a week for the next 6 months, for a total of 1 year. The transdermal E2 patch resulted in faster bone accrual at the spine and increased uterine growth compared with the oral conjugated estrogen. There were no significant differences between the two treatment groups

Table 7.5 Studies on puberty induction with EE2

Authors	Age (years)	EE dose	GH Therapy	N° cases	End-point
Martinez et al. [83]	8.6–13.3	100 ng/kg BW/day 2.4 μg/day		9	
Ross et al. [84]	5–15	100 ng/kg BW/day 50 ng/kg BW/day	Yes	39	Leg growth rate
Vanderschueren-Lodeweyckx et al. [85]	5–6.6	25 ng/kg/day	Yes	40	Height increase velocity, bone maturation, breast development
Mauras et al. [86]	7.7±0.5	100 ng/kg BW/day	… No	9	Endogenous Production rate and MCR of GH
Ross et al. [87]	7–9	25 ng/kg/day	Yes		Verbal and non-verbal memory
Johnston et al. [88]	9.1	50–75 ng/kg BW/day (GH after the first year) GH GH + EE	Yes	58	Height increase
Ross et al. [89]	5–12.5	Double placebo EE alone + placebo injection GH +oral placebo EE+ GH	Yes	149	Adult height
Perry et al. [90]	7–13	Year 1: 1–2 μg/day Year 2: 2–4 μg/day Year 3: 6–8/10 μg/day × 4 months	yes	92	Height increase velocity, bone maturation Pubertal progression
Quigley et al. [82]	5–12.5	25 ng/kg/day, ages 5–8 years 50 ng/kg/day, ages >8–12 years Escalating EE2 doses after age 12 years, starting at a nominal dosage of 100 ng/kg/day. Reduction by 50 % placebo/EE2 dosages for Breast development < 12 years, Vaginal bleeding <14 years, or Undue advance in bone age.	GH placebo	149	Childhood low-dose EE2 (as early as age 5 years) Followed by Individualized pubertal induction regimen starting after age 12 and escalating to full replacement over 4 years

Table 7.6 Conjugated estrogens, oral estradiol and transdermal estradiol equivalents [93]

Conjugated estrogens (mg)	Oral estradiol (mg)	Transdermal estradiol (μg)
0.3–0.45	0.5–1	25–37.5
0.625	1–2	

regarding high-density lipoprotein, low-density lipoprotein, triglycerides, or growth rate over time [92] (Table 7.6).

7.3.8 Progesterone and/or Progestin Addition

It is important to add progesterone or a progestin when estrogen therapy is administered to balance the estrogenic stimulation of the endometrium. Moreover, recent findings permit us to hypothesize that progesterone has an effect on human osteoblasts. One meta-analysis showed that postmenopausal women treated with combined hormone replacement therapy presented a 1.7 % increase yearly in bone mineral density (BMD) compared to the 1.3 % increase yearly in BMD in women using unopposed estrogens; associated administration of progestogen increased BMD by an additional 0.4 % yearly [94]. Progesterone is usually added to the treatment schedule either after 2 years of estrogen therapy, when breakthrough bleeding occurs, or when breast Tanner B3 is reached [95].

7.3.8.1 Micronized Progesterone for Oral Administration

Efficient oral delivery of progesterone is achieved by using a micronized form of the hormone [96] in suspension in oil and packaged in a gelatin capsule [97]. The mean plasma levels achieved with oral progesterone doses of ≥100 mg are at least as high as luteal phase levels. Maximum concentration is reached within 3 h. The concentration remains significantly elevated for up to 12 h and does not return to baseline level until at least 24 h after administration [98]. We note, however, that studies on the endometrium of post-menopausal women undergoing hormonal replacement therapy demonstrated that 200/300 mg per day did not induce uniform endometrial secretory features. There is sufficient evidence that when given orally progesterone is metabolized in the liver to pregnenolone and pregnanediol, but the high concentrations of progesterone metabolites produced during the first liver pass might result in artificially high concentrations of progesterone in serum [99] due to laboratory methodology [100]. In addition, the metabolites produced may cause side effects such as nausea and sleepiness. The half-life for 100–300 mg doses of oral micronized progesterone are:

Single daily dose	Half-life after (h)
100 mg	18.3 ± 3.5
200 mg	16.8 ± 2.3
300 mg	16.2 ± 2.7

With two doses daily (100 mg in the morning + 200 mg in the evening), progesterone plasma concentration remains significantly elevated for 24 h [101].

Vaginal administration of micronized progesterone avoids the first-pass metabolism in the gastro-intestinal tract and liver and it produces sustained plasma concentrations [102]. This method does not present any important objective side effects, but it does entail problems of compliance in younger patients who generally do not accept vaginal administration, especially before first intercourse, and in girls and women of any age in some cultures. In addition, this method of administration can have unpleasant effects such as vaginal discharge, vulvar edema, and irritation, as mentioned in numerous reports on the internet but not in the professional literature [103]. This situation has led to the alternative administration of progestins during hormonal replacement therapy.

7.3.8.2 Progestins

Four types of active oral synthetic progestins are available: progesterone derivatives, 19-nor progesterone derivatives, 19-nor testosterone derivatives, and spironolactone derivative (Drospirenone). All four exercise progestational action and some also have tissue antiestrogenic effects. Depending on their individual chemical structures, they may act as weak androgens or antiandrogens, glucocorticoids or antimineral corticoids (Table 7.7).

Table 7.7 Endocrine characteristics of principal progestins

Derivatives of progesterone	Androgenic	Progestogenic	Estrogenic	Gluco-corticoid	Mineral-corticoid
Derivatives of progesterone					
Dydrogesterone	00	+++	+	0	+
17-OH Progesterone					
Cyproterone acetate	0/–	+++	0	+	+
MAP	+	+++	0	+	+
19-nor progesterone Nomegestrol acetate	––	+++	0	0	0
Derivatives of progesterone					
Estranes (13-methyl gonanes)					
Norethisterone acetate	++	+++	++	+	0
Norethisterone	+++	+++	++	+	+
Gonanes (13-ethyl gonanes)					
Levonorgestrel	+++	+++	0	0/+	0
Desogestrel	+	+++	0	0/+	0
Gestodene	+	+++	0	+	0/–
Dienogest	–––	+++	0	0	0

0 = neutral; –,––,––– = antagonist; +,++,+++,++++ = agonist [74]

Dydrogesterone, included in the group of Pregane derivatives, is a retroprogesterone formed from progesterone by UV light exposure; it is commercially available, does not have clinically relevant androgenic, estrogenic, glucocorticoid, or mineralcorticoid effects, and it resembles progesterone mainly in its progestogenic effects [104]. The metabolite half-life is 17 h, and it has a 75 % relative binding affinity for progesterone receptor; the configuration of metabolites remain stable also after oral administration [105]. These are the reasons why dydrogesterone can be considered an ideal oral supplement progestogen in hormone replacement therapy. Other considerations are that it has minimal side effects, as demonstrated in a recent review in the literature [103]; its beneficial effects and safety in hormone replacement therapy have been widely confirmed [106]; and it has been used as support therapy in the second phase of the menstrual cycle in place of micronized progesterone [107, 108].

There are many reasons for choosing non-androgenic progestins in hormone replacement therapy. Androgenic progestins antagonize the favorable cardiovascular effect of estrogens, whereas non-androgenic progestins do not impair, and may even enhance, the beneficial effect of estrogens [109]. Data on progestins in menopausal hormone therapy demonstrated that MPA Medroxyprogesterone acetate, but not oral micronized progesterone or other progestins, increase monocyte cell endothelium adhesion; MPA and the association MPA/E2 have negative effects on the brain, whereas the progesterone/E2 combination has neuroregenerative effects [110] (Table 7.8).

7.3.9 Special Considerations in Choosing Hormone Replacement Therapy

Turner's syndrome patients may present particular cardiovascular anomalies (structural defects and various cardiovascular risk factors, including arterial hypertension, hyperlipidemia, obesity, and diabetes mellitus), autoimmune conditions (such as hypothyroidism, celiac disease) and altered brain structure and function [64, 112, 113]. These subjects present a 4.7 % prevalence of metabolic syndrome associated with visceral obesity; fatty liver was observed in Turner's syndrome patients with metabolic syndrome and insulin resistance [114]. Although insulin resistance in Turner's syndrome adolescents undergoing GH treatment is comparable to that of obese patients, their overall metabolic risk factors seem to be lower [115].

Table 7.8 Metabolic effects of Dydrogesterone, MPA, and Norethisterone [111]

Type of effects	Dydrogesterone	MPA	Norethisterone (Norethindrone)
Androgenic	No	Mild	Yes
Estrogenic	No	No	Metabolites
Glucocorticoid	No	Yes	No
HDL cholesterol	No effect	↓ (reduces E effect)	↓↓ androgen effect
Glucose metabolism	No effect	↓ glucose tolerance	↓ glucose tolerance

7.3.10 Effects of Hormone Replacement Therapy

Mammary gland development to stage B4 within 2 years is the primary criterion for successful puberty induction. Normal breast development up to B5 is generally mimicked, but with a 2-year delay in one series [77]. Another series found incomplete breast development in women with 45,X (54.3 % breast, Tanner Stage 5) and 45,X/46,XY karyotype (50.0 % breast, Tanner Stage 5), whereas 75 % of women with 45,X/46,XX karyotype presented complete breast development [116].

Uterus development is generally suboptimal in Turner subjects treated with oral estrogens (Table 7.9).

Bone Mineral Density Whatever the cause, ovarian insufficiency with onset in fertile aged women comports reduced bone mass density (BMD). The problem is particularly important when it occurs before the individual reaches peak bone mass. It is well known that the highest individual levels of bone mass are conditioned by genetic and ethnic factors, nutrition and physical activity, as well as

Table 7.9 Oral estrogen treatment and uterus development in Turner's syndrome

Authors	Estrogen	N° cases (age in years)	Results (uterus)
Paterson et al. [117]	EE	56 (13.5–18)	Incomplete uterus development in 50 %
Doerr et al. [116]	EE CEE E2V COC	75 (15.8–30.8)	Normal uterus sizes in women with karyotype 45,X/46,XX Uterus length <22 SDS in 26 % of TS women with karyotype 45,X Uterus volume <22 SDS in 18 %
Bakalov et al. [118]	E2 (12 %) CEE (32 %) COC (31 %) No ERT (20 %) Other 5 %	86 (28–45)	24.4 % fully developed size and shape of uterus 44.2 % transitional uterus 31.4 % immature "cylindrical shaped" uterus No correlation between age at first exposure to estrogens and uterus size
Nabhan et al. [92]	CEE TD E2	12 (14.0 ± 1.7)	Increased uterine growth after 1 year TD-E2; 66 % in TD-E2 group vs. 0 % in CEE group
Snajderova et al. [119]	E2	57 (18.1–41.5)	Suboptimal uterine development in most patients.
Bannink et al. [77]	E2	56 (19.2)	⇩Uterus volume vs. controls (subnormal uterus dimensions in women aged nearly 20 years)
Cleemann et al. [79]	E2	41 (17 ± 3.3, range 11.2–24.9)	Mean uterus volumes lower than controls
Kim et al. [120]	E2V	19 (13–17)	Better uterine development with 1 mg E2V than 0.5 mg starting dose

sex steroid levels. In Turner's syndrome BMD is present in the cortical bone with osteopenia or osteoporosis, increased risk of fractures, and it is most evident in childhood and after age 45 years [121–124]. The increased risk of fractures is due to the specific characteristics of the bones in Turner's syndrome, e.g., small bones, altered bone geometry, and greater risk of falls and trauma related to hearing impairment [125, 126] as well as to the sedentary lifestyle of many of these subjects.

It has been known for many years that Turner patients have low bone mineralization, documented by standard X-ray examination [127]. Studies on bone fragility in Turner's syndrome using quantitative ultrasonography (QUS), measuring speed of sound, and two dimensional DXA of radius and tibia evidenced low speed of sound (indicating high bone fragility), but the DXA did not evidence lower bone mass density compared to controls [128]. We note that since the two-dimensional nature of DXA scanning gives an area value of BMD, it gives lower measures of BMD in Turner's syndrome patients. Corrected to size, the quantitative DXA findings show normal volumetric BMD in these patients [128].

Subsequent investigations evidenced reduced cortical bone density with normal trabecular bone density in girls with Turner's syndrome, with bone mineral apparent density (BMAD) of the femoral neck together with reduced cortical bone density of the radius (the trabecular bone was spared) [129, 130]. Other studies using the same method of high-resolution peripheral quantitative computed tomography (HR-pQCT) demonstrated higher cortical thickness with lower cortical porosity in radius of Turner's syndrome patients; trabecular integrity was compromised with lower bone volume per tissue volume (BV/TV) (27 % in radius, 22 % in tibia, both $p<0.0001$), trabecular number (27 % in radius, 12 % in tibia, both $p<0.05$), and higher trabecular spacing (54 % in radius, 23 % in tibia, both $p<0.01$) [131]. However, it is an open question. Recently some of the same investigators affirmed that cortical BMD is not decreased in the radius in Turner's syndrome subjects, and that the artificially low cortical bone mineral density is due to the partial volume effect [132]. In addition, a group of 32 TS girls with an average age of 16.7 years (range 12.4–20.2) had lower BMAD ((g/cm^3) at the lumbar spine than an age- and sex-matched population [133].

The altered mechanical strength of the skeleton in Turner's syndrome is probably related to haploinsufficiency due to certain genes located on the X-chromosome; one candidate gene is SHOX, on the distal portion of Xp [134]. Skeletal growth is also impaired by the presence of smaller than normal bones and bones with altered geometry. Recently, Faienza et al. [135] demonstrated for the first time high osteoclastogenic potential both in girls and young women with Turner's syndrome. This seems to be associated with elevated FSH serum levels before hormone replacement therapy and high RANKL levels during the therapy, irrespective of karyotype. A genetic defect related to vitamin D receptor gene polymorphism (genotype BsmI or FokI) could aggravate the hormonal deficit [136] as well as conditions such as celiac disease and thyroid disorders. In summary, various mechanisms contribute to reduced bone mass in Turner's syndrome [137]. Turner's syndrome related mechanisms are:

- Puberty delay
- Estrogen deficiency which persists throughout life
- Low intake of vitamin D
- Vitamin D receptor gene polymorphisms
- Hormonal factors (i.e., thyroid disorders)
- Autoimmune diseases

7.3.10.1 Treatment to Improve Bone Mineral Density in Turner's Syndrome

A study on longitudinal changes in bone mineral density in Turner's syndrome and related changes in biochemical parameters in 54 TS women (22–65 years, mean 37) after conventional hormonal replacement therapy with 17β-estradiol (E2, 2 mg) for the entire cycle and norethisterone (1 mg), medroxyprogesterone (10 mg), or levonorgestrel (0.25 mg) for 10 days each cycle showed only slight longitudinal changes in bone mass density in the 5.9-year study period. No changes in bone formation markers were seen during the study, but bone resorption markers decreased in Turner's syndrome patients who were all encouraged to maintain a healthy lifestyle and take calcium and vitamin D [78].

Good results were achieved with transdermal E2 administration in a randomized controlled study using conjugated oral estrogen (0.3 mg daily for the first 6 months followed by alternating 0.3 mg and 0.625 mg daily for the second 6 months) versus transdermal E2 (0.025-mg patch twice a week for 6 months followed by 0.0375 mg patch twice a week for the second 6 months) for 1 year [92]. Another study using ECE (0.625 mg + dihydrogesterone 10 mg/day for 11 days) indicated that estrogen therapy may be effective in increasing BMD in young TS patients if initiated before age 18 years [138].

7.4 Hormonal Therapy in POI with Post-menarche Onset

In POI with post-menarcheal onset, therapy is targeted at recuperation of normal endocrine asset both to treat unpleasant menopause-related symptoms (e.g., vasomotor symptoms and vaginal atrophy) and to prevent the adverse effects of estrogen deficiency. The therapy involves protecting the cardiovascular system, maintaining and optimizing bone mass, sexuality, quality of life, and even preparing patients for assisted reproduction techniques. Subjects with POI are at higher than normal risk for cardiovascular problems, as evidenced by the numerous reports of death risk due to vascular events [139–146], especially women who underwent ovariectomy before age 45 years in a Mayo Clinic Cohort Study on 4780 women [147] and a Nurses' Health Study on 30,000 women [148]. These data have been confirmed in recent meta-analyses [149, 150]. Women ovariectomized before natural menopause are at increased risk of cognitive impairment or dementia [151] and Parkinsonism [152]. In addition, women with premature ovarian failure (or premature menopause) present early onset vascular endothelial dysfunction, associated with sex steroid deficiency [153, 154]. Circulating EPCs, CIMT, and diastolic function are significantly affected in young women with POF. We note that also healthy women in the transitional phase to menopause [155] and young women in menopause due to surgery [147, 156] present altered endothelial function related to estrogen deficit. The data regarding risk of ischemic stroke in POI patients is controversial: some investigators have reported increased risk [157], others found no changes [158], and others reported increased mean arterial pressure (94 ± 10 vs. 86 ± 5 mmHg) despite normal endothelial and autonomic modulation of vasculature [159]. Increased risk of venous thromboembolism (VTE) was also reported in these patients [58].

Natural estrogens can be administered in oral (17β-estradiol, estradiol valerate, conjugated estrogens) and transdermal (patch, gel, cream) preparations, and synthetic estrogen is also now available for administration in oral and vaginal preparations for use in hormonal replacement therapy. Conjugated estrogens purified from pregnant mare urine have been used in estrogen hormone replacement therapy since 1942, but only recently were the steroidal components of the product fully identified [160]. In Italy, conjugated estrogens are currently available only in 0.3 mg doses combined with 1.5 mg MAP. A synthetic estrogen (EE2) is also available for administration in both oral and vaginal preparations for use in hormonal replacement therapy.

Transdermal E2 is, from a metabolic point of view, the best choice treatment in adult women with POI. Various investigators have seen that oral estrogens can cause increase in C-reactive protein, decreased IGF-I and IGF binding protein-3 levels, increased SHBG, and triglyceride enrichment of low- and high-density lipoprotein particles [70, 74, 161, 162]. A study comparing administration of oral or transdermal E2 (41 women, age 49 +/− 6 years, hysterectomized and oophorectomized) demonstrated statistically significant reduction in tissue factor pathway inhibitor and plasminogen activator inhibitor-1 levels with oral administration without significant changes in D-dimer levels [163]. The metabolic profile of ethinyl estradiol differs from that of natural estrogen primarily with transdermal administration. Ethinyl estradiol is present in many contraceptive preparations, and it has a stronger hepatic impact than natural estradiol on estrogen dependent markers, such as liver proteins, as listed here below [73].

Effects of ethinyl-estradiol on proteins produced in the liver

↑ SHBG
↑ HDL-C
↑ VLDLk
↑ Angiotensinogen
± Modification of certain estrogen-dependent clotting factors

There is growing observational evidence that transdermal E2 therapy may be associated with lower risk of deep vein thrombosis, stroke, and myocardial infarction [164, 165].

In 64 postmenopausal women randomly assigned to receive either oral or transdermal hormonal replacement therapy (HRT), transdermal HRT (estradiol combined with NETA) exerted favorable or neutral effects on serum lipids and hs-CRP in postmenopausal women, including decrease in serum triglyceride and Lp(a) levels and increased HDL-2 cholesterol concentration. Therapy with the oral combination was associated with a significant decrease in serum LDL cholesterol and a significant increase in hs-CRP, but no change in serum triglyceride levels [55].

The American College of Obstetricians and Gynecologists has published an opinion on adolescent health care suggesting the use of estradiol-17β delivered via transdermal patch with doses of 100 μg (or 0.625–1.25 mg/day oral conjugated estrogen or 2 mg/day oral E2) associated with 10 mg oral medroxyprogesterone acetate daily for 12–14 days every 30–60 days (or 200 mg oral micronized progesterone daily for12–14 days every 30–60 days). The postpubertal patient treatment options proposed include combined hormone contraception [166].

The addition of natural progesterone or synthetic progestagens is essential for prevention of endometrial hyperplasia during estrogen replacement therapy regimens. Micronized progesterone seems to be neutral from a metabolic point of view [167]. Oral dydrogesterone in combination with transdermal estradiol showed no elevation in VTE compared to non-HRT users [168] and may be the preferred when considering thromboembolic risk [106]. The synthetic progestogens differ in their affinity with different steroid receptors and may have some negative impact on cardiovascular risk factors [169] (See section on Progesterone and/or Progestin Addition, 7.3.8).

All patients with POI under treatment with hormonal replacement therapy must be made aware that they have a 5–10% possibility of conceiving [170]; thus they must use barrier contraceptive methods, such as a condom or intrauterine devices. *Combined oral contraception* appears to be acceptable for adolescents undergoing hormonal replacement therapy if peak bone mass has been achieved and there are no contraindications. It can also be considered for young women, especially when contraceptive cover is necessary or requested by the patient, especially considering the benefits of hormonal contraception in regard to both prevention and therapy.

7.4.1 Bone Mineral Density in POI with Post-menarche Onset

Young women with primary ovarian insufficiency have significantly reduced bone mineral density compared to regularly menstruating women [171–175]. Bone health was the primary endpoint in a few studies. The results of an open-label, randomized, controlled, crossover trial involving 34 women with POF who were randomized to a 4-week treatment with either TD E2 plus vaginal progesterone or 30 μg EE plus 1.5 mg NETA (for 1/3 weeks) demonstrate a beneficial effect on bone mass acquisition on the lumbar spine over 12 months of therapy, mediated by increased bone formation and decreased bone resorption [176]. HRT in those with early menopause does appear to reduce the risk of fracture when administered for at least 3 years [177]. The principal studies on HRT in POI with post-menarche onset involve patients 19–40 years old. All patients received the same dose without variations in relation to age or peak bone mass acquisition; the dose was higher than that normally considered standard for HRT in natural menopause (Table 7.10).

Table 7.10 Studies on HRT in POI with post-menarcheal onset [181]

Investigators	Intervention/comparison	Population	Outcomes	Results
Guttmann et al. [178]	ECE (0.625 mg) for 28 days MPA (5 mg) for the last 14 days	N° 17 young TS	Bone turnover, uterine and cardiac variables	
Panay and Kalu [5]	E2 TD patch (75–100 mg) or estrogel 0.06 % twice daily Cyclical progesterone/progestogen (at least 12 days each month)]	Proposals for POI treatment	Short term: maintenance of quality of life Long term: avoidance of sequelae of POI	Need for confirmation from randomized trials
Langrish et al. [59]	pSSR: E2 TD patch (100mcg) for 1 week followed by E2 TD patch (150 mcg) for 3 weeks Cyclical progesterone 200 g twice daily for weeks 3 and 4 or dydrogesterone 10 mg twice daily sHRT: EE (30 mcg) for weeks 1–3 and NETA [0.5 mg] for weeks 1–3	N° 42 POI Age 19–39 years (chemo/radiotherapy, surgery, Turner's syndrome)	Blood pressure and arterial stiffness	
Crofton et al. [176]	pSSR: phonological sex-steroid replacement sHRT: standard hormone replacement therapy	N° 18 POI Age 19–39 years	Bone mass acquisition and turnover	Only with pSSR increase in bone formation markers
O'Donnel et al. [179]	Open-label, randomized, controlled, crossover trial (reported in Langrish 2009): all participants received both treatments (pSSR and sHRT)	N° 34 POF Age 19–40 years (idiopathic, surgery, following cancer treatment, Turner's syndrome)	Uterine volume and ET, uterine blood flow, non-uterine end-points: bone & cardiovascular	
Popat et al. [180]	3-year prospective, double-blind, randomized, placebo-controlled clinical trial. E2 TD patch (100 μg/day) + MAP 10 mg/day (12 d/mo) or Transdermal estradiol (100 μg/d) + oral medroxyprogesterone acetate 10 mg/day (12 d/mo) + testosterone	N° 145 (spontaneous, 46 XX POI and 70 controls)	Change in BMD at the femoral neck measured by DEXA	BMD restored to normal control levels with E2/MAP therapy; no further benefit with T addition

Modified from Gambacciani and Levancini [181]

The optimal dose for patients with POI onset after age 30 years remains to be established. Hormonal replacement therapy regimens must be based on individual patient symptoms and bone mineral density at the time of first observation. HRT must be continued until the patient reaches the age of average normal menopause. Five years ago, a committee of the American College of Obstetricians and Gynecologists proposed bone density monitoring by dual-energy X-ray absorptiometry (DEXA) once a year to document peak bone mass achievement during early- to mid-puberty, and then once every 2 years through late adolescence [166].

Evidence statements regarding eight prospective cohort studies (sample sizes ranging from over 300 to 100,000 women) showed that the risk of any non-vertebral, vertebral, hip and/or wrist fracture was significantly lower for current HRT users than either women not currently using HRT or who had never used HRT [181, 182] (Table 7.11).

7.4.2 Cognitive Function in POI

Most available data on cognitive function in POI refer to women over 40 years old, prevalently women who have undergone oophorectomy before menopause. Premenopausal oophorectomy (unilateral and bilateral) increases the risk of cognitive impairment, dementia and/or Parkinsonism [151, 152]. The younger the patient is at the time of oophorectomy the higher the risk of such problems.

7.4.3 Psychological Consequences of POI

We emphasize that diagnosis of primary ovarian insufficiency can be emotionally traumatic for the patient and even the family. Women with spontaneous hypergonadotropic hypogonadism have the perception of receiving less social support and have less self-esteem than control women. Specific strategies targeted at alleviating such psychological discomforts could help these women overcome their disappointment and dismay regarding the life altering diagnosis of spontaneous POI [183]. Also parents need assistance in learning how to help their daughters understand and live with the diagnosis in a way that allows for healthy growth and development [184].

Table 7.11 Estrogen dosages routinely administered for bone protection in HRT

	Oral estradiol (mg)	Conjugated estrogens (mg)	Transdermal estradiol (mcg)	Tibolone (mg)
Standard	2	0.625	50	2.5
Low dose	1	0.45	25	1.25
Ultra-low dose	0.5	0.30	12.5	

Modified from Gambacciani and Levancini [181]

7.4.4 Androgen Deficiency in POI

We know that after menopause both the ovaries and the adrenal glands continue to produce androstenedione and testosterone. Total testosterone concentrations are decreased in women with spontaneous POI or iatrogenic menopause, as pointed out in data from a meta-analysis of 206 articles regarding spontaneous POI and 1358 on iatrogenic menopause [185]. Hypoandrogenism was evidenced in cases with diminished functional ovarian reserve in 140 women under 38 years old, with premature ovarian aging, occult primary ovarian insufficiency, and abnormally low functional ovarian reserve measured by age-specific FSH and/or anti-Müllerian hormone levels and 166 women over 40, with diminished ovarian reserve; the 49 control patients, under 38 years old, demonstrated normal functional ovarian reserve indicated by FSH and/or AMH levels [186].

Regarding dehydroepiandrosterone (DHEA), the limited findings available show that in POI hematic levels are not significantly different from those found in fertile aged normal women, but they are elevated compared to those of postmenopausal women [187, 188]. In a study on 67 women with Hashimoto thyroiditis, only those who tested positive for antithyroid antibody showed comparatively low, but within normal limits, DHEA levels [189].

There is ongoing debate about the repercussions of androgenic deficiency on bone mineral density, sexual desire, quality of life, self-esteem, and mood. Women with POF tend to have a lower sense of sexual wellbeing than normal women; they experience less sexual arousal and thus have more unsatisfactory sex lives, with less frequent sexual intercourse, reduced lubrification and increased genital pain. Although total testosterone and androstenedione levels are lower in women with POF, this is only one of the factors to be considered among the many that may play an important independent role in the various aspects of sexual functioning [190]. The treatment of low/hypoactive sexual desire disorder is multifaceted and should include a combination of both pharmacological treatments able to maximize the biological signals that drive sexual response as well as individualized psychosocial therapies to help patients overcome personal and relational difficulties [191].

7.4.5 Testosterone Replacement Therapy

Administration of testosterone replacement in POI is controversial, and it has been studied only in the context of surgical menopause [192]. Regarding repercussions on bone mineral content, in a double-blind, randomized, placebo-controlled clinical trial involving patients with iatrogenic POI, administration of testosterone did not modify bone mineral density at the femoral neck, evidenced by DEXA. The patients in this study received transdermal testosterone (150 μg/day) and transdermal estradiol (100 μg/day) plus oral medroxyprogesterone acetate (10 mg/day, 12 days/

month) for 3 years [180]. Another trial investigating the efficacy of physiologic testosterone replacement in hormonal replacement therapy with E2 T(100 μg/d)+ MAP (10 mg/day) also evaluated quality of life, self-esteem, and depressive symptoms in patients. After 12 months of treatment, there were no differences between treatment groups regarding changes in quality of life, self-esteem, and/or mood symptoms [193].

7.4.6 DHEA Therapy

Dehydroepiandrosterone (DHEA) and its sulfate ester (DHEAS) are the most abundant steroid hormones in humans. DHEA is produced mainly by the adrenal cortex and to a limited extent by the ovaries, and is rapidly sulfated by sulfotransferases into DHEAS [194]. Large amounts of DHEA and DHEAS are produced during fetal development; the production falls sharply after birth and remains low for several years; during adrenarche (age 6–8 years) synthesis resumes and high levels are maintained throughout adult life, providing substrates for conversion into potent androgens and estrogens in peripheral tissues [195–197]. An age-dependent decline in DHEA and DHEAS levels begins by the third decade and progresses with advancing age, by around 2–5 % per year, such that by menopause the DHEA level has decreased by 60 %.

"DHEA and its unconjugated and sulfated metabolites participate in various physiological and pathophysiological processes, including management of GnRH cyclic release, regulation of glandular and neurotransmitter secretions, maintenance of glucose homeostasis [...] and insulin insensitivity [...], control of skeletal muscle and smooth muscle activities including vasoregulation, promotion of tolerance to ischemia and other neuroprotective effects." [198] The biological actions of DHEA(S) in the brain involve neuroprotection, neurite growth, neurogenesis and neuronal survival, apoptosis, catecholamine synthesis and secretion, as well as antioxidant, anti-inflammatory, and antiglucocorticoid effects. In addition, DHEA affects neurosteroidogenesis and endorphin synthesis/release [199]. DHEA is also a precursor of estrogen receptor beta (ERβ) ligands [200].

Several studies have explored the role of DHEA in sexual function in women, and replacement therapy with DHEA in women with androgen insufficiency and sexual dysfunction appears to have some beneficial effects on sexual desire, arousal, activity, interest, fantasy and drive, and relationships, but further studies are necessary [201].

The role of DHEA/DHEAS in POI therapy is intriguing. The basic question is whether or not DHEA supplementation is useful in POI. This is a relatively recent therapeutic addition to the management of female infertility, in particular for women with diminished ovarian reserve. The mechanism of action of DHEA on the ovaries is not clear. DHEA has been found to be a prehormone of the follicular fluid testosterone during the administration of gonadotropins for ovulation induction which leads to the formation of estradiol. Androgen has been proposed to be a metabolic precursor for steroid production and acts as a ligand for androgen receptors, thus influencing follicular growth in ovaries. Another hypothesis is that the beneficial effect of DHEA may be due to an increase in insulin-like growth factor-I. In fact studies on rhesus monkeys showed that androgen treatment (testosterone and dihydrotestosterone) can promote IGF 1 and IGF 1 receptor gene expression in the primate ovary [202]. Finally, some investigators have postulated that DHEA has a beneficial effect on oocyte quality and mitochondrial function [203].

The effectiveness and safety of DHEA and testosterone as adjuncts to androgen replacement therapy in women undergoing assisted reproduction have been investigated. Treatment with DHEA and testosterone appeared to improve the live birth/ongoing pregnancy rate and clinical pregnancy rate in women identified as poor responders [204]. However, when studies with a high risk of bias in sensitivity analyses are excluded the effects of DHEA and T treatment are no longer statistically significant, also given the variable lengths of treatment. In addition there is scarce proof of the safety of DHEA and testosterone treatment, and evidence to date is limited by generally small sample sizes and inadequately reported study methodologies.

A Task Force appointed by the Endocrine Society, American Congress of Obstetricians and Gynecologists (ACOG), American Society for Reproductive Medicine (ASRM), European Society of Endocrinology (ESE), and International Menopause Society (IMS) commissioned two systematic reviews of published data, meta-analyses, and trials on DHEA and T replacement therapy. The Endocrine Society continues its strong recommendation against the general use of testosterone in treating infertility, sexual dysfunction (except for a specific diagnosis of hypoactive sexual desire, and only for 3–6 months), cognitive, cardiovascular, metabolic and bone health, or general well-being as well as against the routine use of DHEA for women due to limited data concerning its effectiveness and safety in normal women or those with adrenal insufficiency. The Task Force recommends against routine prescription of testosterone or dehydroepiandrosterone for women with low androgen levels due to hypopituitarism, adrenal insufficiency, surgical menopause, pharmacological glucocorticoid administration, or other conditions associated with low androgen levels because the data supporting improvement in signs and symptoms with these therapies are limited and there are to date no long-term studies of risk [205]. Another two recent meta-analyses also confirm the need for further investigations to clarify the effects of DHEA exposure in assisted reproduction technology [206, 207].

On the other hand, all the scientific societies recommend use of hormonal therapy or oral contraception until the median age of natural menopause with periodic reassessment for all women with POI. A fundamental part of that therapy is psychological support to help patients address the issues associated with early menopause, including loss of fertility, changes in self image, and sexual dysfunction [208]. Early initiation of HRT is, however, always necessary to optimize metabolic parameter and enhance bone, mass [209].

References

1. Albright F, Smith PH, Fraser RA (1942) A syndrome characterized by primary ovarian insufficiency and decreased stature: report of 11 cases with a diagnosis on hormonal control of axillary and pubic hair. Am J Med Sci 204:625–648
2. Welt CK (2008) Primary ovarian insufficiency: a more accurate term for premature ovarian failure. Clin Endocrinol (Oxf) 68:499–509
3. Coulam CB, Adamson SC, Annegers JF (1986) Incidence of premature ovarian failure. Obstet Gynecol 67:604–606
4. Qin Y, Jiao X, Simpson JL et al (2015) Genetics of primary ovarian insufficiency: new developments and opportunities. Hum Reprod Update 21:787–808
5. Panay N, Kalu E (2009) Management of premature ovarian failure. Best Pract Res Clin Obstet Gynaecol 23(1):129–140
6. Rebar R, Connolly H (1990) Clinical features of young women with hypergonadotropic amenorrhea. Fertil Steril 53:804–810
7. Nelson LM (2009) Primary ovarian insufficiency. N Engl J Med 360(6):606–614
8. Aittomäki K, Lucena JL, Pakarinen P et al (1995) Mutation in the follicle-stimulating hormone receptor gene causes hereditary hypergonadotropic ovarian failure. Cell 82(6):959–968
9. Lussiana C, Guani B, Mari C et al (2008) Mutations and polymorphisms of the FSH receptor (FSHR) gene: clinical implications in female fecundity and molecular biology of FSHR protein and gene. Obstet Gynecol Surv 63(12):785–795
10. Ebrahimi M, Asbagh FA (2011) Pathogenesis and causes of premature ovarian failure: an update. Int J Fertil Steril 5:54–65
11. Goswami D, Conway GS (2005) Premature ovarian failure. Hum Reprod Update 11:391–410
12. Bricaire L, Laroche E, Bourcigaux N et al (2013) Insuffisances ovariennes prématurées. Presse Med 42:1500–1507
13. Tartaglia NR, Howell S, Sutherland A et al (2010) A review of trisomy X (47, XXX). Orphanet J Rare Dis 5:8. doi:10.1186/1750-1172-5-8
14. Pouresmaeili F, Fazeli Z (2014) Premature ovarian failure: a critical condition in the reproductive potential with various genetic causes. Int J Fertil Steril 8:1–12
15. Cordts EB, Christofolini IDM, dos Santos AA et al (2001) Genetic aspects of premature ovarian failure: a literature review. Arch Gynecol Obstet 283:635–643
16. Chapman C, Cree L, Shelling AN (2015) The genetics of premature ovarian failure: current perspectives. Int J Womens Health 7:799–810
17. Rizzolio F, Pramparo T, Sala C et al (2009) Epigenetic analysis of the critical region I for premature ovarian failure: demonstration of a highly heterochromatic domain of the long arm of the mammalian X chromosome. J Med Genet 46:585–592
18. De Vos M, Devroey P, Fauser BCJM (2010) Primary ovarian insufficiency. Lancet 376:911–921
19. Rege G, Foidart JM, Nisolee M et al (2012) Insuffisance ovarienne prématurée: de la génétique à la clinique. Rev Med Liege 67:413–419
20. Fridovich-Keil JL, Gubbels CG, Spencer JB et al (2011) Ovarian function in girls and women with GALT-deficiency galactosemia. J Inherit Metab Dis 2:357–366
21. Bilgin EM, Kovanci E (2015) Genetics of premature ovarian failure. Curr Opin Obstet Gynecol 27(3):167–174
22. Dragojević-Dikić S, Marisavljević D, Mitrović A (2010) An immunological insight into premature ovarian failure (POF). Autoimmun Rev 9:771–774
23. Silva CA, Yamakami LYS, Aikawa NE et al (2014) Autoimmune primary ovarian insufficiency. Autoimmun Rev 13(4–5):427–430
24. Falorni A, Laureti S, Candeloro P et al (2002) Steroid-cell autoantibodies are preferentially expressed in women with premature ovarian failure who have adrenal autoimmunity. Fertil Steril 78:270–279

25. Chernyshov VP, Radysh TV, Gura IV et al (2001) Immune disorders in women with premature ovarian failure. Am J Reprod Immunol 46:220–225
26. La Marca A, Brozzetti A, Sighinolfi G et al (2010) Primary ovarian insufficiency: autoimmune causes. Curr Opin Obstet Gynecol 22:277–282
27. Jin M, Yu YQ, Huang HF (2012) An update on primary ovarian insufficiency. Sci China Life Sci 55:677–686
28. Yan G, Schoenfeld D, Penney C (2000) Identification of premature ovarian failure patients with underlying autoimmunity. J Womens Health Gend Based Med 9:275–287
29. Shelling AN (2010) Premature ovarian failure. Reproduction 140:633–641
30. Iorio R, Castellucci A, Ventriglia G et al (2014) Ovarian toxicity: from environmental exposure to chemotherapy. Curr Pharm Des 20:5388–5397
31. Wo JY, Viswanathan AN (2009) The impact of radiotherapy on fertility, pregnancy and neonatal outcomes of female cancer patients. Int J Radiat Oncol Biol Phys 73:1304–1312
32. Wallace WH, Thomson AB, Saran F et al (2005) Predicting age of ovarian failure after radiation to a field that includes the ovaries. Int J Radiat Oncol Biol Phys 62:738–744
33. Leal de Assumpção CR (2014) Falência ovariana precoce. Arq Bras. Endocrinol Metab 58:132–143
34. Ohl J, Partisani M, Demangeat C et al (2010) Alteration of ovarian reserve tests in human immunodeficiency virus (HIV)-infected women. Gynecol Obstet Fertil 38:313–317
35. Hoyer PB, Keating AF (2014) Xenobiotic effects in the ovary: temporary versus permanent infertility. Expert Opin Drug Metab Toxicol 10:511–523
36. Klein P, Serje A, Pezzullo JC (2001) Premature ovarian failure in women with epilepsy. Epilepsia 42:1584–1589
37. Deligeoroglou E, Athanasopoulos N, Tsimaris P et al (2010) Evaluation and management of adolescent amenorrhea. Ann N Y Acad Sci 1205:23–32
38. Petraglia F, Hartmann B, Luisi S et al (1998) Low levels of serum inhibin A and inhibin B in women with hypergonadotropic amenorrhea and evidence of high levels of activin a in women with hypothalamic amenorrhea. Fertil Steril 70:907–912
39. Messina MF, Aversa T, Salzano G (2015) Inhibin B in adolescents and young adults with Turner syndrome. J Pediatr Endocrinol Metab 28(11–12):1209–1214. doi:10.1515/jpem-2014-0229
40. Welt CK, Hall JE, Adams JM et al (2005) Relationship of estradiol and inhibin to the follicle-stimulating hormone variability in hypergonadotropic hypogonadism or premature ovarian failure. J Clin Endocrinol Metab 90(2):826–830
41. Weenen C, Laven JS, Von Bergh AR et al (2004) Anti-Mullerian hormone expression pattern in the human ovary: potential implication for initial and cyclic follicle recruitment. Mol Hum Reprod 10:77–83
42. Visser JA, Themmen AP (2005) Anti-Müllerian hormone and folliculogenesis. Mol Cell Endocrinol 234(1–2):81–86
43. Leader B, Baker VL (2014) Maximizing the clinical utility of antimüllerian hormone testing in women's health. Curr Opin Obstet Gynecol 26(4):226–236
44. Harlow SD, Gass M, Hall JE et al (2012) Addressing the unfinished agenda of staging reproductive aging. Fertil Steril 97(4):843–851
45. Alipour F, Rasekhjahromi A, Maalhagh M et al (2015) Comparison of specificity and sensitivity of AMH and FSH in diagnosis of premature ovarian failure. Hindawi Publishing Corporation Disease Markers, Article ID 585604, 4 pages. doi:org/10.1155/2015/585604
46. Göksedef BP, Idiş N, Görgen H et al (2010) The correlation of the antral follicle count and serum anti-Mullerian hormone. J Turk Ger Gyneocol Assoc 11(4):212–215
47. Knauff E, Eijkemans M, Lambalk CB et al (2009) Anti-Mullerian hormone, inhibin B, and antral follicle count in young women with ovarian failure. J Clin Endocrinol Metab 94:786–792
48. Ebrahimi M, Asbagh FA (2015) The role of autoimmunity in premature ovarian failure. Iran J Reprod Med 13(8):461–472

49. Fierabracci A, Bizzarri C, Palma A et al (2012) A novel heterozygous mutation of the AIRE gene in a patient with autoimmune polyendocrinopathy-candidiasis-ectodermal dystrophy syndrome (APECED). Gene 511(1):113–117
50. Davenport ML (2010) Approach to the patient with Turner syndrome. J Clin Endocrinol Metab 95(4):1487–1495
51. Negreiros LP, Bolina ER, Guimarães MM (2014) Pubertal development profile in patients with Turner syndrome. J Pediatr Endocrinol Metab 27(9–10):845–849
52. Bondy CA (2007) Care of girls and women with Turner syndrome: a guideline of theTurner syndrome Study Group. J Clin Endocrinol Metab 92:10–25
53. Taboada M, Santen R, Lima J et al (2011) Pharmacokinetics and pharmacodynamics of oral and transdermal 17-estradiol in girls with Turner syndrome. J Clin Endocrinol Metab 96(11):3502–3510
54. Mauras N, Torres-Santiago L, Taboada M (2012) Estrogen therapy in Turner syndrome: does the type, dose and mode of delivery matter? Pediatr Endocrinol Rev 9(suppl 2):718–722. Review
55. Strandberg TE, Ylikorkala O, Tikkanen MJ (2003) Differing effects of oral and transdermal hormone replacement therapy on cardiovascular risk factors in healthy postmenopausal women. Am J Cardiol 92:212–214
56. Tremollieres F, Brincat M, Erel CT et al (2011) Managing menopausal women with a personal or family history of VTE. Maturitas 69:195–198
57. L'Hermite M (2013) HRT optimization, using transdermal estradiol plus micronized progesterone, a safer HRT. Climacteric 16(suppl 1):44–53. doi:10.3109/13697137.2013.808563
58. Canonico M, Plu-Bureau G, O'Sullivan MJ et al (2014) Age at menopause, reproductive history, and venous thromboembolism risk among postmenopausal women: the Women's Health Initiative Hormone Therapy Clinical Trials. Menopause 21(3):214–220
59. Langrish JP, Mills NL, Bath LE et al (2009) Cardiovascular effects of physiological and standard sex steroid replacement regimens in premature ovarian failure. Hypertension 53:805–811
60. Jospe N, Orlowski CC, Furlanetto RW (1995) Comparison of transdermal and oral estrogen therapy in girls with Turner's syndrome. J Pediatr Endocrinol Metab 8(2):111–116
61. Isotton AL, Osorio Wender MC, Casagrande A (2012) Effects of oral and transdermal estrogen on IGF1, IGFBP3, IGFBP1, serum lipids, and glucose in patients with hypopituitarism during GH treatment: a randomized study. Eur J Endocrinol 166:207–213
62. Ankarberg-Lindgren C, Elfving M, Wikland KA et al (2001) Nocturnal application of transdermal estradiol patches produces levels of estradiol that mimic those seen at the onset of spontaneous puberty in girls. J Clin Endocrinol Metab 86:3039–3044
63. Ankarberg-Lindgren C, Kriström B, Norjavaara E (2014) Physiological estrogen replacement therapy for puberty induction in girls: a clinical observational study. Horm Res Paediatr 81(4):239–244
64. Davenport ML (2008) Moving toward an understanding of hormone replacement therapy in adolescent girls looking through the lens of Turner syndrome. Ann N Y Acad Sci 1135:126–137
65. Piippo H, Lenko P, Kainulainen P et al (2004) Estradiol gel for induction of puberty in girls with Turner syndrome. J Clin Endocrinol Metab 89(7):3241–3247
66. Rosenfield RL, Fang VS (1974) The effects of prolonged physiologic estradiol therapy on the maturation of hypogonadal teenagers. J Pediatr 85:830–837
67. Rosenfield RL, Perovic N, Devine N et al (1998) Optimizing estrogen replacement treatment in Turner syndrome. Pediatrics 102(2 Pt 3):486–488
68. Rosenfield RL, Devine N, Hunold JJ et al (2005) Salutary effects of combining early very low-dose systemic estradiol with growth hormone therapy in girls with Turner syndrome. J Clin Endocrinol Metab 90(12):6424–6430
69. Weinstein I, Soler-Argilaga C, Wener HV et al (1979) Effects of ethynyloestradiol on the metabolism of [1–14C]oleate by perfused livers and hepatocytes from female rats. Biochem J 180:265–271

70. Ockner RK, Lysenko N, Manning JA et al (1980) Sex steroid modulation of fatty acid utilization and fatty acid binding protein concentration in rat liver. J Clin Invest 65:1013–1023
71. O'Sullivan AJ, Crampton LJ, Freund J et al (1998) The route of estrogen replacement therapy confers divergent effects on substrate oxidation and body composition in postmenopausal women. J Clin Invest 102:1035–1040
72. O'Sullivan AJ, Ho KK (2000) Route-dependent endocrine and metabolic effects of estrogen replacement therapy. J Pediatr Endocrinol Metab 13(Suppl 6):1457–1466
73. Sitruk-Ware R, Nath A (2013) Characteristics and metabolic effects of estrogen and progestins contained in oral contraceptive pills. Best Pract Res Clin Endocrinol Metab 27(1):13–24
74. Kuhl H (2005) Pharmacology of estrogens and progestogens: influence of different routes of administration. Climacteric 8(Suppl 1):3–63
75. Naeraa RW, Gravholt CH, Kastrup KW et al (2001) Morning versus evening administration of estradiol to girls with Turner syndrome receiving growth hormone: impact on growth hormone and metabolism. A randomized placebo-controlled crossover study. Acta Paediatr 90(5):526–531
76. Gravholt CH, Hjerrild BE, Naeraa RW et al (2005) Effect of growth hormone and 17beta-oestradiol treatment on metabolism and body composition in girls with Turner syndrome. Clin Endocrinol (Oxf) 62(5):616–622
77. Bannink EM, van Sassen C, van Buuren S et al (2009) Puberty induction in Turner syndrome: results of oestrogen treatment on development of secondary sexual characteristics, uterine dimensions and serum hormone levels. Clin Endocrinol (Oxf) 70(2):265–273
78. Cleemann L, Hjerrild BE, Lauridsen A et al (2009) Long-term hormone replacement therapy preserves bone mineral density in Turner syndrome. Eur J Endocrinol 161:251–257
79. Cleemann L, Holm K, Fallentin E et al (2011) Uterus and ovaries in girls and young women with Turner syndrome evaluated by ultrasound and magnetic resonance imaging. Clin Endocrinol (Oxf) 74(6):756–761
80. Mauras N, Shulman D, Hsiang HY (2007) Metabolic effects of oral versus transdermal estrogen in growth hormone-treated girls with Turner syndrome. J Clin Endocrinol Metabol 92(11):4154–4160
81. Torres-Santiago L, Mericq V, Taboada M et al (2013) Metabolic effects of oral versus transdermal 17β-estradiol (E_2): a randomized clinical trial in girls with Turner syndrome. J Clin Endocrinol Metab 98(7):2716–2724
82. Quigley CA, Wan X, Garg S et al (2014) Effects of low-dose estrogen replacement during childhood on pubertal development and gonadotropin concentrations in patients with Turner syndrome: results of a randomized, double-blind, placebo-controlled clinical trial. J Clin Endocrinol Metab 99(9):1754–1764
83. Martínez A, Heinrich JJ, Domené H et al (1987) Growth in Turner's syndrome: long term treatment with low dose ethinyl estradiol. J Clin Endocrinol Metab 65(2):253–257
84. Ross JL, Cassorla F, Carpenter G et al (1988) The effect of short term treatment with growth hormone and ethinyl estradiol on lower leg growth rate in girls with Turner's syndrome. J Clin Endocrinol Metab 67(3):515–518
85. Vanderschueren-Lodeweyckx M, Massa G, Maes M et al (1990) Growth-promoting effect of growth hormone and low dose ethinyl estradiol in girls with Turner's syndrome. J Clin Endocrinol Metab 70(1):122–126
86. Mauras N, Rogol AD, Veldhuis JD (1990) Increased hGH production rate after low-dose estrogen therapy in prepubertal girls with Turner's syndrome. Pediatr Res 28(6):626–630
87. Ross JL, Roeltgen D, Feuillan P et al (2000) Use of estrogen in young girls with Turner syndrome: effects on memory. Neurology 54(1):164–170
88. Johnston DI, Betts P, Dunger D et al (2001) A multicentre trial of recombinant growth hormone and low dose oestrogen in Turner syndrome: near final height analysis. Arch Dis Child 84(1):76–81
89. Ross JL, Quigley CA, Cao D et al (2011) Growth hormone plus childhood low-dose estrogen in Turner's syndrome. N Engl J Med 364(13):1230–1242

90. Perry RJ, Gault EJ, Paterson WF et al (2014) Effect of oxandrolone and timing of oral ethinylestradiol initiation on pubertal progression, height velocity and bone maturation in the UK Turner study. Horm Res Paediatr 81(5):298–308
91. Chernausek SD, Attie KM, Cara JF et al (2000) Growth hormone therapy of Turner syndrome: the impact of age of estrogen replacement on final height. (Genentech Inc Collaborative Study Group). J Clin Endocrinol Metab 85(7):2439–2445
92. Nabhan ZM, Di Meglio LA, Qi R (2009) Conjugated oral versus transdermal estrogen replacement in girls with Turner syndrome: a pilot comparative study. J Clin Endocrinol Metab 94(6):2009–2014
93. Mashchak CA, Lobo RA, Dozono-Takano R et al (1982) Comparison of pharmacodynamic properties of various estrogen formulations. Am J Obstet Gynecol 144(5):511–518
94. Seifert-Klauss V, Prior JC (2010) Progesterone and bone: actions promoting bone health in women. J Osteoporos. doi:10.4061/2010/845180
95. Heinz M (2010) Hormonal development therapy (HDT) in hypogonadism in long-term view. Best Practice & Research. Clin Obstet Gynaecol. doi:10.1016/j.bpobgyn.2009.11.013
96. Maxson WS, Hargrove JT (1985) Bioavailability of oral micronized progesterone. Fertil Steril 44:622–626
97. Hargrove JT, Maxson WS, Wentz AC (1989) Absorption of oral progesterone is influenced by vehicle and particle size. Am J Obstet Gynecol 161:948–951
98. Fitzpatrick LA, Good A (1999) Micronized progesterone: clinical indications and comparison with current treatments. Fertil Steril 72(3):389–397
99. Nahoul K, Dehennin L, Scholler R (1987) Radioimmunoassay of plasma progesterone after oral administration of micronized progesterone. J Steroid Biochem 26:241–249
100. Nahoul K, De Ziegler D (1994) "Validity" of serum progesterone levels after oral progesterone. Fertil Steril 61:790–796
101. Simon JA, Robinson DE, Andrews MC et al (1993) The absorption of oral micronized progesterone: the effect of food, dose proportionality, and comparison with intramuscular progesterone. Fertil Steril 60:26–33
102. Tavaniotou A, Smitz J, Bourgain C et al (2000) Comparison between different routes of progesterone administration as luteal phase support in infertility treatments. Hum Reprod Update 6(2):139–148
103. Carp HJ (2015) Progestogens in the threatened miscarriage. In: Carp HJA (ed) Progestogens in obstetrics and gynecology, Chapter 4. Springer International Publishing, Switzerland, pp 53–64
104. Rižner TL, Brožič P, Doucette C et al (2011) Selectivity and potency of the retroprogesterone dydrogesterone in vitro. Steroids 76(6):607–615. doi:10.1016/j.steroids.2011.02.043) (Epub2011Mar3
105. Scholer HF, Reerink EH, Westerhof P (1960) The progestational effect of a new series steroids. Acta Physiol Pharmacol Neerl 9:134–136
106. Stevenson JC, Panay N, Pexman-Fieth C (2013) Oral estradiol and dydrogesterone combination therapy in postmenopausal women: review of efficacy and safety. Maturitas 76(1):10–21
107. Barbosa MW, Silva LR, Navarro PA et al (2015) Dydrogesterone versus progesterone for luteal-phase support: systematic review and meta-analysis of randomized controlled trials. Ultrasound Obstet Gynecol. doi:10.1002/uog.15814
108. Tomic V, Tomic J, Klaic DZ et al (2015) Oral dydrogesterone versus vaginal progesterone gel in the luteal phase support: randomized controlled trial. Eur J Obstet Gynecol Reprod Biol 186:49–53
109. Rosano GM, Vitale C, Silvestri A et al (2003) Metabolic and vascular effect of progestins in post-menopausal women. Implications for cardioprotection. Maturitas 46(Suppl 1):S17–S29
110. Prior JC (2015) Progesterone or progestin as menopausal ovarian hormone therapy: recent physiology-based clinical evidence. Curr Opin Endocrinol Diabetes Obes 22(6):495–501
111. Schindler AE (2015) Pharmacology of progestogens. In: Carp HJA (ed) Progestogens in obstetrics and gynecology, Chapter 2. Springer International Publishing, pp 33–40

112. Poprawski K, Michalski M, Ławniczak M et al (2009) Cardiovascular abnormalities in patients with Turner syndrome according to karyotype. Own experience and literature review. Pol Arch Med Wewn 119(7–8):453–460
113. Mullaney R, Murphy D (2009) Turner syndrome: neuroimaging findings: structural and functional. Dev Disabil Res Rev 15:279–283
114. Calcaterra V, Brambilla P, Maffè GC et al (2014) Metabolic syndrome in Turner syndrome and relation between body composition and clinical, genetic, and ultrasonographic characteristics. Metab Syndr Relat Disord 12(3):159–164
115. Wojcik M, Janus D, Zygmunt-Gorska A (2015) Insulin resistance in adolescents with Turner syndrome is comparable to obese peers, but the overall metabolic risk is lower due to unknown mechanism. J Endocrinol Invest 38(3):345–349
116. Doerr HG, Bettendorf M, Hauffa BP et al (2005) Uterine size in women with Turner syndrome after induction of puberty with estrogens and long-term growth hormone therapy: results of the German IGLU follow-up study (2001). Hum Reprod 20(5):1418–1421
117. Paterson WF, Hollman AS, Donaldson MD (2002) Poor uterine development in Turner syndrome with oral oestrogen therapy. Clin Endocrinol (Oxf) 56(3):359–365
118. Bakalov VK, Shawker Ceniceros I, Bondy CA (2007) Uterine development in Turner syndrome. J Pediatr 151(5):528–531
119. Snajderova M, Mardesic T, Lebl J et al (2003) The uterine length in women with Turner syndrome reflects the postmenarcheal daily estrogen dose. Horm Res 60(4):198–204
120. Kim NY, Lee DY, Kim MJ et al (2012) Estrogen requirements in girls with Turner syndrome; how low is enough for initiating puberty and uterine development? Gynecol Endocrinol 28(2):130–133
121. Ross JL, Long LM, Feuillan P et al (1991) Normal bone density of the wrist and spine and increased wrist fractures in girls with Turner's syndrome. J Clin Endocrinol Metab 73:355–359
122. Davies MC, Gulekli B, Jacobs HS (1995) Osteoporosis in Turner's syndrome and other forms of primary amenorrhea. Clin Endocrinol (Oxf) 43:741–746
123. Landin-Wilhelmsen K (1999) Osteoporosis and fractures in Turner syndrome – importance of growth promoting and oestrogen therapy. Clin Endocrinol (Oxf) 51:497–502
124. Gravholt CH, Vestergaard P, Hermann AP et al (2003) Increased fracture rates in Turner's syndrome: a nationwide questionnaire survey. Clin Endocrinol (Oxf) 59:89–96
125. Han TS, Cadge B, Conway GS (2006) Hearing impairment and low bone mineral density increase the risk of bone fractures in women with Turner's syndrome. Clin Endocrinol (Oxf) 65(5):643–647
126. El-Mansoury M, Barrenäs ML, Bryman I et al (2009) Impaired body balance, fine motor function and hearing in women with Turner syndrome. Clin Endocrinol (Oxf) 71(2):273–278
127. Finby N, Archibald RM (1963) Skeletal abnormalities associated with gonadal dysgenesis. Am J Roentgenol Radium Ther Nucl Med 89:1222–1235
128. Zuckerman-Levin N, Yaniv I, Schwartz T et al (2007) Normal DXA bone mineral density but frail cortical bone in Turner's syndrome. Clin Endocrinol (Oxf) 67(1):60–64. (Epub 2007 Apr 16)
129. Holroyd CR, Davies JH, Taylor P et al (2010) Reduced cortical bone density with normal trabecular bone density in girls with Turner syndrome. Osteoporos Int 21(12):2093–2099
130. Soucek O, Lebl J, Snajderova M et al (2011) Bone geometry and volumetric bone mineral density in girls with Turner syndrome of different pubertal stages. Clin Endocrinol (Oxf) 74(4):445–452
131. Hansen S, Brixen K, Gravholt CH (2012) Compromised trabecular microarchitecture and lower finite element estimates of radius and tibia bone strength in adults with Turner syndrome: a cross-sectional study using high-resolution-pQCT. J Bone Miner Res 27(8):1794–1803
132. Soucek O, Schönau E, Lebl J et al (2015) Artificially low cortical bone mineral density in Turner syndrome is due to the partial volume effect. Osteoporos Int 26(3):1213–1218
133. Nadeem M, Roche EF (2014) Bone mineral density in Turner's syndrome and the influence of pubertal development. Acta Paediatr 103(1):38–42
134. Ross JL, Scott C Jr, Marttila P et al (2001) Phenotypes associated with SHOX deficiency. J Clin Endocrinol Metab 86(12):5674–5680

135. Faienza MF, Brunetti G, Ventura A et al (2015) Mechanisms of enhanced osteoclastogenesis in girls and young women with Turner's syndrome. Bone 81:228–236
136. Peralta López M, Miras M, Silvano L et al (2011) Vitamin D receptor genotypes are associated with bone mass in patients with Turner syndrome. J Pediatr Endocrinol Metab 24(5–6):307–312
137. Stagi S, Iurato C, Lapi E et al (2015) Bone status in genetic syndromes: a review. Hormones (Athens) 14(1):19–31
138. Kodama M, Komura H, Kodama T et al (2012) Estrogen therapy initiated at an early age increases bone mineral density in Turner syndrome patients. Endocr J 59(2):153–159
139. Van der Schouw YT, van der Graaf Y, Steyerberg EW et al (1996) Age at menopause as a risk factor for cardiovascular mortality. Lancet 347(9003):714–718
140. Snowdon DA, Kane RL, Beeson WL et al (1989) Is early natural menopause a biologic marker of health and aging? Am J Public Health 79(6):709–714
141. Jacobsen BK, Nilssen S, Heuch I et al (1997) Does age at natural menopause affect mortality from ischemic heart disease? J Clin Epidemiol 50(4):475–479
142. Jacobsen BK, Heuch I, Kvåle G (2003) Age at natural menopause and all-cause mortality: a 37-year follow-up of 19,731 Norwegian women. J Clin Epidemiol 157(4):923–929
143. Cooper GS, Sandler DP (1998) Age at natural menopause and mortality. Ann Epidemiol 8(4):229–235
144. De Kleijn MJ, van der Schouw YT, Verbeek AL et al (2002) Endogenous estrogen exposure and cardiovascular mortality risk in postmenopausal women. Am J Epidemiol 155(4):339–345
145. Mondul AM, Rodriguez C, Jacobs EJ (2005) Age at natural menopause and cause-specific mortality. Am J Epidemiol 162(11):1089–1097
146. Shuster LT, Rhodes DJ, Gostout BS et al (2010) Premature menopause or early menopause: long-term health consequences. Maturitas 65(2):161–166
147. Rocca WA, Grossardt BR, de Andrade M (2006) Survival patterns after oophorectomy in premenopausal women: a population-based cohort study. Mortality findings from the Mayo Clinic Cohort Study of Oophorectomy and Aging. Lancet Oncol 7:821–828
148. Parker WH, Broder MS, Chang E et al (2009) Ovarian conservation at the time of hysterectomy and long-term health outcomes in the Nurses' Health Study. Obstet Gynecol 113:1027–1037
149. Roeters van Lennep JE, Heida KY, Bots ML et al (2016) Cardiovascular disease risk in women with premature ovarian insufficiency: A systematic review and meta-analysis. Eur J Prev Cardiol 23(2):178–186
150. Tao XY, Zuo AZ, Wang JQ et al (2016) Effect of primary ovarian insufficiency and early natural menopause on mortality: a meta-analysis. Climacteric 19(1):27–36
151. Rocca WA, Bower JH, Maraganore DM et al (2007) Increased risk of cognitive impairment or dementia in women who underwent oophorectomy before menopause. Neurology 69:1074–1083
152. Rocca WA, Bower JH, Maraganore DM et al (2008) Increased risk of Parkinsonism in women who underwent oophorectomy before menopause. Neurology 70:200–209
153. Kalantaridou SN, Nelson LM (2000) Premature ovarian failure is not premature menopause. Ann N Y Acad Sci 900:393–402
154. Kalantaridou SN, Naka KK, Bechlioulis A et al (2006) Premature ovarian failure, endothelial dysfunction and estrogen-progestogen replacement. Trends Endocrinol Metab 17:1–9
155. Moreau KL, Hildreth KL, Meditz AL et al (2012) Endothelial function is impaired across the stages of the menopause transition in healthy women. J Clin Endocrinol Metab 97(12):4692–4700
156. Virdis A, Ghiadoni L, Pinto S et al (2000) Mechanism responsible for endothelial dysfunction associated with acute estrogen deprivation in normotensive women. Circulation 101:2258–2263
157. Rocca WA (2012) Premature menopause or early menopause and risk of ischemic stroke. Menopause 19(3):272–277

158. Roeters van Lennep JE, Heida KY, Bots ML et al (2014) Cardiovascular risk management after reproductive disorders. Cardiovascular disease risk in women with premature ovarian insufficiency: a systematic review and meta-analysis. Eur J Prev Cardiol 23(2):178–186
159. Goldmeier S, De Angelis K, Rabello Casali K et al (2013) Cardiovascular autonomic dysfunction in primary ovarian insufficiency: clinical and experimental evidence. Am J Trans Res 6(1):91–101
160. Levy MJ, Boyne MT, Rogstad S et al (2015) Marketplace analysis of conjugated estrogens: determining the consistently present steroidal content with LC-MS. AAPS J 17(6):1438–1445
161. Leung H, Wang JJ, Rochtchina E et al (2004) Does hormone replacement therapy influence retinal microvascular caliber? Microvasc Res 67:48–54
162. Vrablik M, Fait T, Kovar J et al (2008) Oral but not transdermal estrogen replacement therapy changes the composition of plasma lipoproteins. Metabolism 57:1088–1092
163. Fait T, Vrablik M, Zizka Z et al (2008) Changes in hemostatic variables induced by estrogen replacement therapy: comparison of transdermal and oral administration in a crossover-designed study. Gynecol Obstet Invest 65(1):47–51
164. Roach RE, Lijfering WM, van Hylckama VA (2013) The risk of venous thrombosis in individuals with a history of superficial vein thrombosis and acquired venous thrombotic risk factors. Blood 122:4264–4269
165. Canonico M (2015) Hormone therapy and risk of venous thromboembolism among postmenopausal women. Maturitas 82(3):304–307
166. Committee ACOG (2011) Primary ovarian insufficiency in the adolescent. (Opinion no. 502). Obstet Gynecol 118(3):741–745
167. Simon JA (2012) What's new in hormone replacement therapy: focus on transdermal estradiol and micronized progesterone. Climacteric 15(Suppl 1):3–10
168. Canonico M, Oger E, Plu-Bureau G et al (2007) Hormone therapy and venous thromboembolism among postmenopausal women: impact of the route of estrogen administration and progestogens: the ESTHER study. Circulation 115:840–845
169. Mittal M, Savvas M, Arya R (2013) A randomized controlled trial comparing the effects of micronized progesterone to medroxyprogesterone acetate on cardiovascular health, lipid metabolism and the coagulation cascade in women with premature ovarian insufficiency: study protocol and review of the literature. Menopause Int 19(3):127–132
170. De Caro JJ, Dominguez C, Sherman SL (2008) Reproductive health of adolescent girls who carry the FMR1 premutation: expected phenotype based on current knowledge of fragile X associated primary ovarian insufficiency. Ann N Y Acad Sci 1135:99–111
171. Anasti JN, Kalantaridou SN, Kimzey LM et al (1998) Bone loss in young women with karyotypically normal spontaneous premature ovarian failure. Obstet Gynecol 91:12–15
172. Uygur D, Sengul O, Bayar D et al (2005) Bone loss in young women with premature ovarian failure. Arch Gynecol Obstet 273:17–19
173. Francucci CM, Romagni P, Camilletti A (2008) Effect of natural early menopause on bone mineral density. Maturitas 59(4):323–328
174. Popat VB, Calis KA, Vanderhoof VH et al (2009) Bone mineral density in estrogen deficient young women. J Clin Endocrinol Metab 94(7):2277–2283
175. Amarante F, Vilodre LC, Maturana MA et al (2011) Women with primary ovarian insufficiency have lower bone mineral density. Brazilian J Med Biol Res 44:78–83
176. Crofton PM, Evans N, Bath LE et al (2010) Physiological versus standard sex steroid replacement in young women with premature ovarian failure: effects on bone mass acquisition and turnover. Clin Endocrinol (Oxf) 73:707–714
177. Van der Klift M, de Laet CE, McCloskey EV et al (2004) Risk factors for incident vertebral fractures in men and women: the Rotterdam Study. J Bone Miner Res 19:1172–1180
178. Guttmann H, Weiner Z, Nikolski E et al (2001) Choosing an oestrogen replacement therapy in young adult women with Turner syndrome. Clin Endocrinol (Oxf) 54:159–164
179. O'Donnel P, Warner RJ, Lee J et al (2012) Physiological sex steroid replacement in premature ovarian failure: randomized crossover trial of effect on uterine volume, endometrial

thickness and blood flow, compared with a standard regimen. Hum Reprod 27(4):1130–1138
180. Popat VB, Calis KA, Kalantaridou SN et al (2014) Bone mineral density in young women with primary ovarian insufficiency: results of a three-year randomized controlled trial of physiological transdermal estradiol and testosterone replacement. JCEM 99:3418–3426
181. Gambacciani M, Levancini M (2014) Hormone replacement therapy and the prevention of postmenopausal osteoporosis. Prz Menopauzalny 13(4):213–220
182. National Collaborating Centre for Women's and Children's Health (UK) (2015) Menopause: full guideline. London: National Institute for Health and Care Excellence (UK)
183. Orshan SA, Ventura JL, Covington SN (2009) Women with spontaneous 46, XX primary ovarian insufficiency (hypergonadotropic hypogonadism) have lower perceived social support than control women. Fertil Steril 92(2):688–693
184. Covington SN, Hillard PJ, Sterling EW et al (2011) A family systems approach to primary ovarian insufficiency. J Pediatr Adolesc Gynecol 24(3):137–141
185. Janse F, Tanahatoe SJ, Eijkemans MJ et al (2012) Testosterone concentrations, using different assays, in different types of ovarian insufficiency: a systematic review and meta-analysis. Hum Reprod Update 18(4):405–419
186. Gleicher N, Kim A, Weghofer A et al (2013) Hypoandrogenism in association with diminished functional ovarian reserve. Hum Reprod 28:1084–1091
187. Hartmann BW, Kirchengast S, Albrecht A et al (1997) Androgen serum levels in women with premature ovarian failure compared to fertile and menopausal controls. Gynecol Obstet Invest 44(2):127–131
188. Bennati-Pinto CL, Bedone AJ, Magna LA (2005) Evaluation of serum androgen levels in women with premature ovarian failure. Fertil Steril 83:508–510
189. Ott J, Pecnik P, Promberger R et al (2014) Dehydroepiandrosterone in women with premature ovarian failure and Hashimoto's thyroiditis. Climacteric 17:92–96
190. Van der Stege JG, Groen H, van Zadelhoff SJ et al (2008) Decreased androgen concentrations diminishes general and sexual well-being in women with premature ovarian failure. Menopause 15:23–31
191. Pluchino N, Carmignani A, Cubeddu A (2013) Androgen therapy in women: for whom and when. Arch Gynecol Obstet 288(4):731–737
192. Davies MC, Cartwright B (2012) What is the best management strategy for a 20-year-old woman with premature ovarian failure? Clin Endocrinol (Oxf) 77:182–186
193. Guerrieri GM, Martinez PE, Klug SP et al (2014) Effects of physiologic testosterone therapy on quality of life, self-esteem, and mood in women with primary ovarian insufficiency. Menopause 21(9):952–961
194. Labrie F, Bélanger A, Luu-The V et al (1998) DHEA and the intracrine formation of androgens and estrogens in peripheral target tissues: its role during aging. Steroids 63:322–328
195. Traish AM, Kang P, Saad F et al (1998) DHEA and the intracrine formation of androgens and estrogens in peripheral target tissues: its role during aging. Steroids 63:322–328
196. Traish AM, Kang P, Saad F et al (2011) Dehydroepiandrosterone (DHEAS) – a precursor steroid or an active hormone in human physiology. J Sex Med 8:2960–2982
197. Labrie F, Bélanger A, Luu-The V et al (2011) Dehydroepiandrosterone (DHEAS) – a precursor steroid or an active hormone in human physiology. J Sex Med 8:2960–2982
198. Hill M, Duskovà M, Stàrka L (2015) Dehydroepiandrosterone, its metabolites and ion channels. J Steroid Biochem Mol Biol 145:293–314
199. Pluchino N, Drakopulos P, Bianchi-Demicheli F (2015) Neurobiology of DHEA and effects on sexuality, mood and cognition. J Steroid Biochem Mol Biol 145:273–280
200. Warner M, Gustafsson JA (2015) DHEA- a precursor of ERβ ligands. J Steroid Biochem Mol Biol 145:245–247
201. Lois K, Kassi E, Prokopiou M et al (2000–2014) Adrenal androgens and aging. In: De Groot LJ, Beck-Peccoz P, Chrousos G et al (eds) Endotext [Internet]. MDText.com, Inc., South Dartmouth

202. Vendola K, Zhou J, Wang J et al (1999) Androgens promote insulin-like growth factor-I and insulin-like growth factor-I receptor gene expression in the primate ovary. Hum Reprod 14(9):2328–2332
203. Narkwichean A, Maalouf W, Campbell BK et al (2013) Efficacy of dehydroepiandrosterone to improve ovarian response in women with diminished ovarian reserve: a meta-analysis. Reprod Biol Endocrinol 11:44. doi:10.1186/1477-7827-11-44
204. Nagels HE, Rishworth JR, Siristatidis CS et al (2015) Androgens (dehydroepiandrosterone or testosterone) for women undergoing assisted reproducion (Review). Cochrane Database Syst Rev 11, CD009749
205. Wierman ME, Arlt W, Basson R et al (2014) Androgen therapy in women: a reappraisal: an Endocrine Society clinical practice guideline. J Clin Endocrinol Metab 99:3489–3510
206. Qin JC, Fan L, Qin AP (2016) The effect of dehydroepiandrosterone (DHEA) supplementation on women with diminished ovarian reserve (DOR) in IVF cycle: evidence from a meta-analysis. J Gynecol Obstet Biol Reprod (Paris). doi:10.1016/j.jgyn.2016.01.002
207. Zhang M, Niu W, Wang Y et al (2016) Dehydroepiandrosterone treatment in women with poor ovarian response undergoing IVF or ICSI: a systematic review and meta-analysis. J Assist Reprod Genet. (Epub ahead of print)
208. Faubion SS, Kuhle CL, Shuster LT, Rocca WA (2015) Long-term health consequences of premature or early menopause and considerations for management. Climacteric 18(4):483–491. doi:10.3109/13697137.2015.1020484. Epub 2015 Apr 7. Review
209. Nakamura T, Tsuburai T, Tokinaga A, Nakajima I, Kitayama R, Imai Y, Nagata T, Yoshida H, Hirahara F, Sakakibara H (2015) Efficacy of estrogen replacement therapy (ERT) on uterine growth and acquisition of bone mass in patients with Turner syndrome. Endocr J 62(11): 965–970

Functional Hypothalamic Amenorrhea as Stress Induced Defensive System

8

Alessandro D. Genazzani, Giulia Despini, Riccardo Bonacini, and Alessia Prati

8.1 Introduction

Usually amenorrhea defines the absence or abnormal cessation of the menstrual cyclicity [1], and it is defined as primary or secondary amenorrhea depending from the occurrence of amenorrhea before or after menarche, respectively. Most of the causes of primary and secondary amenorrhea are similar. Timing of the evaluation of primary amenorrhea recognizes the trend to earlier age at menarche and is therefore indicated when there has been a failure to menstruate by age 15 in the presence of normal secondary sexual development (two standard deviations above the mean of 13 years), or within 5 years after breast development if that occurs before age 10 [2].

Failure to initiate breast development by age 13 (two standard deviations above the mean of 10 years) also requires investigation [2]. In women with regular menstrual cycles, a delay of menses for as little as 1 week may require the exclusion of pregnancy; secondary amenorrhea lasting 3 months, and oligomenorrhea involving less than 9 cycles a year require investigation.

The prevalence of amenorrhea not due to pregnancy, lactation, or menopause is approximately 3–4 % [3, 4]. Although the list of potential causes of amenorrhea is long, the majority of cases can be restricted to four conditions: polycystic ovary syndrome, hypothalamic amenorrhea, hyperprolactinemia, and ovarian failure. Other causes can involve diseases that are typical for internal medicine or endocrinologycal diseases such as diabetes, adrenal gland or thyroid diseases and where amenorrhea is not really related to a typical reproductive problem but is related to an unbalanced endocrine control of organs or systems that can induce an abnormal control of the hypothalamus-pituitary-ovarian axis.

A.D. Genazzani (✉) • G. Despini • R. Bonacini • A. Prati
Center for Gynecological Endocrinology, Department of Obstetrics and Gynecology, University of Modena and Reggio Emilia, Modena, Italy
e-mail: algen@unimore.it

C. Sultan, A.R. Genazzani (eds.), *Frontiers in Gynecological Endocrinology*, ISGE Series, DOI 10.1007/978-3-319-41433-1_8

Primary amenorrhea is not so common, in our Centre for Gynecological Endocrinology only 8–10 patients per annum are diagnosed a primary amenorrhea, while higher number of patients is diagnosed with secondary amenorrhea [5–7]. The World Health Organization (WHO) has logically recognized specific groups of amenorrheic patients: WHO group I: no evidence of endogenous estrogen production, normal or low FSH (Follicle Stimulating Hormone) levels, normal prolactin levels, and no evidence of a lesion in the hypothalamic-pituitary region; WHO group II: evidence of estrogen production and normal levels of prolactin and FSH; WHO group III: elevated serum FSH levels indicating gonadal failure [8, 9].

Whatever are the causes, the patients affected by functional hypothalamic amenorrhea (FHA) belong to the WHO group II, that is, they show evidence of low estrogen production, FSH secretion and PRL levels normal or within the upper limit of normality.

8.2 Functional Hypothalamic Amenorrhea (FHA)

Though functional hypothalamic amenorrhea (FHA) is classified in the WHO group I, it is considered as a hypogonadotropic hypogonadism related to a severe change of the pulsatile release of gonadotropin-releasing hormone (GnRH) from the hypothalamus [10–12]. The disturbances of the hypothalamic-pituitary-ovarian axis in FHA may be very broad and includes from low to the complete absence of LH pulses in presence of normal level of FSH [12]. Because of this, there are low or very low estradiol plasma levels due to a reduced estradiol production in the ovary. The disturbed hypothalamic-pituitary-ovarian axis in FHA cases is associated typically with stress, weight loss, and/or excessive physical exercise and is one of the most common causes of secondary amenorrhea [12]. Depending on the triggering factor, there are three typologies of FHA: weight loss related, stress related, and exercise related [13]. However, it is relevant to state that though the trigger might be one of these three, usually all of them result to be tightly interconnected and regardless of the specific trigger, a complex state of hypoestrogenism, other endocrinologycal aberrations, and metabolic abnormalities due to FHA may affect the whole body homeostasis [14].

8.3 Epidemiology and Diagnosis

Classically, secondary amenorrhea is defined when there is at least an interval of 3 months of absence of menstruation, and usually occurs in approximately 3–5 % of women after menarche. FHA can be recognized in 20–35 % of secondary amenorrhea cases and in 3 % of FHA cases of primary amenorrhea that is in those cases where menarche does not occur at the right time but later than expected and no other cause is recognized as causal factor for such situation of delayed menarche [15]. Hypothalamic amenorrhea is very frequent among athlete women. In fact, it has been estimated [16] that approximately 50 % of women who exercise regularly experience menstrual disorders and approximately 30 % of them experience amenorrhea. Several of them show the triad of distorted eating, amenorrhea, and osteoporosis, first described in 1997 and is known as female athlete triad [17].

Functional hypothalamic amenorrhea can be differentiated from the other forms of primary or secondary amenorrhea on the basis of the anamnesis as well as from the assessment of low or very low gonadotropins and estradiol plasma levels [12]. In patients with FHA, the GnRH stimulation test shows the LH and FSH response, thus distinguishing FHA from pituitary diseases, where hypogonadism is also characteristic [13, 15]. Once the hypothalamic origin has been found, it is important to exclude eventual rare genetic and organic diseases such as Kallman syndrome (characterized by anosmia, specific mutations), Prader-Willi syndrome (with characteristic hyperorexia, obesity, retardation), and other rare syndromes with idiopathic hypogonadotropic hypogonadism [12, 15, 18]. Obviously, features such as delayed puberty, primary amenorrhea, and the presence of additional symptoms (anosmia, mental retardation, extreme obesity, facial dysmorphia, and malabsorption) are suggestive of congenital diseases [15, 18].

8.4 Neuroendocrine Dysfunctions of FHA

As it can be argued from what is reported in the previous section, FHA [19–21] is a model of reproductive dysfunction characterized by the fact that there is no organic disease to trigger it. Indeed, FHA is classically characterized by a hypoestrogenic condition as a result of several neuroendocrine aberrations, which occur after a relatively long period of exposure to a repetitive and/or chronic stressor(s) that negatively affect the neuroendocrine hypothalamic activity [10, 22] as well as the release of several hypophyseal hormones [23]. In these patients, the reproductive axis is severely impaired and both the opioid and dopaminergic systems are involved as potential mediators of stress-related amenorrhea in humans [24, 25]. As demonstrated in experimental animals, the EOPs exert an inhibitory effect on the episodic release of both GnRH and LH also in humans [26]. Naloxone infusion is able to induce the increase of LH plasma levels only during the late follicular and luteal phases of the menstrual cycle but not during the early follicular phase [27, 28], and such response was recorded also in postmenopausal women only after hormonal replacement therapy [29]. All these reports sustain the fact that estrogens modulate the opioidergic blockade and when naltrexone cloridrate is administered in FHA, LH plasma levels start to increase within few weeks [30]. In the last two decades, it has been demonstrated that also dopaminergic and serotoninergic pathways are deeply involved in the mechanisms that link stress-induced amenorrhea and reproductive function in FHA [24, 31, 32]. In addition, most of the patients that suffer really for a FHA show an elevation of the cortisol plasma levels close to the upper limits of normality, while in other amenorrheic conditions (i.e., hyperprolactinemic or hyperandrogenic amenorrhea) cortisol shows normal levels [33].

At the basis of the mechanism of stress, there is the perfect combination and overlapping of various independent situations that occur whenever the stressant condition(s) is long lasting or chronic. Psychological, metabolic, and physical stressors are the relevant ones that negatively impact on the brain and on the neurovegetative systems as well as on the neuroendocrine pathways. The central structure for the reproductive control is the hypothalamus where GnRH is synthetized and released. GnRH secretion is under a specific control of various other hypothalamic nuclei that are all around the paraventricular and sopraoptic nuclei where GnRH is secreted. These other nuclei control satiety, glucose, water, and salt levels, and they also receive inputs from the cortex and from other subcortical areas of the brain deeply connected on whatever refers to information coming from the environment in terms of sounds, sights, metabolism, and danger. Practically the hypothalamus is informed on whatever is going on inside and outside the human body. Whatever event changes the perfect equilibrium of all these elements, it results to be able to activate a reaction by the hypothalamus so that to counteract such adverse environmental change and to predispose a defensive condition. Such hypothalamic activation parallel the occurrence of stressant situations, more frequent is the stress, more repetitive activation of the hypothalamic reaction leads to the significant changes that are observed under chronic stressant situations. The block that occurs on the reproductive axis is mainly exerted by the significant reduction of the amount of GnRH secreted by the hypothalamic nuclei (sopraoptic and paraventricular) that reduce the gonadotropin episodic discharge with the concomitant reduction of mean plasma concentrations of LH, FSH, and of ovarian steroids.

8.5 Stress as Defensive System

From what is described above, it appears evident that hypothalamus acts as a "computer" that takes care of all inputs and defines specific outputs to monitor/modulate/regulate a lot of other biological functions such as sleep, glucose control, heart function, feeding, reproduction, and many others. This happens also in males, but it is incredibly active and sensitive in females. Nowadays, weight control, physical activity, and a healthy choice of our food are primary elements of our everyday life. These are relevant issues since our western civilization is becoming even more overweight up to obese! Indeed, at least in Italy, progression of obesity has been up to 25 % in 25 years and the higher occurrence of obese-related diseases, such as diabetes, hypertension, stroke, has stimulated a part of the population to keep weight and feeding under control. Within this last decade, a higher amount of women started to exercise more than 20 years ago and a certain percentage of them realized that they could move from simple physical activity to a more serious training. It is clear that physical activity is absolutely a healthy element in our everyday life, but the excess of training can frequently occur and this can induce negative effects of the reproductive ability of young girls as well of adult women [34]. These negative effects have been identified in a lower fertility rate due to a higher anovulatory condition. Moreover, it is relevant to note that the pregnancy rate of patients that attend IVF programs are incredibly lower for those women that train too much or have an agonistic training [35–37] and that the more is the training the higher is the infertility risk (3.2 fold than controls) [37].

Abnormal or irregular menstrual cyclicity is always possible and it is considered normal to have an irregular event per year but those that train or perform an intense physical activity usually experience such irregular cycles more frequently and it has been demonstrated to be correlated to the reduced BMI [38]. The causal factors of this are clear: the beginning of the follicular phase is slowed by the physically induced stress on the hypothalamic areas, these triggers a difficulty in gaining an optimal ovulation so that the following luteal phase results to be insufficient in terms of progesterone released. All this induces an abnormal menstrual cycle in terms of length and/or frequency. Such mechanism can replicate frequently (one cycle after the other) or rarely, but in case the physical stress is furthermore enriched by psychological factors (i.e., working or familiar problems, school failure, etc.); it might evolve to a menstrual cycle blockade. It is important to observe that in such conditions, even though a pregnancy starts, there are higher chances that it stops prematurely within the first 2–4 weeks. The reason of this relies on the fact that a lower estrogen secretion and later a reduced progesterone secretion do not prepare adequately the endometrial tissue to the embryo implantation. An inadequate endometrial tissue that is too thin (below 8–9 mm) is frequently unable to support the embryo implantation.

It is important to consider that physical activity is a positive activity but while it is important to reduce weight in overweight or obese women, for other women, usually with normal BMI, it represents a sort of "running away" from life problems and everyday life. If this is the case, stress of physical activity becomes a sort of "drug" that initially cures the stress cumulated, but after some time it becomes an additional stress on the stressant situations that are still pressing those women. For some time, biology tries to face the adverse conditions (everyday life and physical activity), but if the training becomes too much (i.e., too much hours of sport/gym every week), the neuroendocrine blockade is quite certain.

Not all these events are a real disease, they all belong to a sort of biological attempt to protect those women. Something dated back more or less 30 thousand years ago. For that time, reproduction was probably the less important function since a human being (or a primate) could perfectly survive without reproduction, and the survival of the single human being could not be guaranteed if reproduction hits its goal (i.e., the occurrence of a pregnancy) especially during seasons/periods during which no food was available or a strenuous energy consumption was ongoing (migration), as well as psychological stressors (fear to die). For those times, a pregnancy in the wrong moment might mean an incredibly higher risk to die. To avoid this and to avoid losing that single human being, the hypothalamus developed the ability to block the reproductive axis in reversible way to avoid ovarian function (i.e., ovulation), with the chance to restart it only when the external conditions might be improved and more adequate.

Life in this twenty-first century is not like that many thousand years ago, but there are always many stressful events that can trigger our hypothalamus and homeostatic system(s) and induce a blockade of reproduction. Although this has to be considered an incredibly well designed defensive system, unfortunately, it might be activated in peculiar period such as during pubertal development, inducing a delayed menarche/puberty. Indeed, when intensive sport training or recreational activity is started at a prepubertal age, it is not so rare to observe a significant delay in the occurrence of pubertal maturation up to 2–4 years [3, 38]. The meaning of this observation is obvious since it indicates that if energy consumption and physical stressors are too much, growth and reproductive axis maturation might not occur in the same time. In fact, most of the girls who suffer from this condition recover into normal development and/or menstrual cyclicity as soon as training is significantly reduced or suspended.

The presence of the right amount of fat is fundamental for pubertal development since it is considered as a specific and obliged reserve of energy that the body might need to have stored in case a pregnancy occurs within the very first ovarian cycles [38, 39]. Nowadays, this reserve of fat is important just for the beginning of the menstrual cyclicity (i.e., menarche) since pregnancy during pubertal age is not so common in Western countries (more frequent in underdeveloped countries), but it is important to consider this biological aspect every time we study a girl who wants to start or has just started any kind of physical activity. Physical activity has not to be strenuous or stressful to avoid any conflict with the maturation/activation of her reproductive axis. A delay in such event might induce reduced bone mass peak, osteopenia, and then reduced bone mass density during fertile life, exposing the girl to damages of the skeleton and of the muscle activity. Hypoestrogenism during adolescence, with no menarche and/or menstrual cyclicity and with a sub-normal development of sex-steroid-dependent tissues (fat distribution, breast development), might be responsible also for an abnormal or conflicting self-image.

What has to be pointed out is that our biology is for sure a perfect system that controls our homeostasis, but we are always forgetting that nowadays, this biology is still working as 30 thousand years ago. Since in those times food was scarce, our biology developed systems/pathways that permitted a fast and optimal way to store the energetic elements derived from food (i.e., glucose, lipids) and a not so fast system to download energetic substances once stored (i.e., lipids from fat cells). Doing so our biology was sure to accumulate at least a minimum of the energy introduced as food, putting the basis of the fact that in the presence of relevant amount of food (as in our times), our homeostatic system would have stored the great part of that energy as fat, inducing overweight up to obesity. It is well clear that we all have to take care of the right amount and quality of food. Even though today we can access to whatever kind of food, we always have to keep feeding under control. That is why the amount of overweight/obese people is a growing social problem and a health issue in all Western countries.

The right amount of food is crucial, not too much and not too low. Quality is essential since it permits a good maintenance and better performances of whatever organ/homeostatic system of our biology. Excess in restriction or excess in feeding induces only abnormal behavior(s) of our homeostatic systems, that in general create the predisposition to reproductive and health concerns.

References

1. Thomas Lathrop S (2000) Stedman's medical dictionary, 27th edn. Lippincott Williams & Wilkins, Philadelphia, p 56
2. Herman-Giddens ME, Slora EJ, Wasserman RC, Bourdony CJ, Bhapkar MV, Koch GG et al (1997) Secondary sexual characteristics and menses in young girls seen in office practice: a study from the Pediatric Research in Office Settings network. Pediatrics 99:505–512
3. Pettersson F, Fries H, Nillius SJ (1973) Epidemiology of secondary amenorrhea. I. Incidence and prevalence rates. Am J Obstet Gynecol 117:80–86
4. Bachmann G, Kemmann E (1982) Prevalence of oligomenorrhea and amenorrhea in a college population. Am J Obstet Gynecol 144:98–102
5. Reindollar RM, Byrd JR, McDonough PG (1981) Delayed sexual development: a study of 252 patients. Am J Obstet Gynecol 140:371–380
6. Reindollar RH, Novak M, Tho SP, McDonough PG (1986) Adult-onset amenorrhea: a study of 262 patients. Am J Obstet Gynecol 155:531–543
7. Mashchak CA, Kletzky OA, Davajan V, Mishell DR (1981) Clinical and laboratory evaluation of patients with primary amenorrhea. Obstet Gynecol 57:715–721
8. Insler V (1988) Gonadotophin therapy: new trends and insights. Int J Fertil 33:85–97
9. Doody KM, Carr BR (1990) Amenorrhea. Obstet Gynecol Clin North Am 17:361–387
10. Berga SL, Mortola JF, Girton L, Suh B, Laughlin G, Pham P, Yen SS (1989) Neuroendocrine aberrations in women with functional hypothalamic amenorrhea. J Clin Endocrinol Metab 68:301–308
11. Gordon MC (2010) Functional hypothalamic amenorhea. N Engl J Med 363:365–371
12. Genazzani AD (2005) Neuroendocrine aspects of amenorrhea related to stress. Pediatr Endocrinol Rev 2:661–668
13. Meczekalski B, Podfigurna-Stopa A, Warenik-Szymankiewicz A, Genazzani AR (2008) Functional hypothalamic amenorrhea: current view on neuroendocrine aberrations. Gynecol Endocrinol 24:4–11
14. Harlow SD (2000) Menstruation and menstrual disorders : the epidemiology of menstruation and menstrual dysfunction. In: Goldman MB, Katch M (eds) Women and health. Academic, San Diego, pp 99–113
15. Practice Committee of the American Society for Reproductive Medicine (2006) Current evaluation of amenorrhea. Fertil Steril 86:S148
16. De Souza MJ et al (2009) High prevalence of subtle and severe menstrual disturbances in exercising women: confirmation using daily hormone measures. Hum Reprod 25:491–503
17. Otis CL et al (1997) American college of sports medicine position stand. The female athlete triad. Med Sci Sports Exerc 29:1–9
18. Valdes-Socin H, Rubio Almanza M, Tomé Fernández-Ladreda M, Debray FG, Bours V, Beckers A (2014) Reproduction, smell, and neurodevelopmental disorders: genetic defects in different hypogonadotropic hypogonadal syndromes. Front Endocrinol (Lausanne) 5:109
19. Cannavò S, Curtò L, Trimarchi F (2001) Exercise-related female reproductive dysfunction. J Endocrinol Invest 24:823–832
20. American Psychiatric Association (1995) Diagnostic and statistical manual of mental disorders, 4th edn. American Psychiatric Association, Washington, DC
21. Genazzani AD, Petraglia F, Fabbri G, Monzani A, Montanini V, Genazzani AR (1990) evidence of luteinizing hormone secretion in hypothalamic amenorrhea associated with weight loss. Fertil Steril 54:222–226
22. Vigersky RA, Andersen AE, Thompson RH, Lauriaux DL (1977) Hypothalamic dysfunction in secondary amenorrhea associated with simple weight loss. N Engl J Med 297:1141–1146
23. Genazzani AD, Gastaldi M, Volpe A, Petraglia F, Genazzani AR (1995) Spontaneous episoidc release of adenohypophyseal hormones in hypothalamic amenorrhea. Gynecol Endocrinol 9:325–334

24. Quigley ME, Sheehan KL, Casper RF, Yen SSC (1980) Evidence for increased dopaminergic and opioid activity in patients with hypothalamic hypogonadotropic amenorrhea. J Clin Endocrinol Metab 50:949–954
25. Petraglia F, Panerai AE, Rivier C, Cocchi D, Genazzani AR (1988) Opioid control of gonadotropin secretion. In: Genazzani AR, Montemagno U, Nappi C, Petraglia F (eds) Brain and female reproductive function. The Parthenon Publishing Group, Carnforth, pp 65–72
26. Petraglia F, D'Ambrogio G, Comitini G, Facchinetti F, Volpe A, Genazzani AR (1985) Impairment of opioid control of luteinizing hormone secretion in menstrual disorders. Fertil Steril 43:535–540
27. Quigley ME, Yen SSC (1980) The role of endogenous opiates on LH secretion during the menstrual cycle. J Clin Endocrinol Metab 51:179–181
28. Snowden UE, Khan-Dawood SF, Dawood MY (1984) The effect of naloxone on endogenous opioid regulation of pituitary gonadotropins and prolactin during the menstrual cycle. J Clin Endocrinol Metab 59:292–296
29. Remorgida V, Venturini PL, Anserini P, Salerno E, De Cecco L (1990) Naltrexone in functional hypothalamic amenorrhea and in the normal luteal phase. Obstet Gynecol 76:1115–1120
30. Genazzani AD, Gastaldi M, Petraglia F, Battaglia C, Surico N, Volpe A, Genazzani AR (1995) Naltrexone administration modulates the neuroendocrine control of luteinizing hormone secretion in hypothalamic amenorrhea. Hum Reprod 10:2868–2871
31. Yen SSC (1984) Opiates and reproduction: studies in women. In: Delitala G (ed) Opioid modulation of endocrine function. Raven, New York, pp 191–199
32. Kalra SP, Kalra PS (1984) Neural regulation of luteinizing hormone secretion in the rat. Endocr Rev 4:311–351
33. Genazzani AD, Chierchia E, Santagni S, Rattighieri E, Farinetti A, Lanzoni C (2010) Hypothalamic amenorrhea: from diagnosis to therapeutical approach. Ann Endocrinol 71:163–169
34. Olive DL (2010) Exercise and fertility: an update. Curr Opin Obstet Gynecol 22:259–263
35. Chavarro JE, Rich-Edwards JW, Rosner BA, Willett WC (2007) Diet and lifestyle in the prevention of ovulatory disorder infertility. Obstet Gynecol 110:1050–1058
36. Morris SN, Misssmer SA, Cramer DW et al (2006) Effects of lifetime exercise on the outcome of in vitro fertilization. Obstet Gynecol 108:938–945
37. Gudmundsdottir SL, Flanders WD, Augestad LB (2009) Physical activity and fertility in women: the North-Trondelag health study. Hum Reprod 24:3196–3204
38. Loucks AB (2001) Physical health of the female athlete: observations, effects, and causes of reproductive disorders. Can J Appl Physiol 26(Suppl):S179–S185
39. Fourman LT, Fazeli PK (2015) Neuroendocrine causes of amenorrhea – an update. J Clin Endocrinol Metab 100:812–824

9 Amenorrhoea and Anorexia Nervosa in Adolescent Girls

Sebastien Guillaume, Laurent Maimoun, Charles Sultan, and Patrick Lefebvre

Anorexia nervosa (AN) is characterized by an intense fear of becoming fat despite an obvious thinness and extreme behaviours for weight loss, such as food restriction with or without self-induced vomiting or use of laxatives. The result is a massive weight loss and pathological thinness. The 12-month prevalence of AN among young females is approximately 0.4 %. The presence of AN dramatically affects quality of life both of people with AN and their relatives, and people with eating disorders have particularly high utilization rate of health services [29]. AN is a multifactorial disorder currently conceptualized with biopsychosocial model. There is a strong genetic component, since the heritability is about 60 %. These genetic factors are likely to predispose to vulnerability via endophenotype such as perfectionist traits, lack of cognitive flexibility, facilitating the secretion of opioids during fasting, etc. [23, 29]. These factors will be expressed in a specific environmental context and will lead to emergence of disorders, adolescence being a period of particular vulnerability. The main environmental factors favouring the emergence of disorders include idealization of thinness and performance of our western societies, a focused education on the ideal of thinness or food rigidity and the presence of trauma including early trauma. Management of AN is difficult and few treatments have shown efficacy. Cares are usually multidisciplinary and aims to restore normal weight, a suitable and relaxed behaviour with food, improve social and interpersonal relationships, as well as self-perception of patients. Despite these supports, approximately 30 % of patients will not curc from thcir discasc. This crcatcs an cxccss mortality in AN. Mortality increases over time, and is estimated to be 5 % per decade of illness [25]. Thus, AN is the psychiatric disorder with the highest mortality rates. From people who will cure, the recover process will take several months to years. In this short review we will discuss three points: what are the features of amenorrhoea in AN, why amenorrhoea has been removed as a criteria of AN and the therapeutics issues of amenorrhoea in AN.

S. Guillaume (✉) • L. Maimoun • C. Sultan • P. Lefebvre
Lapeyronie Hospital, CHRU Montpellier, and University of Montpellier, Montpellier, France
e-mail: s-guillaume@chu-montpellier.fr

C. Sultan, A.R. Genazzani (eds.), *Frontiers in Gynecological Endocrinology*, ISGE Series, DOI 10.1007/978-3-319-41433-1_9

9.1 Features of Amenorrhoea in AN

Amenorrhoea in AN is related to a functional hypothalamic disorder (FHA) which is a condition characterized by the absence of menses due to the suppression of the hypothalamic-pituitary-ovarian axis, in which no anatomical or organic disease is identified. The decreased pulses of gonadotropins and the lack of LH surges lead to the absence of follicular development, anovulation and low estradiol levels. Variable neuroendocrine patterns of LH secretion can be seen [9, 24] including a lower mean frequency of LH pulses, the complete absence of LH pulsatility, as well as a normal-appearing secretion pattern and higher mean frequency of LH pulses. Serum concentrations of FSH often exceed those of LH, similar to the pattern in prepubertal girls in the early stage and as the disease is more advanced both are very low. The wide spectrum of hypothalamic-pituitary disturbances may reflect different stages of the disease and/or genetic susceptibility. In patients with anorexia nervosa, secretion of gonadotropin releasing hormone (GnRH) is also reduced which leads to anovulation and causes a functional hypothalamic amenorrhoea. Several factors are involved in the GnRH dysfunction in AN who share a lot of common characteristics of women with FHA without AN criteria (Table 9.1). The disturbed hypothalamic-pituitary-ovarian axis in FHA cases is usually associated typically with weight loss, stress and/or excessive physical exercise and is one of the most common causes of secondary amenorrhoea. According to the eliciting factor, there are three classes of FHA: weight loss related, stress related and exercise related. The precise mechanisms underlying the pathophysiology of FHA are complex and unclear. Attention should be paid to such substances as kisspeptin, neuropeptide Y (NPY), ghrelin, leptin, corticotropin-releasing hormone (CRH), β-endorphin and allopregnanolone. An energy deficit (which can occur independently of body weight) appears to be the critical factor in both weight-loss and exercise-induced forms of hypothalamic amenorrhoea.

Some of the behavioural features of AN have a direct impact on amenorrhoea:

- Weight loss of between 10 and 15 % of normal weight disrupts the menstrual cycle in most women [15]. The value of oestrogen is reduced according to BMI and in patients where the BMI are lower to 15 kg/m^2, plasma estradiol was not

Table 9.1 Common characteristics in FHA and AN

Characteristics	Functional Hypothalamic Amenorrhoea (FHA)	Anorexia nervosa (AN)
Body weight	Normal or low	Very low to normal
Body fat	Normal or low	Very low to normal
Intake of calories or fat	Normal or low	Low
Strenuous exercise	Frequent	Hyperactivity
Eating disorders	Variable	Restriction
Leptin	Low	Very low to normal
Emotional stress	Variable	Variable

detected [13]. However, amenorrhoea may precede weight loss in up to 20% of women with AN. Although a minority of women with AN maintains some menstrual activity even at significantly low weights, this should not falsely reassure clinicians or patients that weight restoration is not necessary. Weight gain usually restores normal menstrual cycles. The time course and amount of weight required for resumption of menses has varied among different studies but a goal of attaining 90% of ideal body weight in order to restore normal menses is often described or the weight at which menstruation ceased [26]. Nevertheless, amenorrhoea persists in about 10–30% of patients with AN despite weight gain, because of ongoing abnormal eating behaviours (binge eating and purging), exercise, or stress.

- Nutritional deficiencies that are not associated with weight loss or hyperactivity may lead also to FHA [5]. In contrast to their menstruating counterparts, the women with amenorrhoea severely restricted their fat consumption and had lower body fat mass.
- Patients with AN experiment high levels of stress. Increased CRH secretion results in an increased secretion of adrenocorticotrophin from the pituitary and cortisol from the adrenal glands, and these phenomena are linked to a reduced GnRH drive. Elevated serum and also cerebrospinal cortisol concentrations have been reported in FHA [27]. For patients distressed by persistent amenorrhoea, eventual recovery of menstrual periods may occur following psychotherapy [3].

This amenorrhoea has some important consequence on the prognosis of AN. Patients suffering from AN exhibit impaired bone remodelling, which is characterized by a decrease in bone formation and a concomitant increase in bone resorption [19–21]. Oestrogen plays a crucial role on bone mass acquisition and on its maintenance. The effects of oestrogen on bone metabolism have been described as inhibitory for the resorption process, although direct effects on osteoblastic activity have been also described, resulting a reduction of bone turnover [2]. The demonstrated effects of oestrogen on bone metabolism associated with very low values had highly oriented clinicians to claim that the oestrogen deficiency is the major cause of bone loss in AN patients. However, osteopenia is much more severe in AN patients compared to other amenorrhoeic-deficient populations [11]. This suggested that osteopenia/osteoporosis genesis in AN is multifactorial and that other endocrine factors such as IGF-1, cortisol or sclcrostin acting on thc alteration of the bone cell activity [19–21]. By the way, amenorrhoea has clinical utility because it alerts clinicians to potential deficits in bone mineral density (BMD).

Amenorrhoea and level of oestrogen might also impact the phenotype of anorexia also at a psychological level. Behavioural abnormalities as well as depression and anxiety driven by underlying cognitive processes are a prominent feature of AN and suggested directions for developing innovative therapeutic programmes. Oestrogens, acting through oestrogens receptor-β, is anxiolytic in animals [18] and levels of anxiety change across the estrus cycle. Oestrogen may also be involved with perception of body shape, and may account for greater body shape concerns in females than males [22]. Finally, a study suggests that AN people who were in amenorrhoea or had irregular menses showed significant cognitive deficits across a broad range of many cognitive domains [6].

All this aspects suggest than amenorrhoea is a critical issue in AN. Nevertheless, question of this utility as a marker of AN is controversial.

9.2 Amenorrhoea a Criteria of AN ?

Until the last revision, one of necessary criteria for the diagnosis of AN was amenorrhoea. The fourth edition of the *Diagnostic and Statistical Manual of Mental Disorder* (DSM-IV) specifies the diagnostic criterion for amenorrhoea in AN as "the absence of at least three consecutive menstrual cycles (a woman is considered to have amenorrhoea if her periods occur only following hormone)". In the updated edition fifth edition (DSM-5) as well as in the upcoming International classification of disease (ICD-11), amenorrhoea has been removed from diagnostic criteria for AN. Several arguments have been advanced for this removal. The first is the lack of specificity of amenorrhoea regarding AN. Indeed, in comparison of groups of patients with AN according to DSM IV criteria and of patients who meet all the criteria with the exception of the amenorrhoea, there are no differences in behavioural phenotype or on any aspects of the psychopathological and neuropsychological functioning between [28]. Moreover, in a latent class analysis amenorrhoea is not linked to AN but distributed in all lower weight classes [4]. We currently do not have markers of anorexia specific enough beings used for diagnostic purposes, but some adipocytokines such as leptin or ghrelin seems to have a higher specificity towards anorexia than amenorrhoea [23]. Another argument is the clinical utility of amenorrhoea as a marker of malnutrition. Amenorrhoea is no more predictive of physical complications and somatic consequences (including bone remodelling) of AN than current BMI and lowest BMI lifetime [1]. On a biological level, the most predictive somatic marker of complications related to under nutrition is the prealbumin [8]. Also, the requirement of amenorrhoea is irrelevant in some subgroups of patients with AN such as women under contraceptive medication, men or menopausal women. Finally, a recurrent critical made to DSM-IV diagnosis was the proportion of patients not responding to a specified disorder (AN, bulimia nervosa). Without amenorrhoea but with all the others features of the disease, AN patients were switched to a category called Eating Disorders Not Otherwise Specified (EDNOS). Up to 60 % of eating disorders were classified in this category [7]. This heterogeneous category initially designed to include residual disorders, was actually a wastebasket class of no interest to identify a clinical description and guide treatment. By relaxing the criteria of AN and bulimia nervosa, and including a new category the binge eating disorders as a separate diagnosis, as well as a number of smaller sub-diagnoses, the DSM-5 aims to reduce numbers of EDNOS. All these arguments therefore logically led to moving amenorrhoea from a mandatory diagnosis criterion to an associated features supporting diagnosis.

9.3 Therapeutics Implications

The weight restoration with a return of menstruation is considered the prerequisite to an improvement of the disease. The global aim of care is to restore normal weight, a suitable and relaxed behaviour with food, improve social and interpersonal relationships, as well as self-perception of patients. Given alterations in gonadal function usually observed in patients suffering from AN, it has been proposed to compensate low oestrogens levels by introduction of substitution therapy. Several studies hypothesised that replacement might be effective in increasing BMD. However, randomized clinical trials using different molecules (Premarin, Provera, ethinyl estradiol, norethindrone) [10, 12, 16] showed no significant benefits on BMD. However, the response to the treatment may depend on various factors. Klibanski et al. [16] reported that patients with the lowest percent ideal body weight had the most significant improvement in spinal BMD during oestrogen administration, suggesting that oestrogen replacement therapy may be beneficial in preventing bone loss in young women with extremely low body weight. It was also probable that the lack of significant BMD gain may be attributed to the dose which is usually too low to have a favourable impact on BMD [17]. A too short duration of prescription as well as a poor compliance might also be in play [14]. Klibanski et al. [16] reported a marked improvement in spinal BMD in patients who spontaneously resumed menses during the study, suggesting that resumption of normal menstrual function has a different effect on bone mass than oestrogen replacement. It was probable that oestrogen treatment alone cannot correct the multiple factors (nutritional or other hormonal variable) contributing to bone loss [16]. From these results, hypoestrogenia may be considered only as a contributing factor to the bone alteration in AN patients, and it may be implicated principally in the reduction of the volumetric BMD, while malnutrition may account for reduced bone size [14]. For a better efficacy, hormonal replacement therapy should be considered soon after diagnosis.

Other studies regarding impact oestrogen in AN are scarce. One study has examined if physiologic oestrogen replacement would ameliorate anxiety and improves eating attitudes [22]. Seventy-two adolescents from 13 to 18 years old were randomized to transdermal estradiol with cyclic progesterone or placebo patches and pills for 18 months. Among the 37 who completed the study, oestrogen replacement improved trait-anxiety (the tendency to experience anxiety), but did not impact eating attitudes or body shape perception. No studies have assessed impact of substitution on cognitive function.

In summary, even if amenorrhoea has been removed from criteria of the disorders, it is an important feature of the disease the clinician has to take into account. The recovery of menstrual function in adolescent patients with AN should be a major treatment goal to prevent severe long-term somatic and psychiatric consequences.

References

1. Attia E, Roberto CA (2009) Should amenorrhea be a diagnostic criterion for anorexia nervosa? Int J Eat Disord 42(7):581–589
2. Audi L, Vargas DM, Gussinye M et al (2002) A clinical and biochemical determinants of bone metabolism and bone mass in adolescent female patients with anorexia nervosa. Pediatr Res 51:497–504

3. Berga SL, Marcus MD, Loucks TL et al (2003) Recovery of ovarian activity in women with functional hypothalamic amenorrhea who were treated with cognitive behavior therapy. Fertil Steril 80:976
4. Bulik CM, Sullivan PF, Kendler KS (2000) An empirical study of the classification of eating disorders. Am J Psychiatry 157(6):886–895
5. Couzinet B, Young J, Brailly S et al (1999) Functional hypothalamic amenorrhoea: a partial and reversible gonadotrophin deficiency of nutritional origin. Clin Endocrinol (Oxf) 50:229
6. Chui HT, Christensen BK et al (2008) Cognitive function and brain structure in females with a history of adolescent-onset anorexia nervosa. Pediatrics 122(2):e426–e437
7. Fairburn CG, Bohn K (2005) Eating disorder NOS (EDNOS): an example of the troublesome "not otherwise specified" (NOS) category in DSM-IV. Behav Res Ther 43(6):691–701
8. Gaudiani JL, Sabel AL, Mehler PS (2014) Low prealbumin is a significant predictor of medical complications in severe anorexia nervosa. Int J Eat Disord 47(2):148–156
9. Genazzani AD (2005) Neuroendocrine aspects of amenorrhearelated to stress. Pediatr Endocrinol Rev 2:661–668
10. Golden NH, Lanzkowsky L et al (2002) The effect of estrogen-progestin treatment on bone mineral density in anorexia nervosa. J Pediatr Adolesc Gynecol 15(3):135–143
11. Grinspoon S, Miller K et al (1999) Severity of osteopenia in estrogen-deficient women with anorexia nervosa and hypothalamic amenorrhea. J Clin Endocrinol Metab 84:2049–2055
12. Grinspoon STL, Miller K, Herzog D, Klibanski A (2002) Effects of recombinant human IGF-I and oral contraceptive administration on bone density in anorexia nervosa. J Clin Endocrinol Metab 87(6):2883–2891
13. Hotta M, Shibasaki T, Sato K, Demura H (1998) The importance of body weight history in the occurrence and recovery of osteoporosis in patients with anorexia nervosa: evaluation by dual X-ray absorptiometry and bone metabolic markers. Eur J Endocrinol 139:276–283
14. Karlsson MK, Weigall SJ, Duan Y, Seeman E (2000) Bone size and volumetric density in women with anorexia nervosa receiving estrogen replacement therapy and in women recovered from anorexia nervosa. J Clin Endocrinol Metab 85:3177–3182
15. Katz MG, Vollenhoven (2000) The reproductive endocrine consequences of anorexia nervosa B BJOG 107(6):707
16. Klibanski ABB, Schoenfeld DA, Herzog DB, Saxe VC (1995) The effects of estrogen administration on trabecular bone loss in young women with anorexia nervosa. J Clin Endocrinol Metab 80(3):898–904
17. Legroux-Gerot I, Vignau J, Collier F, Cortet B (2008) Factors influencing changes in bone mineral density in patients with anorexia nervosa-related osteoporosis: the effect of hormone replacement therapy. Calcif Tissue Int 83:315–323
18. Lund TD, Rovis T, Chung WC, Handa RJ (2005) Novel actions of estrogen receptor-beta on anxiety-related behaviors. Endocrinology 146(2):797–807
19. Maïmoun L, Guillaume S et al (2014) Role of sclerostin and dickkopf-1 in the dramatic alteration in bone mass acquisition in adolescents and young women with recent anorexia nervosa. J Clin Endocrinol Metab 99(4):E582–E590
20. Maimoun L, Guillaume S et al (2016) Is serum serotonin involved in the bone loss of young females with anorexia nervosa? Horm Metab Res 48(3):174–177
21. Maimoun L, Guillaume S et al (2016) Evidence of a link between resting energy expenditure and bone remodelling, glucose homeostasis and adipokine variations in adolescent girls with anorexia nervosa. Osteoporos Int 27(1):135–146
22. Misra M, Katzman DK, Estella NM et al (2013) Impact of physiologic estrogen replacement on anxiety symptoms, body shape perception and eating attitudes in adolescent girls with anorexia nervosa: data from a randomized controlled trial. J Clin Psychiatry 74(8):e765–e771. doi:10.4088/JCP.13m08365

23. Monteleone P, Maj M (2013) Dysfunctions of leptin, ghrelin, BDNF and endocannabinoids in eating disorders: beyond the homeostatic control of food intake. Psychoneuroendocrinology 38(3):312–330
24. Perkins RB, Hall JE, Martin KA (1999) Neuroendocrine abnormalities in hypothalamic amenorrhea: spectrum, stability, and response to neurotransmitter modulation. J Clin Endocrinol Metab 84(6):1905–1911
25. Sullivan PF (1995) Mortality in anorexia nervosa. Am J Psychiatry 152(7):1073–1075
26. Swenne I (2004) Weight requirements for return of menstruations in teenage girls with eating disorders, weight loss and secondary amenorrhoea. Acta Paediatr 93:1449
27. Valdes-Socin H, Rubio Almanza M et al (2014) Reproduction, smell, and neurodevelopmental disorders: genetic defects in different hypogonadotropic hypogonadal syndromes. Front Endocrinol (Lausanne) 5:109
28. Watson TL, Andersen AE (2003) A critical examination of the amenorrhea and weight criteria for diagnosing anorexia nervosa. Acta Psychiatr Scand 108(3):175–182
29. Zipfel S, Giel KE, Bulik CM, Hay P, Schmidt U (2015) Anorexia nervosa: aetiology, assessment, and treatment. Lancet Psychiatry 2(12):1099–111

10 The Long-Term Cardiovascular Risks Associated with Amenorrhea

Tommaso Simoncini, Andrea Giannini, and Andrea R. Genazzani

Amenorrhea is the absence or abnormal cessation of the menses. Primary and secondary amenorrhea describe the occurrence of amenorrhea before and after menarche, respectively. The majority of the causes of primary and secondary amenorrhea are similar. Timing of the evaluation of primary amenorrhea recognizes the trend to earlier age at menarche and is therefore indicated when there has been a failure to menstruate by age 15 in the presence of normal secondary sexual development (two standard deviations above the mean of 13 years), or within 5 years after breast development if that occurs before age 10. Failure to initiate breast development by age 13 (two standard deviations above the mean of 10 years) also requires investigation. In women with regular menstrual cycles, a delay of menses for as little as 1 week may require the exclusion of pregnancy; secondary amenorrhea lasting 3 months and oligomenorrhea involving less than nine cycles a year require investigation. The prevalence of amenorrhea not due to pregnancy, lactation, or menopause is approximately 3–4 %. Although the list of potential causes of amenorrhea is long, the majority of cases are accounted for by four conditions: polycystic ovary syndrome, hypothalamic amenorrhea, hyperprolactinemia, and ovarian failure. Secondary amenorrhea, which is defined as 3 months absence of menstruation, occurs in approximately 3–5 % of adult women [1, 2].

According to the American Society of Reproductive Medicine, Functional Hypothalamic Amenorrhea (FHA) is one of the most common causes of secondary amenorrhea; therefore, it is responsible for 20–35 % of secondary amenorrhea cases and approximately 3 % of cases of primary amenorrhea. There are three types of FHA: weight loss-related, stress-related, and exercise-related amenorrhea therefore, DeSouza et al. estimated that approximately 50 % of women who exercise regularly

T. Simoncini, MD, PhD (✉) • A. Giannini • A. Genazzani
Division of Obstetrics and Gynecology, Department of Experimental and Clinical Medicine, University of Pisa, Via Roma, 67, 56100 Pisa, Italy
e-mail: tommaso.simoncini@med.unipi.it

C. Sultan, A.R. Genazzani (eds.), *Frontiers in Gynecological Endocrinology*, ISGE Series, DOI 10.1007/978-3-319-41433-1_10

experience subtle menstrual disorders and approximately 30 % of women have amenorrhea, for that reason the incidence of FHA is higher in athlete women. The complex of distorted eating, amenorrhea, and osteoporosis was first described in 1997 and is known as female athlete triad. FHA results from the aberrations in pulsatile gonadotropin-releasing hormone (GnRH) secretion, which in turn causes impairment of the gonadotropins (follicle-stimulating hormone and luteinizing hormone). The final consequences of these clinical conditions are complex hormonal changes manifested by profound hypoestrogenism leading to several short and long-term health implications [3].

As it is known, hypoestrogenism can interfere with the cardiovascular system function in many ways, this is the reason why Cardiovascular disease (CVD) is the leading cause of death in women in developed countries and, interestingly, proportionally more women die from CVD than men. Coronary and peripheral vessels contain estrogen receptors that permit estradiol to play a regulatory role in vascular function. Estrogen excites the synthesis of nitric oxide (NO) through both genomic and nongenomic effects, leading to the augmented production of endothelial-derived NO, causing vasodilatation [4]. Estradiol exerts a positive, cardioprotective effect through its influence on the endothelial, myocardial, and vascular function and metabolic parameters [5]. In contrast, hypoestrogenism can lead to endothelial dysfunction, an impaired bioactivity of nitric oxide, perturbation in autonomic function, activation of the rennin–angiotensin system, and lipid profile changes [6]. These physiological and pathological phenomena are reflected in clinical studies. Several investigators have demonstrated a correlation between FHA and endothelial dysfunction. It was clearly shown that the flow-mediated dilation of the brachial artery, which is a precise predictor of coronary endothelial dysfunction, is impaired in women with FHA. It is suggested that the decrease of endothelial NO bioavailability is caused by chronic estrogen deficiency. Moreover, some authors have proved the protective effect of exogenous estrogens in young women against impaired vessels' dilatation. Rickenlund et al. documented significantly increased brachial artery dilatation after 9 months of treatment with low-dose combined contraceptives (30 μg of ethinyl estradiol and 150 μg of levonorgestrel): from 1.42 ± 0.98 % before treatment to 4.88 ± 2.20 % during treatment [7].

A Women's Ischemia Syndrome Evaluation (WISE) study found a significant association between premenopausal angiographic coronary artery disease (CAD) and hypothalamic hypogonadism [8]. O'Donnell et al. recently showed that young athletes with chronic hypoestrogenemia displayed an impaired peripheral vascular function that was combined with lower resting blood pressures and heart rate and reduced ischemic responses to occlusion challenge compared to ovulatory women. Impaired cardiovascular function in hypothalamic amenorrhea is believed to be linked mainly to hypoestrogenism, but it is also aggravated by negative energy balance and metabolic disturbances [9]. Patients with FHA are characterized by an impaired lipid profile and are at risk of glucose metabolism abnormalities. Women with exercise-related amenorrhea present higher serum total cholesterol, LDL cholesterol, apolipoprotein B and triglyceride concentrations than healthy individuals [10]. On the other hand, premenopausal women with hypoestrogenism of hypothalamic origin present an increased frequency of diabetes mellitus. Moreover, Ahmed et al. showed that coronary artery disease (detected in coronarography) has an increased prevalence and extent among women with diabetes and hypothalamic hypoestrogenism in comparison to women with diabetes alone. These observations substantiate the importance of cyclic ovarian function as an indicator of cardiovascular health. However, the influence of hypoestrogenism in young women of hypothalamic origin on cardiovascular health requires further studies. Especially the issue of the long-term consequences of FHA on CVD risk needs to be cleared to possibly minimize the risk of cardiovascular events in this group of women [11].

Despite the large number of studies investigating the effects of menopause on cardiovascular outcomes and endothelial function, currently, little is known about the cardiovascular effects of Premature Ovarian Failure (POF) in young women. Flow mediated vasodilatation (FMD) of the brachial artery is the most common method in the assessment of endothelial function and measures the changes in arterial diameter in response to increased blood flow by stimulating endothelial nitric oxide production. It has been shown previously that endothelial function assessed by FMD is impaired in patients with POF; in particular it has been found that FMD was significantly lower in women with POF. New findings suggested that Circulating Endothelial Progenitor cells (EPC) originate from the bone marrow and play an important role in vascular homeostasis for both repair and regeneration of damaged endothelium. This line of progenitor cells has recently been recommended as a novel biomarker of endothelial function showing a close relationship with FMD. Circulating EPCs may have an important contribution to estrogen-induced cardiac protection but they have not been studied in POF previously. Also decreased EPCs may lead to accelerated vascular remodeling like increased carotid intima media thickness (CIMT) due to chronic impairment of endothelial maintenance [12]. Remarkably, polycystic ovary syndrome (PCOS) patients who have chronic anovulation and hyperandrogenism have been shown to have decreased EPC counts and increased CIMT. In this view, Kalantaridou et al. evaluated endothelial dysfunction in a patient group including 18 patients with POF compared to age-matched premenopausal women investigating the relationship between POF and EPC, endothelial function, carotid intima media thickness (CIMT), and left ventricular diastolic function [13, 14].

This group of research found lower FMD in patients with POF compared to healthy age-matched controls. Furthermore, there was a significant correlation between estradiol and FMD, consistent with previous studies where low levels of estradiol were associated with endothelial dysfunction. The association between EPCs and endothelial function has been evaluated in different previous studies, suggesting that EPCs may play a critical role in maintaining endothelial function in mature blood vessels in addition to mature endothelial cells. In this study, it has been demonstrated for the first time a lower circulating number of EPCs in patients with POF. It has been also found that there is a significant correlation between estradiol level and EPC which may be one of the mechanisms impairing endothelial function. In this view, Kalantaridou and colleagues demonstrated that hormone replacement restored endothelial function within 6 months of treatment among patients with POF.

The same group investigated the endothelium-dependent and -independent vascular function by measuring flow-mediated dilation (FMD) and nitrate-mediated dilation in the brachial artery in patients affected by PCOS. Women with PCOS showed significant endothelial dysfunction at an early age (i.e., early 20s) and largely independent of obesity, but in this study, there were no modifications on the hormonal status of the patients and any therapy was administered. This evidences suggested that women with PCOS are at increased risk for early onset cardiovascular disease and may gain particular benefit from measures to improve endothelial function, as well as women with POF have high risk of premature death from cardiovascular causes, therefore, early recognition or diagnosis may provide clinical significance. However, whether these findings might translate into clinical benefit requires further prospective studies [13, 14].

Many reports associate cardiovascular disease and mortality with age of menopause (within the healthy age range, premature, or following oophorectomy). The relation between late menopause and a reduced cardiovascular disease (CVD) risk is well established. Observational studies have shown a reduced risk of cardiovascular disease, fewer calcifications in the aorta, and less extensive atherosclerosis in women with later menopause, moreover, age at menopause is associated with carotid atherosclerosis as assessed with ultrasonography [15, 16].

Menopausal state has been added to the Framingham risk function for estimating absolute cardiovascular disease risk in women. The postmenopausal use of estradiol seems to reduce progression of CVD although studies about postmenopausal hormone therapy and cardiovascular risk are inconclusive [17]. The risk of cardiovascular mortality was significantly higher for women with natural early compared with late menopause (age-adjusted hazard ratio [HR] 0.98, 95 % CI 0.97–0.99, $p = 0.01$ for every year menopause is delayed) in a cohort of 12,000 postmenopausal women. A meta-analysis showed the association between postmenopausal hormonal status and cardiovascular disease was pronounced for women with an artificial menopause (age-adjusted HR 2.62, 95 % CI 2.05–3.35) following bilateral oophorectomy. Investigators of the same cohort showed that a long overall survival occurred in women with late menopause [18, 19]. A small but significant inverse correlation between age of natural menopause and all-cause mortality was established in both a 37-year follow-up study in almost 20,000 women from Norway and a 20-year follow-up in 68,000 women from the USA [20, 21]. Increased cardiovascular mortality was also noted after bilateral oophorectomy before 45 years of age (HR 1.67, 95 % CI 1.16–2.40, $p = 0.006$) with increased overall mortality in women who did not have estrogen therapy until they were aged 45 years or more (1.84, 1.27–2.68, $p = 0.001$) [22, 23]. A 24-year follow-up of more than 16,000 women who had a hysterectomy with or without bilateral oophorectomy (from a cohort of 30,000 women in the Nurses' Health Study) had the following long-term health outcomes, after adjustment for the use of estrogens: an HR of 1.12 (95 % CI 1.03–1.21) for total mortality, 1.17 (1.02–1.35). for coronary heart disease, 1.26 (1.02–1.56) for lung cancer, and 1.14 (0.98–1.33) for stroke [24]. Knauff and colleagues showed small changes in the lipid profile (e.g., raised triglyceride and marginally lowered HDL cholesterol concentrations) in women presenting with ovarian insufficiency [25]. Some data show a cardioprotective effect of estrogen treatment. Steroid replacement results in increased carotid pulsatility index, decreased blood pressure, improved renal function, and lowered activation of the renin-angiotensin system. Although direct evidence of the beneficial effects of estrogen replacement on primary outcomes is limited, hormone replacement therapy is indicated, despite the hazards of this therapy after chemotherapy in young women who have experienced thromboembolic events such as pulmonary embolism or deep vein thrombosis, and in women with breast cancer [26, 27].

Despite the encouraging results of several findings, further studies are needed to exactly elucidate both pathophysiological mechanisms affecting cardiovascular system and new therapies aiming to prevent premature atherosclerotic process of the early and later impact of amenorrhea and subsequent hormonal withdrawal in young women, during menopausal transition and in postmenopausal period.

References

1. Bachmann G, Kemmann E (1982) Prevalence of oligomenorrhea and amenorrhea in a college population. Am J Obstet Gynecol 144:98–102
2. Reindollar RH, Novak M, Tho SP et al (1986) Adult-onset amenorrhea: a study of 262 patients. Am J Obstet Gynecol 155:531–543
3. De Souza MJ et al (2009) High prevalence of subtle and severe menstrual disturbances in exercising women: confirmation using daily hormone measures. Hum Reprod 25:491–503
4. Mendelsohn ME (2002) Protective effects of estrogen on the cardiovascular system. Am J Cardiol 89:12E–17E
5. Reckelhoff JF (2005) Sex steroids, cardiovascular disease, and hypertension: unanswered questions and some speculations. Hypertension 45:170–174
6. O'Donnell E, Goodman JM, Harvey PJ (2011) Clinical review: cardiovascular consequences of ovarian disruption: a focus on functional hypothalamic amenorrhea in physically active women. J Clin Endocrinol Metab 96:3638–3648
7. Rickenlund A, Eriksson MJ, Schenck-Gustafsson K et al (2005) Oral contraceptives improve endothelial function in amenorrheic athletes. J Clin Endocrinol Metab 90:3162–3167
8. Bairey Merz CN, Johnson BD, Sharaf BL et al (2003) Hypoestrogenemia of hypothalamic origin and coronary artery disease in premenopausal women: a report from the NHLBI sponsored WISE study. J Am Coll Cardiol 41:413–419
9. O'Donnell E, Harvey PJ, Goodman JM et al (2007) Long-term estrogen deficiency lowers regional blood flow, resting systolic blood pressure, and heart rate in exercising premenopausal women. Am J Physiol Endocrinol Metab 292:E1401–E1409
10. Friday KE, Drinkwater BL, Bruemmer B et al (1993) Elevated plasma low-density lipoprotein and high-density lipoprotein cholesterol levels in amenorrheic athletes: effects of endogenous hormone status and nutrient intake. J Clin Endocrinol Metab 77:1605–1609
11. Ahmed B, Bairey Merz CN, Johnson BD et al; WISE Study Group (2008) Diabetes mellitus, hypothalamic hypoestrogenemia, and coronary artery disease in premenopausal women (from the National Heart, Lung, and Blood Institute sponsored WISE study). Am J Cardiol 102:150–154
12. Yorgun H, Tokgözoğlu L, Canpolat U et al (2013) The cardiovascular effects of premature ovarian failure. Int J Cardiol 168:506–510
13. Kalantaridou SN, Naka KK, Papanikolaou E (2004) Impaired endothelial function in young women with premature ovarian failure: normalization with hormone therapy. J Clin Endocrinol Metab 89:3907–3913

14. Kravariti M, Naka KK, Kalantaridou SN et al (2005) Predictors of endothelial dysfunction in young women with polycystic ovary syndrome. J Clin Endocrinol Metab 90:5088–5095
15. Hu FB, Grodstein F, Hennekens CH et al (1999) Age at natural menopause and risk of cardiovascular disease. Arch Intern Med 159:1061–1066
16. Joakimsen O, Bønaa K, Stensland-Bugge E et al (2000) Population based study of age at menopause and ultrasound assessed carotid atherosclerosis: the Tromsø Study. J Clin Epidemiol 53:525–530
17. Rossouw J, Prentice R, Manson J et al (2007) Postmenopausal hormone therapy and risk of cardiovascular disease by age and years since menopause. JAMA 97:146–177
18. van der Schouw Y, van der Graaf Y, Steyerberg E et al (1996) Age at menopause as a risk factor for cardiovascular mortality. Lancet 347:714–718
19. Atsma F, Bartelink M-L, Grobbee D et al (2006) Postmenopausal status and early menopause as independent risk factors for cardiovascular disease: a meta-analysis. Menopause 13:265–279
20. Jacobsen B, Heuch I, Kvåle G (2003) Age at natural menopause and all-cause mortality: a 37-year follow-up of 19,731 Norwegian women. Am J Epidemiol 157:923–929
21. Mondul A, Rodriguez C, Jacobs E et al (2005) Age at natural menopause and cause-specific mortality. Am J Epidemiol 162:1089–1097
22. Rocca WA, Grossardt BR, de Andrade M (2006) Survival patterns after oophorectomy in premenopausal women: a population-based cohort study. Lancet Oncol 7:821–828
23. Lobo R (2007) Surgical menopause and cardiovascular risks. Menopause 14:562–566
24. Parker W, Broder M, Chang E et al (2009) Ovarian conservation at the time of hysterectomy and long-term health outcomes in the nurses' health study. Obstet Gynecol 113:1027–1037
25. Knauff E, Westerveld H, Goverde A et al (2008) Lipid profile of women with premature ovarian failure. Menopause 15:919–923
26. Langrish J, Mills N, Bath L et al (2009) Cardiovascular effects of physiological and standard sex steroid replacement regimens in premature ovarian failure. Hypertension 53:805–811
27. Rees M (2008) Premature menopause: hormone replacement therapy is indeed indicated. BMJ 336:1148

Delayed Puberty: Impact on Female Fertility

11

Martin Birkhaeuser

11.1 Introductory Remarks

Puberty is the period of life that leads to adulthood through complicated and sometimes painful physiological and psychological changes. The hypothalamic-pituitary-gonadal axis undergoes an active phase during foetal and neonatal development and then enters a resting phase that lasts for the rest of childhood until puberty. Puberty begins with an activation of the hypothalamic-pituitary-gonadal system. It occurs today earlier than a century and even earlier than 20 years ago. Delayed puberty may have a dramatic impact on the mental and social development of an adolescent. In the literature, different definitions for "delayed puberty" can be found and there are no guidelines indicating when in the absence of pubertal signs an investigation should be started. Usually, in girls, a first evaluation should be done not later than at the age of 13. However, the initiation of a first evaluation has to be earlier in some cases: it depends on the psychosocial pressure exerted on a child by her personal delay when it is compared to the pubertal development of the pair group of schoolmates and friends. One aspect that quite often worries the patient and her parents the most is the impact of delayed puberty might have on later fertility.

This chapter intends to give a short overview for non-specialized endocrinologists over normal puberty, the practically most important forms of delayed puberty and the measures to be taken.

M. Birkhaeuser
Gynaecological Endocrinology and Reproductive Medicine, University of Berne, Gartenstrasse 67, Basel 4052, Switzerland
e-mail: martin.birkhaeuser@balcab.ch

C. Sultan, A.R. Genazzani (eds.), *Frontiers in Gynecological Endocrinology*, ISGE Series, DOI 10.1007/978-3-319-41433-1_11

11.2 Normal Puberty

11.2.1 Clinical Aspects

The clinical onset of external pubertal development is announced by the appearance of secondary sex characteristics. In females, these signs are the appearance of breast buds and of pubic and axillary hair.

The development of secondary sex characteristics is rated into five stages according to Tanner's criteria [1–5]. They evolve progressively over several years until adulthood is reached and are designated as Tanner stages B1 through B5 for breast development and PH1 through PH6 for pubic hair growth (Figs. 11.1 and 11.2). A detailed description of the Tanner stages can be found in standard textbooks of paediatrics and paediatric or gynaecological endocrinology [1–3].

In girls, pubertal growth spurt occurs during Tanner stages 2 and 3. In girls, it occurs 2 years earlier than in boys. Girls do not show the same slowing down of growth velocity as boys before puberty and increase their growth velocity to 6 cm/year during the first year of puberty, and to 8 cm/year on average during the second year [6].

Menarche A variety of environmental and genetic factors are involved in the regulation of menarche. The first menstrual period (menarche) occurs at an average age of 13.4 years, according to the longitudinal data obtained by Largo et al. [4].

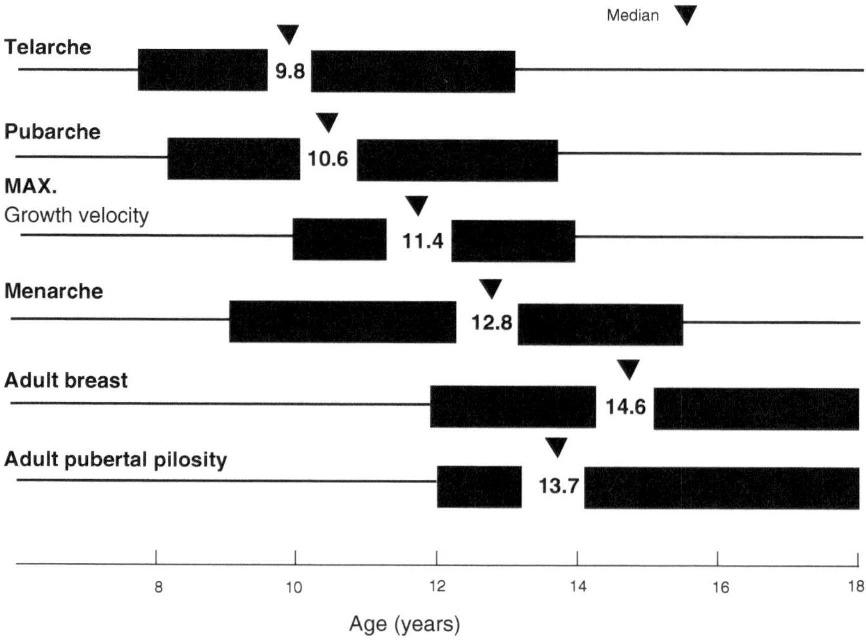

Fig. 11.1 The sequence of events during puberty in girls. Breast bud appearance is usually before pubic hair growth; in the meantime growth velocity increases reaching the peak at Stage 4 of puberty. At this time menarche may appear [4]

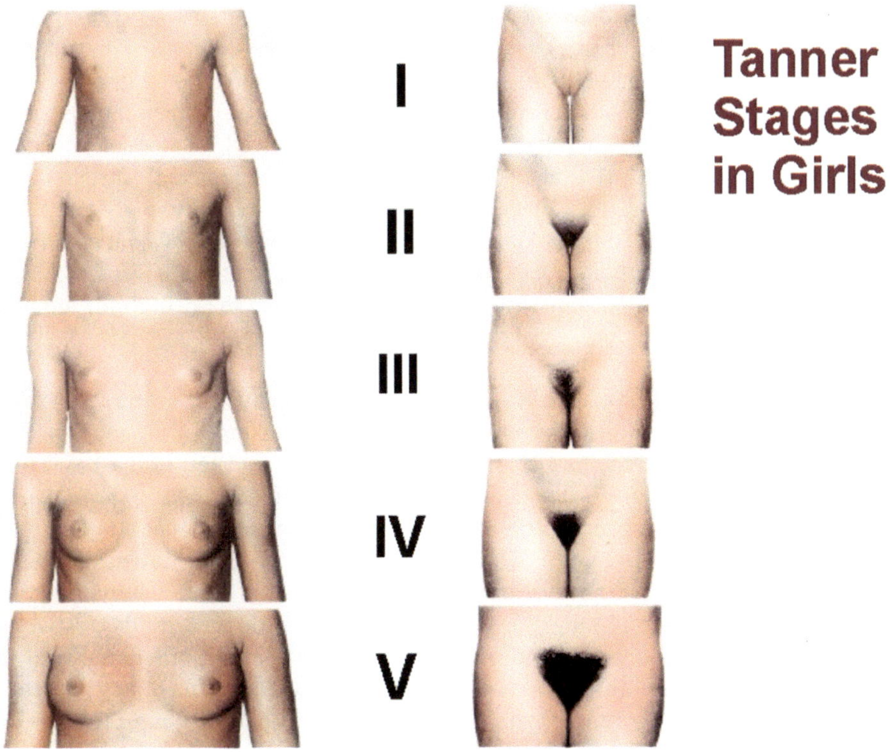

Fig. 11.2 Breast development in girls. The mammary gland grows from a breast bud that can be palpated under the nipple (Tanner stage B2) to a fully developed female breast (Tanner stage B4 or B5) over a period of 3.6 years, on average [4]

Menarche occurs generally at Tanner stage 4. The mean age at menarche is highly correlated within families, between monozygotic twins, and within ethnic groups [7]. Twin analyses suggest that 53–74 % of the variation in age of menarche may be attributed to genetic effects [7].

11.2.2 Endocrinological Aspects of Normal Puberty

11.2.2.1 Adrenarche

Endocrinologically, the first signal for puberty is given by the adrenals (adrenarche). The onset of DHEA-S production from the adrenal zona reticularis leads to the phenomenon of adrenarche.

During infancy and early childhood, adrenal androgens (androstenedione, dehydroepiandrosterone, and dehydroepiandrosterone-sulphate) are secreted in small amounts. Their secretion increases gradually with age. This increase in androgen levels is responsible for the appearance of body odour, pubic hair and axillary hair. Therefore, pubic hair develops independently of the activation of the hypothalamic-pituitary-gonadal pathways.

Adrenarche is marked by the growth of the zona reticularis [8] and a parallel increase in the adrenal androgen levels. This phenomenon is only seen in the human beings and in some old world primates, such as the chimpanzee [9]. Plasma concentrations of the adrenal androgens increase, whereas those of cortisol remain stable, suggesting that factors other than corticotropin are involved. Hormones postulated for this role are the yet undefined androgen-stimulating factor, Corticotrophin Releasing Hormone (CRH) and more recently hormones related to body mass, such as insulin and leptin [10–13]. Although the temporal relation between adrenarche and the onset of puberty suggests that adrenal androgens might have a regulatory influence on the timing of puberty, it is now accepted that the two events are independent processes.

11.2.2.2 Regulation of the Hypothalamo-Hypophyseal-Gonadal Axis

Gonadotropin releasing-hormone Gonadotropin releasing-hormone (GnRH), a decapeptide secreted by approximately 1000 neurons located in the basal forebrain and extending from the olfactory bulbs to the mediobasal hypothalamus, is responsible for the gonadotropin secretion by the pituitary gland. GnRH stimulates the release of LH and FSH from the pituitary which in turn stimulate the gonads. LH and FSH have negative feedback effects on the hypothalamus, whereas testosterone (T) and Androstenedione (A) produced by the testis, and Estradiol (E2) produced by the ovary, inhibit both the hypothalamus and the pituitary gland. Inhibin, activin, and follistatin have also feedback effects at both levels. GnRH secretion by the hypothalamus is under the control of a great amount of central and peripheral signals: excitatory amino acids and other neurotransmitters such GABA, gonadal sex steroids, adrenal and thyroid hormones, the GH-IGF-IGFBP axis, nutrition and related hormones such as leptin and insulin (Fig. 11.3).

Two types of GnRH neurons have been identified to date, GnRH neuron I and II. GnRH neurons II have no known function in humans and are not involved in reproductive function, as inferred from Kallmann's syndrome patients in whom GnRH neurons I only are affected. GnRH neurons I originate in the embryonic period and exhibit an endogenous secretion very early in development. After birth, their activity is "turned-off" by the low circulating levels of androgens/oestrogens released by the gonads, by means of a negative feedback mechanism. At puberty, the reactivation of this "gonadostat" is independent of the effect exerted by the steroids and is related to a reduced sensitivity to their action [14–17].

Transcriptional factors Recently three *transcriptional factors*, Oct-2, TTF-1, and EAP-1, have been identified as potential regulators of the cell network, which controls the GnRH secretion ("Upstream control"). They regulate the expression of genes involved in cell function and cell-cell communication (for details, see [18–21]. In the mammalian, hypothalamic lesions that induce sexual precocity activate both Oct-2 and TGF <61537>expression in astrocytes near the lesion site [18], suggesting that TGF <61537>is one of Oct-2 target.

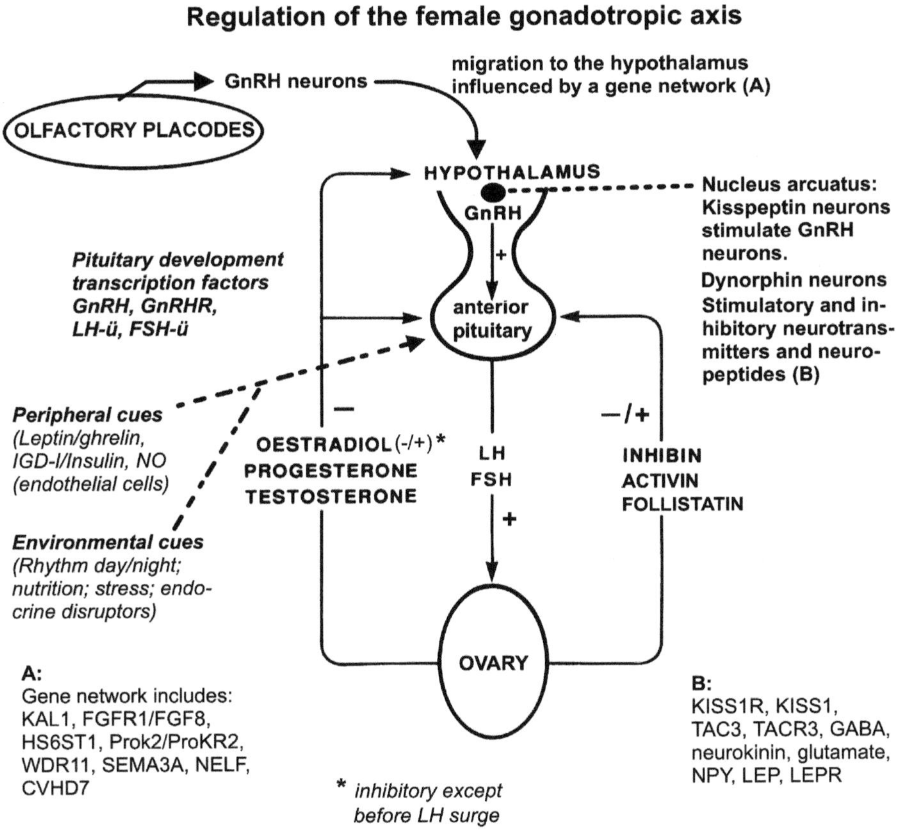

Fig. 11.3 Principals of the development and the regulation of the female gonadotropic axis (see text)

The second candidate is TTF-1 (thyroid transcriptional factor-1), another homeobox gene. After birth, it remains expressed in selected neuronal and glial population of the hypothalamus. At the onset of puberty, TTF-1 enhances GnRH and erbB2 and KiSS-1 gene transcription but inhibits preproenkephalin promoter activity [19].

The third candidate is EAP-1, earlier known as C14ORF4. Like TTF-1, EAP-1 transactivates the promoter of genes involved in facilitating the advent of puberty while suppressing the expression of genes inhibitory to the pubertal process. Knocking down hypothalamic EAP-1 expression causes delayed puberty and disrupted oestrous cyclicity, both in rats and monkeys [20, 21].

KiSS-1/GPR54 system Kisspeptin/metastin (KiSS-1) is a 53-amino-acid-peptide, earlier known as a suppressor of tumour metastases [22, 23]. The proteolitic cleavage of the primary KiSS-1 protein product originates the decapeptide kisspeptin-10 (KiSS-10), whose target is GPR54 receptor. GPR54-containing cells are diffusely distributed [24, 25]. Kiss neurons are important for the gonadal axis. They are located in discrete neuronal subsets of the preoptic area and the nucleus arcuatus [24, 26]. These cells include GnRH neurons and the anterior pituitary [27, 28].

The KiSS-1/GPR54 system has been recognized recently as the director of central functional network and peripheral signals. Genetic, physiological and clinical data strongly indicate that the KiSS-1/GPR system is an essential gatekeeper of GnRH function, and not just one more element in the cascade of signals controlling the gonadotropic axis. It allows the integration of central and peripheral inputs and plays therefore a decisive role in the control of reproductive function [29].

Both in rats and in primates, a marked increase in KiSS-1 and GPR54 mRNA levels coincide with the onset of puberty [24, 30]. Moreover, the sensitivity of GnRH system to kisspeptin is dramatically enhanced in adult versus juvenile mice [42]. Thus, the developmental activation of the GnRH axis by KiSS-1 at puberty reflects a dual phenomenon involving, not only the increase of kisspeptin tone, but also the enhancement of its efficiency to activate GnRH neurons, probably through post-transcriptional changes in GPR54 signalling [31].

Hypothalamic KiSS-1 system also plays an essential role in relaying the negative feedback input of sex steroids onto GnRH neurons. In male and female rats, bilateral gonadectomy evoked a consistent increase in KiSS-1 mRNA at the hypothalamus. Recent studies added further elements to the role of kisspeptin in the feedback control of gonadotropins by showing that negative regulation of hypothalamic KiSS-1 gene expression by oestrogen appears to be restricted to the nucleus arcuatus (Arc), known to be pivotal for negative feedback of sex steroids. In contrast, at the anteroventral periventricular nucleus (AVPN), KiSS-1 mRNA decreased after gonadectomy and increased after sex steroid replacement [32, 33]. AVPN is involved in mediating the positive feedback effects of oestrogen upon GnRH and LH surges. Therefore, via positive regulation of GnRH secretion, KiSS-1 neurons might be involved also in generation of the pre-ovulatory gonadotropin surge.

New strong evidence indicates that hypothalamic KiSS-1 may participate also in delivering information regarding the nutritional status of the organism to GnRH-neurons. Kiss-1 may therefore contribute to the link between energy stores and fertility [34, 35]. It has been shown that the permissive actions of leptin on the reproductive axis are mediated through modulation of GnRH secretion. Because GnRH neurons do not express leptin receptors, [35] kiss peptins might explain badly understood metabolic processes, signalled onto GnRH neurons via peripheral hormones such as leptin. However, several key aspects of the physiology of this system still remain open [36].

In conclusion, KiSS-1 system is an essential downstream element in the negative and (probably) positive feedback loops controlling gonadotropin secretion [37]. In addition, it may participate in the signalling to GnRH neurons of peripheral inputs from hormones such as leptin [38].

Leptin Leptin is a 16-kDa peptide secreted by adipocytes. It is supposed to signal to the brain the critical amount of fat stores necessary for LHRH secretion, which in turn activates the hypothalamic-pituitary-gonadal axis [38]. Leptin was recently shown to suppress neuropeptide Y (NPY) expression in the nucleus arcuatus. NPY stimulates appetite, has an inhibitory effect on the gonadotropin axis and is involved with the inhibition of puberty in conditions of food restriction. Therefore, it has been hypothesized that leptin might exert its effects by acting on NPY. Under favourable nutritional conditions, the rise in leptin levels would suppress NPY, and in turn release the inhibitory effect of NPY neurons on the GnRH-LH/FSH axis, allowing the initiation of puberty [39].

On the other hand, there might be a direct peripheral negative effect of leptin on gonadal function through inhibition of the steroidogenic enzymes [39, 40].

In humans and animals, leptin blood concentrations rise with the onset of puberty. In adolescents of both sexes, the gradual rise in serum leptin levels before puberty together with a decline in circulating levels of soluble leptin receptor suggest that these changes may serve as one of the signals to the central nervous system that metabolic conditions are adequate to support pubertal development and trigger puberty [41].

No gender differences were detected in the relationship between leptin serum levels and fat mass in pre-pubertal and early pubertal subjects. In contrast, at Tanner stages IV and V, the serum hormone concentrations decrease in males and increase in females. In addition, a significant negative correlation between circulating concentrations of testosterone and leptin was described in males only [38].

Finally, it has been shown that normal leptin levels are necessary for the maintenance of menstrual cycles and normal reproductive function in adolescents of both sexes.

In conclusion, leptin seems to exert a positive central effect on the hypothalamic-pituitary-gonadal axis and a negative peripheral one on the gonads. Leptin might signal that the metabolic conditions are adequate to support pubertal development and trigger puberty.

Inhibin, activin, and follistatin Inhibin and follistatin inhibit, and activin stimulates the expression, biosynthesis, and secretion of FSH [42–44]. They are synthesized mainly in the gonads. Inhibin, follistatin and activin are all three involved in the modulation of the hypophyseal-gonadal axis function. Inhibin and follistatin are both negative regulators of FSH secretion.

Inhibin, a heterodimeric glycoprotein, belongs to the TGF-b super family produced by ovarian granulosa cells. It is composed of an alpha and one or two beta subunits. These form two different products, inhibin A and B, respectively. FSH stimulates the synthesis and secretion of inhibins by the gonads, which in turn are involved in the feedback regulation of FSH secretion. In girls, inhibin A concentrations increase between stage 2 and 3 of puberty, remain constant throughout stages 4 and 5, and correlate positively with bone age, inhibin B and oestradiol serum levels [45, 46]. Inhibin B blood concentrations increase further similarly to inhibin A levels, reaching a plateau at 12–18 years. They correlate with oestradiol [45, 46] and FSH serum levels [48].

Blood concentrations of follistatin decrease slightly from stage 1–4 and 5 of puberty in girls [46]. Blood levels of activin A were shown to remain unmodified from stage 1–3 of puberty in females [48].

In conclusion, at puberty the concentrations of the two negative regulators of FSH secretion, inhibin and follistatin, change in opposite directions [46], whereas the blood levels of a positive regulator, activin A, increase, at least in females. All together, these alterations in serum concentrations of FSH-regulatory peptides lead to an increase in FSH secretion.

Melatonin The marked increase in LH amplitude at night observed in early puberty occurs at the same time of melatonin secretion. On the other hand, precocious puberty associated with pineal tumours and due to ectopic secretion of gonadotropins is independent of melatonin [14]. The role of melatonin in puberty is questioned.

Other hormones Growth hormone (GH), insulin, insulin-like growth factor (IGF)-I, and its major binding protein, IGFBP-3, normally rise at puberty [49]. The increase in growth hormone and IGF-I concentrations is probably responsible for most of the metabolic changes observed during puberty, including insulin-resistance, increased beta-cell response to glucose, and growth spurt. GH, and not androgens, may directly affect insulin sensitivity regulating the glucose-insulin homeostasis at the time of puberty [50]. Adiponectin, an adipocytokine with antidiabetic and antiatherogenic effects, were recently shown to progressively decline in parallel with pubertal development in boys [51]. It is inversely related to serum testosterone and dehydroepiandrosterone sulphate levels [51].

11.2.3 Pubertal Maturation of the Hypothalamo-Hypophyseal-Gonadal Axis (Fig. 11.5)

The hypothalamic-pituitary-gonadal axis undergoes an active phase during foetal and neonatal development and then enters a resting phase that lasts for the rest of childhood until puberty.

Puberty begins with an activation of the hypothalamic-pituitary-gonadal system. Changes in GnRH pulsatility during puberty are reflected by the peripheral LH- and FSH-Levels. Qualitative and quantitative changes in LH secretion resulting from pulsatile GnRH secretion, occur approximately 2 years before the appearance of secondary sexual characteristics. At puberty, LH pulsatile secretion is characterized by a 28-fold increase in the pulse amplitude, whereas pulse frequency increases only 1.8-fold. During prepubertal years, both LH and FSH secretions are preponderant during night-time. In the peripubertal period the secretion of gonadotropins increases during sleep, and stimulation with exogenous GnRH shows an enhanced release of LH from the pituitary gland that may be useful in differentiating a pubertal from a pre-pubertal response. Throughout puberty then, gonadotropin pulses further increase becoming apparent during daytime also.

Several studies have been published suggesting that the mechanisms underlying the onset of puberty are different in girls and boys, and different modes of transmission of induction of puberty in boys and girls were revealed [52]. Among other differences, in girls, FSH levels increase during the early stages, and LH levels during the later stages of puberty with a 100-fold increase in hormone concentrations. In contrast, in boys, FSH levels rise progressively through puberty with an increase in amplitude only, whereas LH levels increase in early puberty reaching a plateau shortly [14, 17].

11.2.4 Acceleration of Puberty

Puberty occurs today earlier than a century and even earlier than half a century or 20 years ago. In Tanner's original report [1, 5] white girls had a mean age at onset of breast development and pubic hair of 11.2 and 11.7 years, respectively. The normal mean age at onset of pubertal characteristics in young girls has been revised in 1997 in a considerable population of 17,000 girls evaluated in a cross-sectional study [53]. It has been shown to vary with race, ethnicity, geographical location, and environmental and nutritional conditions.

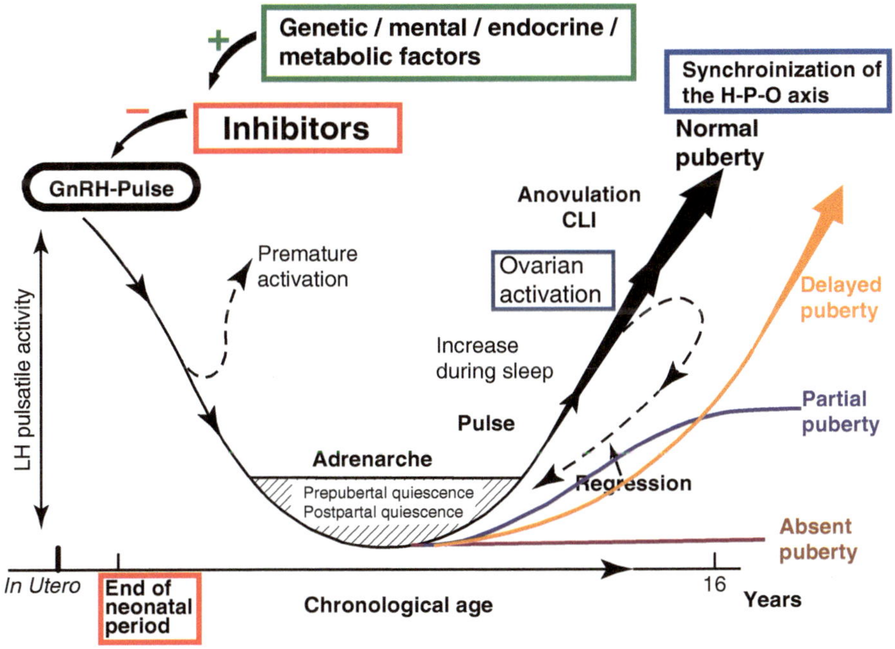

Fig. 11.4 Normal and delayed maturation of the hypothalamo-hypophyseal-gonadal axis (H-P-O-axis). Onset of puberty implies the regression of the inhibitory factors blocking the gonadal axis in childhood. Maturation and activation of the ovarian axis can be interrupted at each stage and may even regress to prepubertal quiescence

Compared to Tanner's original report, pubertal development appears to begin up to 1 year in advance in white and up to 2 years in African-American girls. Breast stage 2 is reported to occur in white girls at 9.96 ± 1.82 years (mean ± SD) with upper and lower limits of 7 and 13 years, and in African-American at 8.87 ± 1.93 years with limits between 6 and 13 years. Pubic hair would occur at 10.51 ± 1.67 and 8.78 ± 2.00 year in white and African-American girls, respectively [54]. In the US white girls puberty would begin by 10 years of age on average, and African American between 8 and 9 years [1, 5, 54, 55].

The age of menarche has been shown to decrease significantly since the nineteenth century. With respect to the first data published by Tanner [5] and Largo [4] 50 and 30 years ago, respectively, it continues to decrease. Menarche seems to occur earlier in white British girls (13.5 years) in 2004 [56] than in 1962 [5] and is reported to occur at 12.88 ± 1.2 years in white and at 12.16 ± 1.21 year in African-American girls [54]. In 2006, a large German survey found the median age at menarche to be 12.8 years [57], suggesting that the secular trend to an earlier menarche is continuing.

11.3 Delayed Puberty

11.3.1 Definition

Puberty is the period of life that leads to adulthood through complicated and sometimes painful physiological and psychological changes. Delayed puberty may have a dramatic impact on the mental and social development of an adolescent.

In the literature, different definitions for "delayed puberty" can be found.

The classical endocrinological definition and the current paediatric definition are identical for girls, but slightly different for boys:

Endocrinological definition (Grumbach and Styne [42])

Delayed puberty is defined as the absence of signs of puberty in healthy girls at age 13 years and in healthy boys at the age 13.5 years (2 SD above the mean age at start of puberty).

Paediatric definition: Delayed puberty is defined as the absence of signs of sexual maturation by an age more than 2–2.5 SD values above the mean of the population (traditionally breast development by 13 years in girls and testicular development by 14 years in boys) (Marshall and Tanner [1]; Lee [2]; Brämswig and Dübbers [55]).

11.3.2 Incidence

Delayed puberty is a rare condition, occurring in only approximately 2.5 % of the population. [1, 2, 42, 55]. The relative incidence of the different forms of hypogonadism in delayed puberty is shown on Table 11.1. In the series of Reindollar et al. [58], hypogonadotropic hypogonadism is found in 31 %, hypergonadotropic

Table 11.1 Relative incidence of observed hypogonadism in delayed puberty [58]

Hypogonadotropic Hypogonadismus	*31 %*
Idiopathic	10 %
GnRH-deficiency	7 %
Anorexia	3 %
Other endocrinopathies	4 %
Organic	13 %
Hypergonadotropic Hypogonadismus	*43 %*
Abnormal karyotype	26 %
Normal karyotype	17 %
Eugonadotropic hypogonadism[a]	*26 %*
Rokitansky-Kuster and similar	17 %
Testicular feminization	1 %

[a]Primary amenorrhea in presence of partial or complete development of secondary sex characteristics

hypogonadism in 43 % and eugonadotropic hypogonadism leading to primary amenorrhea in presence of partial or complete development of secondary sex characteristics in 26 %.

11.3.3 When and How to Investigate?

There are no guidelines indicating when in the absence of pubertal signs an investigation should be started. Following both definitions listed above, in girls, a first evaluation should be done not later than at the age of 13.

Important is empathetic counselling to counteract the mostly deep anxiety due to the fact of being different from other girls at the same age. The child and the parents have to be fully and accurately informed and reassured that an underlying pathological process is rare and that the delay of the onset of puberty is mostly due to a benign, often familiar, deviation from the normal time course.

In most recommendations, a precise diagnostic evaluation is recommended in girls with persisting absence of the onset of puberty at the age of 14.5 years (mean + 3 standard deviations). However, a further evaluation is recommended earlier if a girl without onset of puberty starts to suffer because she becomes socially isolated among her classmates because of her physical retardation. Therefore, acceleration of puberty has to be taken into account for the decision when to start clinical evaluation in absence of pubertal signs.

In conclusion, investigation has to be started earlier than it has been recommended 20 years ago. It depends on the psychosocial pressure exerted on a child by the pubertal development of the pair group of schoolmates and friends.

Figure 11.5 presents a simplified flow chart of the assessment of delayed female puberty. It describes schematically the process for the investigation of adolescent girls presenting with lack of spontaneous pubertal development. Shaded boxes show the major differential diagnoses of constitutional delay of growth and puberty,

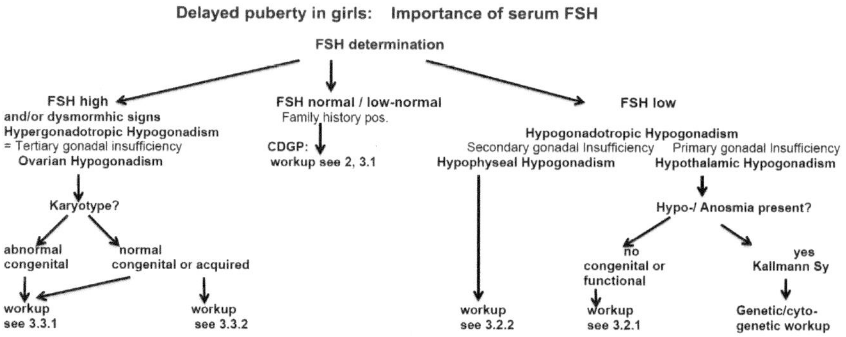

Fig. 11.5 The determination of serum FSH, together with family history and clinical signs, allows in a simple way a first preliminary classification of girls suffering from delayed puberty. Workup numbers relate to the chapters of this review

hypogonadotropic hypogonadism, and hypergonadotropic hypogonadism. However, no clinical algorithm can fully meet the requirements of all individual cases. Thus, adapted clinical decision–making is important at each stage.

11.3.3.1 Hormone Measurements

Gonadotropins

- Basal levels of FSH and LH are low in patients with HH or constitutionally delayed puberty and elevated in hypergonadotropic hypogonadism.
- Levels of FSH and LH remain low after one GnRH injection in hypothalamic and in hypophyseal hypogonadism.
- Levels of LH and FHS increase in hypothalamic hypogonadism with intact pituitary function (but not in hypophyseal hypogonadism) after repeated pulsatile administration of GnRH (0.1 mg GnRH per injection).
- When 0.1 mg of GnRH is injected, pubertal onset is characterized by LH/FSH >1.

Oestradiol

In girls, at pubertal onset, oestradiol levels are >40 ng/ml (<10 ng/ml before puberty).

Inhibin B and Anti-Müllerian Hormone (AMH)

The distinction between constitutional delay of growth and puberty (CDGP) and idiopathic hypothalamic or hypophyseal hypogonadism (IHH) is still a difficult clinical issue. Harrington and Palmer conclude that basal inhibin B may offer a simple, discriminatory test if results from recent studies are replicated: very low levels indicate a high likelihood of IHH [59]. However, current literature does not allow today for recommendation of any diagnostic test for routine clinical use. This applies, too, to the clinical use of AMH in the investigation of delayed puberty [60].

Other Hormones to be Checked
Pituitary deficits should be evaluated by measuring IGF-I, T4, TSH and cortisol.

11.3.3.2 Bone Age

A bone age <11 years in girls with growth failure is encountered in constitutionally delayed puberty.

Bone ages >11 years in girls require further investigation to eliminate hypogonadism.

11.3.3.3 Pelvic Abdominal Ultrasonography

In case of hypergonadotropic hypogonadism, gonads may be small or absent. At the onset of puberty, the ovaries develop follicular cysts long before menarche. Multicystic ovaries with more than six cysts are a normal phenomenon and are already observed in the early stages of puberty [61, 62]. At that stage, these normal cysts should not be confounded with an early expression of a later PSO-syndrome. If ovarian volume is >2 ml and the uterus >35 mm, puberty is imminent [63].

The uterine volume increases at first without, and then with, a visible layer of uterine mucosa. This mucosa layer is induced by the slowly increasing oestrogen secretion.

11.3.3.4 Karyotype

Independent of dysmorphic features suggestive of Turner syndrome, a karyotype should be performed in hypergonadotropic hypogonadism if the patient's history (e.g., chemotherapy, X-ray treatment) cannot explain the gonadal pathology.

11.3.3.5 Brain Magnetic Resonance Imaging (MRI)

In presence of unexplained low levels of LH and FSH, organic pituitary or hypothalamic disease should be eliminated. MRI is the most efficient imaging examination. Agenesis of the olfactory bulbs is typical for Kallmann syndrome. Measurement of the pituitary and pituitary stalk is fundamental.

An elaborate discussion of the investigational process is presented by the specialized literature [55, 59, 64, 65].

11.4 Impact on Fertility of the Different Forms of Delayed Puberty

11.4.1 Constitutional Delay of Growth and Puberty

Constitutional delay of growth and puberty (CDGP) is the most common cause of delayed puberty in girls with 30 % of cases, as it is in boys [66]. CDGP is defined as a delay of growth occurring in otherwise healthy adolescents with stature reduced for chronological age, but generally appropriate for bone age and stage of pubertal development, both of which are usually delayed. It is more frequent in boys than in girls with a 10:1 ratio and is the most common cause of delayed puberty (80–90 %).

In most cases delayed puberty is not due to any underlying pathology, but instead represents an extreme end of the normal spectrum of pubertal timing, a developmental pattern referred to as constitutional delay of growth and maturation [66]. The characteristically retarded linear growth occurs during the early years of life and is followed by regular growth paralleling the normal growth curve throughout the rest of prepubertal years. Pubertal growth spurt is attenuated and occurs after the usual expected time. In girls, exclusive maternal inheritance seems to be the major mode of inheritance whereas for boys the mode of inheritance is almost equally maternal, paternal or bilineal [52]. The majority of cases (70–80 %) are familial. Sedlmyer & Palmert classified family histories of pubertal timing among primary relatives in 95 of 122 of the CD and in 25 of 45 of the functional hypogonadotropic hypogonadism (FHH) cases. Analysis revealed at least a tendency to pubertal delay in 77 % of the CDGP and in 64 % of the FHH families and a diagnosis of delay in 38 % of the CDGP and 44 % of the FHH families. Both parents contributed to the positive family histories. The rates of positive family histories among the CDPD and FHH groups were approximately twice those seen among the other subjects in our case series [66]. Bone mineral density can be compromised by the low serum steroid concentrations measured [67, 68]. Specifically, the attainment of peak bone mass may be impaired, although recent data do not indicate significant changes in volumetric bone mineral density in young men with previous CDGP compared with appropriate controls [69].

The sleep-related increase in LH concentrations that characterizes the onset of puberty, is normally present in CDGP children. As a consequence of inadequate production of gonadal steroids, acute provocative tests may show a GH response wrongly consistent with partial GH deficiency [70]. Pre-treatment with oestrogens in girls results as expected in the normalization of the GH responses. The LH response to the LH-RH analogue leuprolide acetate is intermediate between that of hypogonadal patients and normal pubertal children, and is therefore useful in differentiating CDGP from hypogonadotropic hypogonadism. Recently, a critical appraisal of available diagnostic tests has been published [59].

Supportive care is essential. Although no specific treatment is required, the psychosocial problems faced by CDGP children may force physicians to substitute [55, 64, 71]. In girls, oestrogen therapy is recommended only after statural considerations have been carefully taken into account. Ethinylestradiol should be avoided. The administration of oestrogen, even in small amounts, leads to progressive skeletal maturation, and ultimately to epiphyseal fusion. The use of anabolic steroids or growth hormone to stimulate growth is highly controversial [72–75] and is not recommended in most reviews [66].

The inheritance patter of CDGP has been recently analysed by Winter et al. [52]. In girls, exclusive maternal inheritance seems to be the major mode of inheritance.

Impact on fertility There are no published data suggesting that compared to children with normal puberty, fertility may be decreased in adulthood in individuals who had lived a constitutionally delayed puberty.

11.4.2 Other Forms of Hypogonadotropic Delay of Growth and Puberty

Table 11.1 lists the most important causes of delayed puberty other than constitutional delay of puberty and growth. These causes are usually grouped in four categories:

- Delayed puberty due to congenital hypothalamic hypogonadotropic hypogonadism
- Delayed puberty due to functional hypothalamic hypogonadotropic hypogonadism
- Delayed puberty due to hypophyseal hypogonadotropic hypogonadism
- Delayed puberty due to congenital or acquired hypergonadotropic hypogonadism

The characteristic endocrine pattern for hypothalamic hypogonadotropic, hypophyseal hypogonadotropic and hypergonadotropic hypogonadism is presented on Fig. 11.6.

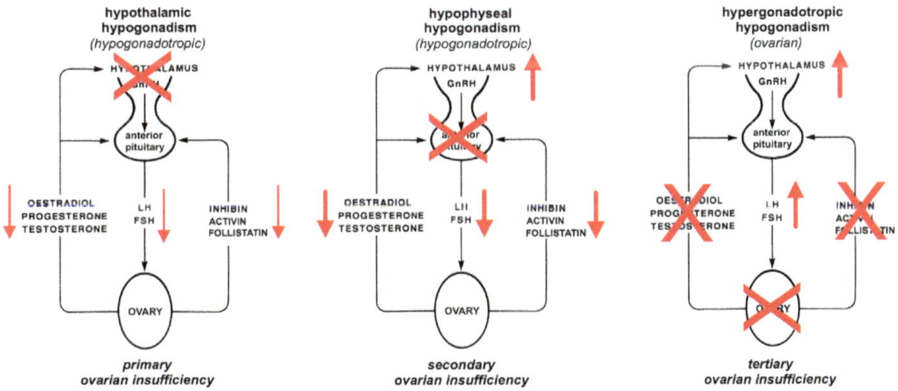

Fig. 11.6 Schematic presentation of the classical endocrine defects in primary, secondary and tertiary ovarian insufficiency

11.4.2.1 Hypothalamic Hypogonadotropic Hypogonadism (Primary Ovarian Insufficiency)

Delay of Puberty in Organic Hypothalamic Hypogonadotropic Hypogonadism (HH) (Table 11.2a)

In girls, HH is proposed when plasma gonadotropins are normal or low, with lack of pubertal signs at 13 years of age. Puberty is absent or partial (congenital and early acquired forms), or arrested in an intermediate stage (acquired forms), depending on the appearance of the pathology in relation to the onset of puberty. Serum gonadotropin levels are low or inappropriately low-normal, sex steroids are low.

Isolated GnRH Deficiency

Congenital isolated hypothalamic hypogonadism (CHH) is clinically characterized by a partial or complete lack of puberty and a primary infertility due to a deficient GnRH-induced gonadotropin secretion, in the absence of anatomical abnormalities in the hypothalamic and pituitary region, and by normal basal and reserve testing of the remaining pituitary hormones.

Biologically, CHH is defined by low or normal serum levels of LH and FSH in the setting of low sex steroids. All other hypophyseal functions are normal as is the

Table 11.2a Classical causes of Hypothalamic Hypogonadism (primary ovarian insufficiency) [55, 64, 65, 77, 80]

Congenital (permanent) hypothalamic hypogonadism
Isolated GnRH deficiency
With ansomia (Kallmann syndrome)
Without ansomia
Associated with a syndrome such as
Prader-Willi
Laurence–Moon
Bardet–Biedl
etc.
Acquired hypothalamic hypogonadism
CNS tumours (cranyopharngeoma, germinoma etc.)
Metastases from non-CNS-tumours
Infections of the central nervous system
Systemic infections, such as tuberculosis, syphilis, Trypanosomiasis
Infiltrating processes ans storage diseases such as haemochromatosis (Thalassaemia major!), histocytosis, granulomas,sarcoidosis, M. Wilson
Multiple sclerosis
Head injury
Stroke, rupture of anevrysm
Cerebral surgery
Chemotherapy/radiotherapy

imaging of the hypothalamo–pituitary region. Patients with CHH typically present in adolescence or early adulthood with delayed onset of puberty, primary amenorrhea, poorly developed sexual characteristics, and/or infertility.

There exist two clinical variants of congenital GnRH deficiency: the form without anosmia and the GnRH deficiency with anosmia. When CHH is associated with anosmia or hyposmia it is termed Kallmann syndrome [76–78]. The Kallmann syndrome is the classic example of congenital hypothalamic hypogonadism. The first description of the so-called Kallmann syndrome has been published by de Morsier [79]. It is due to an impairment of the normal migration of the GnRH neurons from the region of the olfactory nerve to the ventral hypothalamus through the cribriform plate (Fig. 11.4). The clinical features of Kallmann syndrome are variable, with X-linked and autosomal-dominant and -recessive causes and variable penetrance described. Renal anomalies and syncynesia may exist. Its prevalence is 1/8000–1/10,000 in men and 1:50,000 in women. MRI confirms aplasia or hypoplasia of the olfactory bulbs.

Most cases of Kallmann syndrome seem to be sporadic as a consequence of mutations in at least two autosomal genes.

Mostly, genetic mutations are responsible for CHH [55, 64, 80, 81]. Mutations in the KAL1 gene on the short arm of the X chromosome (Xp22.3) are responsible for the X-chromosomal recessive form, while mutations in the FGFR1 (fibroblast growth factor receptor 1) gene on the short arm of chromosome 8 (8p11.2–p11.1) are responsible for the autosomal dominant form (e12). At present, in human, the only type of hypothalamic hypogonadism attributed to a single gene defect is the alteration of GPR54 [76] where KiSS-1 is involved (see above). Subjects with mutations in the human leptin receptor gene have no pubertal development. Table 11.2b lists the classical genetic mutations leading to permanent hypothalamic hypogonadism, with and without anosmia. Gene mutations with normosmic congenital hypogonadal hypodonadism are shown on Table 11.3. In all six listed

Table 11.2b Gene mutations leading to congenital permanent hypogonadal hypogonadism [55, 64, 76, 80–83]

Migration disorder of the GnRH neurons (Kallmann syndrome) due to mutations in (e12):
The KAL1 gene (chromosome Xp22.3)
The fibroblast growth factor receptor 1 (FGFR-1) gene (chromosome 8p11.2–p11.1)
The prokineticin 2 gene (e13)
The prokineticin 2 receptor gene
Nasal embryogenic LHRH factor (NELF)
Disturbances of GnRH secretion without anosmia or hyposmia (e19)
Mutations of the GnRH receptor gene
Mutations of the leptin gene
Mutations of the leptin receptor gene
Mutations of the G-coupled protein receptor 54 gene (GPR54) (e18)

mutations, heredity is recessive. This explains why expression of the anomaly is rare although the frequency of the abnormal gene GnRH1 in Europe is quite high (1/50) [80].

Additional developmental anomalies can occur with CHH including unilateral renal agenesis, synkinesia (mirror movements), cleft lip and/or palate, sensorineural hearing loss, dental agenesis, and skeletal malformations [81]. In some forms of CHH, additional defects are observed. These specific phenotypes are known as syndromes with CHH and additional abnormalities such as coloboma, heart defect, atresia of nasal choanae, retarded growth/development or genital abnormalities. The best known of these clinical syndromes are the Prader-Willi, the Laurence-Moon and the Bardet-Biedl syndrome. CHH and ear abnormalities up to deafness is known as the CHARGE syndrome [82, 83].

Delay of Puberty in Functional Hypogonadal Hypogonadism (Primary Ovarian Insufficiency)

It has been estimated that 10–20% of all women suffer at least once in their life from functional hypothalamic disorders, mostly stress [17]. If such a functional disorder occurs before the normal age of puberty, puberty may be delayed.

Transient hypogonadal hypogonadism is seen in systemic conditions such as anorexia starting before or around puberty, excessive exercise (athletic triad) in

Table 11.3 Genes responsible, frequency and phenotype in normosmic hypothalamic hypogonadism. Heredity is in all six listed mutations *recessive* [80]

Gene responsible of hypogonadism	Frequency of gene	Phenotype
GnRH1	Europe: 1/50	Complete HH
	USA: 1/310	
GnRH-R	40% of cases of familial normosmic HH	Complete HH
	Sporadic mutations: 6–17% of cases of hypogonadism	
KiSS-1	Rare, no sporadic mutations described	Severe gonadotropic deficiency, absence of puberty
KiSS-R	Rare, sporadic or familial idiopathic HH: 26 cases from 9 different families described	Severe gonadotropic deficiency, absence of puberty
TAC3 neurokinin B	Rare, no sporadic mutations described	2 of the 4 sisters with TAC3 mutations had spontaneous pregancies, another has regular cycles and the forth had an early miscarriage
TAC3-R	Rare, no sporadic mutations but rare variant described in sporadic cases	6 of the 7 males and 4 of the 5 females demonstrated evidence for reversibility of their hypogonadism

pubertal girls, in severe chronic diseases of any origin, in malnutrition and in emotional deprivation [66, 84–88]. Sedlmeyer et al. [66] and other groups [84, 85] listed over 25 different underlying chronic diseases in their analysis of children investigated for functional delayed puberty. Among them, in addition to eating disorders and intense exercise, endocrine diseases (GH deficiency, hyperprolactinemia (see above), hypothyroidism), diabetes mellitus, cystic fibrosis, Crohn's disease, celiac disease, severe asthma, nephrotic syndrome, rheumatoid arthritis, systemic lupus erythematodes, sickle cell disease and thalassemia major, congenital heart disease, focal segmental glomerulosclerosis, glycogen storage disease type 1A, several oncological diseases (Hodgkin's disease, leukaemia etc.), CNS disorders (particularly seizure disorders) and poor nutrition.

Acquisition of fat mass is involved in pubertal development. During starvation, in stress-induced amenorrhea with weight loss, in subjects with anorexia nervosa, and in strenuously exercising athletes, leptin and E2 levels fall concomitantly. By limiting the apposition of adipose tissue, chronic diseases affect the development of puberty and fertility by the same mechanism relayed through the hypothalamus, apart from the specific impact of their molecular alteration. As the effect of the drugs used to treat chronic diseases (e.g., corticosteroids) are undistinguishable from the chronic disease itself, pharmacological side effects have to be considered, too [85].

As long as these conditions persist, the onset of puberty remains blocked or its normal continuation stays arrested. In severe cases, a functional regression to prepuberty equivalent with the prepubertal quiescence of the ovarian axis may occur (see Fig. 11.4).

11.4.2.2 Delay of Puberty in Hypophyseal Hypogonadotrophic Hypogonadism (Secondary Ovarian Insufficiency)

Congenital or permanent hypophyseal hypogonadism is rare (Table 11.4). Intracranial tumour is a common cause of acquired hypogonadism in adolescence. Among these, craniopharyngeoma, a typical CNS tumour in adolescents, may lead to destructions in the hypothalamo-hypophyseal region [89]. If the pituitary stalk is compressed which is not rare in extrapituitary tumours such as craniopharyngeomas or metastases from non-CNS-tumours, other hypothalamo-hypophyseal axes in addition to the gonadal axis are affected. Neurosurgery for craniopharyngeoma is mostly followed by radiotherapy. In some other tumours, too, surgical resection may be complemented with radiotherapy and/or chemotherapy leading to secondary damage [90, 91].

In presence of an adenoma of the pituitary including makroprolactinoma, hypogonadotropic hypogonadism can result from the compression of pituitary tissue. In the case of prolactinoma or Cushing's disease, delayed puberty may be secondary to the inhibition of GnRH secretion by the hormones secreted by the endocrine active hypophyseal adenoma, even it is small.

Table 11.4 Classical causes of hypophyseal hypogonadotrophic hypogonadism (secondary ovarian insufficiency)

A. Congentital or permanent hypophyseal hypogonadism
Classical congenital forms are:
Isolated LH and FSH deficiency ("idiopathic isolated gonadotropin deficiency")
Panhypopuitarism (complete or partial)
Congenital (genetic, "idiopathic")
Associated with a lesion of the midline/Rathke's pouch
Syndromes, such as CHARGE syndrome: combined pituitary hormone deficiency (coloboma, heart defect, atresia of nasal choanae, retarded growth/development, genital abnormalities, and ear abnormalities/deafness)
B. Acquired hypophyseal hypoginadotropic hypogonadism
Panhypopituitarism (partial or complete)
CNS tumours, such as craniopharyngioma, hamartoma, germinoma etc.
Metastases from non-CNS-tumours
Prolactinomas
Non-prolactin secreting pituitary adenomas
Hypophysitis
Infections, such as tuberculosis, syphilis, trypanosomiasis
Sarcoidosis
Eosinophilic granuloma
Haemochromatosis (Thalassaemia major!)
Multiple sclerosis
Trauma
Chemotherapy/radiation therapy

A rare cause of hypophyseal hypogonadotropic hypogonadism is the empty sella syndrome. Primary ES occurs when CSF enters the sella through a rent in the sellar diaphragm that may or may not be associated with increased intracranial pressure. Secondary ES is a result of an injury to the pituitary itself or the consequence of surgical or radiation treatment. The incidence of ES in children varies greatly depending on the population surveyed, ranging from 1.2 % (children without endocrine symptoms) to 68 % (children with known endocrinopathy) in the survey of Lenz and Root [92].

In adenomas of the pituitary, in empty sella and in craniopharyngeoma, clinically, visual disturbance or headaches may accompany pubertal arrest. It is essential that all patients with intra- or extrahypophyseal tumours undergo a complete evaluation of anterior and posterior pituitary function.

11.4.2.3 Impact on Fertility

Hypogonadotropic hypogonadism due to congenital hypothalamic disorders have very rarely and only in very light partial forms the chance to get later spontaneously pregnant. However, with the adequate treatment, the possibility to live later a normal pregnancy is excellent even in complete forms of hypothalamic hypogonadism (see below).

Hypogonadotropic hypogonadism resulting from hyperprolactinaemia can be treated medically by dopamin agonists [93]. Because the normalization of prolactin secretion by dopamin agonists allows not only the onset of normal pubertal development but also the uptake of a normal fertility, adolescents have to be informed that in case of intercourse without the desire of a child they need an adequate and efficient contraception.

In non-prolactin-secreting adenomas of the pituitary and in most other CNS tumours, surgical intervention is the usual first line treatment [94–96], followed frequently by radiotherapy or chemotherapy. These treatments per se may lead in survivors to permanent hypogonadism [90, 91]. Later spontaneous fertility depends on the destructions left by the tumour itself or by its treatments. As long as the ovaries are intact and have not suffered by chemotherapy or radiotherapy, the chances to become pregnant through ovulation induction remain intact.

In women, where the delay of puberty has been due to functional hypothalamic hypogonadism, the successful treatment of the underlying disease decides on later fertility. Particularly, in women with eating disorders, a complete remission is the *conditio sine qua non* if normalization of fertility is intended. However, the few longitudinal studies on later fertility show that the risk of a subnormal fertility pattern remains increased, as it has been observed in the "*Avon Longitudinal Study of Parents and Children Fertility and prenatal attitudes towards pregnancy in women with eating disorders*" [97]. In this study, Singleton and live births were included across four groups of women suffering from lifetime eating disorders:

- Lifetime anorexia nervosa (AN; $n = 171$)
- Lifetime bulimia nervosa (BN; $n = 199$)
- Lifetime anorexia nervosa and bulimia nervosa (AN + BN; $n = 82$)
- General population ($n = 10{,}636$).

The results show that women with AN (OR 1.6, 95 % CI 1.1–2.5; $P < 0.021$) and women with AN + BN (OR 1.9, 95 % CI 1.1–3.4; $P < 0.020$) were more likely to have seen a doctor for lifetime fertility problems than women from the general population. Furthermore, women with AN + BN were also more likely to take >6 months to conceive (OR 1.9, 95 % CI 1.0–3.5; $P < 0.04$) and to have conceived the current pregnancy with fertility treatment.

All eating disorders groups experienced more frequently negative feelings upon discovering their pregnancy. Negative feelings remained still higher in the AN + BN group at 18 weeks of gestation. Finally, in spite of the longer time the AB women needed to get pregnant, unplanned pregnancies were more common in the AN group compared with the general population. This points to the persistence of an increased ambivalence against pregnancy in women with eating disorders. These last two findings have been confirmed by a second study [98, 99].

Women with lifetime AN had a higher prevalence of twin births compared with those without the disorder (3.5 versus 1 %), as did women with BN and women with AN+BN, albeit to a lesser extent [99]. All eating disorders taken together were associated with increased odds of having twins (OR 2.7, 95 % CI 1.0–7.9; $P=0.06$). These associations persisted after adjustment for potential confounding factors such as lifetime AN, OR 2.7, 95 % 1.0–8.0, lifetime BN, OR 2.7 (95 % CI 1.1–6.4) and lifetime AN+BN, OR 3.9, (95 % CI 1.3–11.1). Interestingly enough, women with other lifetime psychiatric disorders had similar odds as women without psychiatric disorders.

11.4.2.4 Profertile Measures: Ovulation Induction in Hypogonadotropic Hypogonadism (Primary and Secondary Ovarian Insufficiency)

In the absence of the uptake of normal menstrual cycles, as it is the case in all forms of delayed puberty with permanent hypogonadal hypogonadism, ovulation induction should be used to induce pregnancy. It has to be stressed that the administered hormones have to be considered and handled as a substitution. Therefore, the lowest efficient dose of GnRH/pulse or of HMG resp. FSH/LH per day has to be used to obtain a monofollicular response of the ovary.

To decide on the optimal treatment in hypogonadal hypogonadism, the grading system described by Leyendecker (Table 11.5) is recommended. Finally, it has to be remembered that the administration of pure FSH does not make sense in the absence of endogenous LH secretion.

Considering the risk/benefit ratio, in primary ovarian insufficiency the best results are obtained by the pulsatile administration of GnRH (Table 11.6). The pregnancy rate within 1 year is identical to the one of a healthy fertile couple of the same age with a normal fertility (Fig. 11.8). The incidence of hyperstimulation and the number of multiple pregnancies are close to normal. The success rate in patients <35 years is above 90 % [15–17, 100, 101]. However, pregnancy rate is age dependent: Fig. 11.8 lists the results in women aged <35 years, Table 11.7 the results in women with a mean age >35 years (own data). The same age-dependency has been shown for the pregnancy rate with HMG treatment in hypogonadotropic women [102]. The cumulative pregnancy rate has been after six treatment cycles 97 % in women <35 years and 63 % in women >35 years.

Therefore, in women with hypothalamic hypogonadism, first line treatment of infertility is the pulsatile administration of GnRH, with one exception: in partial hypothalamic insufficiency (Table 11.6), the more economic ovulation induction by oral Clomiphene may be used first although its success rate is lower (Fig. 11.7).

Table 11.7 shows the results of ovulation induction by pulsatile GnRH (i.v.) in 17 patients with hypothalamic amenorrhea grade 3c needing a higher dosage of GnRH per pulse (15–20 GnRH µg/pulse). In spite of the severity of the hypothalamic deficiency and a mean age >35 years, the pregnancy rate was 53 %.

Table 11.5 Grading of hypothalamic amenorrhea on the basis of the progestogen, clomiphene, and Gn-RH tests, respectively [156]

1		Clomiphene positive with bleeding following
	1a	Normal luteal phase
	1b	Insufficient luteal phase
	1c	Anovulatory cycle
2		Progestogen positive
		Clomiphene negative
3		Progestogen negative with pituitary response to 100 μg of Gn-RH i.v.
	3a	"Adult response"
	3b	"Prepubertal response"
	3c	No response

Table 11.6 Ovulation induction in hypothalamic and hypophyseal hypogonadism

Wish for a child positive	Grading (see Table 11.3)	Doses
In presence of a potentially normal pituitary function:		
Pulsatile GnRH [15–17, 100, 101]	Grade 1 or 2	5 μg GnRH/pulse every 90 min in the follicular phase
		5 μg GnRH/pulse every 4 h in the luteal phase (or HCG)
Pulsatile GnRH [15–17, 100, 101]	Grade 3	10–20 μg GnRH/pulse every 90 min in the follicular phase
		10–20 μg GnRH/pulse every 4 h in the luteal phase (or HCG)
In presence of normal pituitary and hypothalamic structures:		
Clomiphene [17]	Grade 1	50–100 mg/day day 5–9 after progestin-induced bleeding
Naltrexon [103]	Grade 1–3	25 mg/day in the evening day 1–3, then 50 mg/day in the evening (until pregnancy is confirmed, then stop)
In presence of an absent or deficient gonatropin secretion:		
HMG or FHS/LH		Begin low-dose (37.5–50 IU/day), individual increase of the dose
First line treatment in pituitary hypo-gonadism (secondary ovarian insufficiency)		Ovulation induction: 5000–10,000 IU HCG
Second line treatment in hypothalamic hypo-gonadism (primary ovarian insufficiency)		

In presence of a congenital defect or an acquired lesion of the pituitary, ovulation induction by HMG or FSH/LH has to be used (Table 11.6). To avoid hyperstimulation and multiple pregnancies in ovulation induction by gonadotropins, the classical

Table 11.7 Results of ovulation induction by pulsatile GnRH (i.v.) in hypothalamic amenorrhea grade 3c (15–20 GnRH μg/pulse, own data)

49 treatment cycles in 17 patients (1 Kallmann syndrome, 16 IHH.), mean age 37.2 years (range 32–39 years)	
Spermiograms have been normal in all male partners. All patients had been treated without success by Clomiphene and/or by HMG during a period of at least 1 year.	
Results per cycles:	
Ovulatory cycles	40 cycles (83 %)
Clinical pregnancies	10 cycles (21 %)
Biochemical pregnancies	6 cycles (13 %)
Clinical abortion	1 cycle (2.1 %)
"Take home babies"	9 cycles (18 %)
53 % of all patient became pregnant.	
No patient developed a hyperstimulation syndrome	
No multiple pregnancies have been seen.	
Complications: Two cycles were interrupted due to two superficial phlebitis	

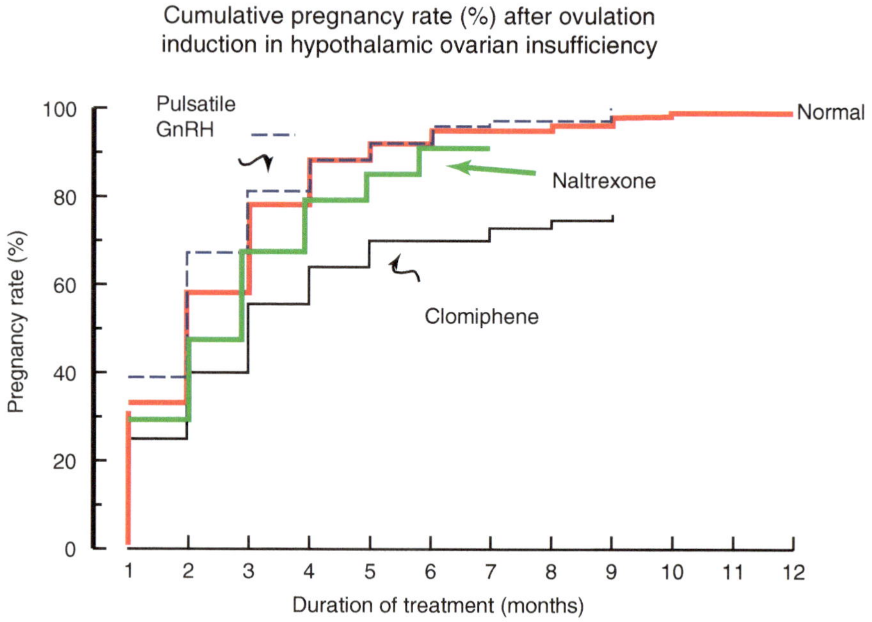

Fig. 11.7 Cumulative pregnancy rate (%) after ovulation induction in hypothalamic ovarian insufficiency by Clomiphene, pulsatile GnRH and Naltrexon compared to normal fertility within 12 months

Doses used:

– Clomiphenen citrate 50–100 mg/day from day 5–9 after a progestin-induced bleeding.

– Pulsatile GnRH s.c.: 5–10 μg/puls every 90 min in the folllicular phase and every 4 h in the luteal phase.

– Naltrexon 25 mg/day in the evening day 1–3, then 50 mg/day in the evening (until pregnancy is confirmed, then stop) (Adapted from Beier et al. [155])

rules have to be observed, meaning administration of the lowest efficient dose and regular supervision by serum oestradiol determination and sonographic control of follicular growth.

Naltrexone, an opioid antagonist, has been used in functional hypothalamic hypogonadism if there was a suspected deregulation of the endogenous opioid system [103]. However, success rate is inferior to pulsatile GnRH (Fig. 11.7); 20–30 % of all patients do not respond sufficiently or at all to Naltrexone. Side effects (mainly nausea, restlessness, sleep problems) are frequent in the first days of treatment.

11.4.3 Delay of Puberty in Hypergonadotropic Hypogonadism (Table 11.8)

11.4.3.1 Congenital Forms

Gonadal Dysgenesis: Phenotypic Female Variants

The term "gonadal dysgenesis" is generally used to describe a variety of clinical conditions. Their common denominator is an abnormal development of the foetal gonads. Gonadal dysgenesis includes Turner syndrome (45/X0, mosaics), mixed gonadal dysgenesis (45X/46, XY), female 46/XY dysgenesis ("pure gonadal dysgenesis, XY type", Swyer's syndrome) and the combination of a normal female sex chromosome constitution and hypergonadotropic hypogonadism (female 46/XX; "pure gonadal dysgenesis, XX type" or "XX gonadal dysgenesis").

Turner Syndrome

Definition, incidence [104] The most frequent disorder in the category of gonadal dysgenesis is Turner syndrome and its variants. Turner syndrome (TS) affects approximately one in 2500–3000 live-born females; in abortions the incidence is 1:270. Girls and women confront the clinician with a challenging array of genetic,

Table 11.8 Delay of puberty in hypergonadotropic hypogonadism

Congenital forms
Turner syndrome
Disorders of sexual development (gonadal dysgenesis and androgen resistance)
Mutations in LH or FSH receptor
Galactosemia
Acquired forms
Chemotherapy/radiotherapy
Endocrine disruptors
Ovarian torsion
Gonadectomy
Autoimmune disease

developmental, endocrine, cardiovascular, psychosocial, and reproductive issues. Intelligence is usually normal, but it may be limited in some cases.

Karyotype All individuals with suspected TS (see below) should have a karyotype performed. A standard 30-cell peripheral blood karyotype is recommended. It identifies at least 10 % mosaicism with 95 % confidence [104]. If there is a strong clinical suspicion of TS, despite a normal blood karyotype, a second tissue, such as skin, may be examined.

TS is a chromosomally determined disorder where complete ovarian agenesis is present with deletion of one X chromosome (karyotype 45 X0). Incomplete forms may be seen in patients with mosaicism (X0/XX, XO/XXX, X0/XX/XXX, 45X0/46XF etc.), in which case the patient may be chromatin positive.

Mosaics may present with a Y chromosome (45X0/46XY). The presence of Y chromosome material is associated with an approximately 12 % risk of a gonadoblastoma which may transform into malignant germ cell neoplasms. Therefore, prophylactic laparoscopic gonadectomy is recommended [105]. The patient and/or her parents should be informed of the finding of Y chromosome material with the utmost sensitivity regarding gender identity issues to minimize psychological harm.

Clinical presentation The phenotype may be oligosymptomatic, dominated by short stature. The diagnosis of TS should be considered in any female with unexplained growth failure or pubertal delay or any constellation of the following clinical findings: oedema of the hands or feet, nuchal folds, left-sided cardiac anomalies, especially coarctation of the aorta or hypoplastic left heart, low hairline, low-set ears, small mandible, short stature with growth velocity less than the 10th percentile for age, markedly elevated levels of FSH, cubitus valgus, nail hypoplasia, hyperconvex uplifted nails, multiple pigmented naevi, characteristic facies, short fourth metacarpal, high arched palate or chronic otitis media.

Absent or delayed puberty Absent pubertal development is one of the most common clinical features of TS, although up to 30 % or more of girls with TS (mosaicisms included) will undergo some spontaneous pubertal development. Ultimately, over 90 % of individuals with TS will have gonadal failure. Therefore, the critical importance of oestrogen treatment for feminization and for bone health during the adult years has to be emphasized. Today, it is accepted that induction of puberty should not be delayed from the age of 12 years until the age of 15 years as recommended earlier to promote statural growth by GnRH treatment first: the positive effect of GnRH administered today to most patients to promote adult height is not hindered by a prudent start of oestrogen substitution at the age of 12 [104].

Impact on fertility Most women with TS are infertile. Only 2–5 %, including forms with mosaicism, achieve spontaneous pregnancy [104]. In a review from 1993 [106], the literature contained reports of 28 spontaneous pregnancies in 16 women with 45, X karyotype and 106 pregnancies in 48 women with mosaicism. Miscarriages, stillbirths and malformations were common. Since then, more spontaneous pregnancies have been known.

Today, various assisted reproductive techniques, particularly egg or embryo donation, are now legally available in many countries for achieving pregnancy. Recent studies show that using these techniques, women with TS become pregnant as easily as women with other types of infertility and carry their pregnancies to term without an increased miscarriage rate [104] if the uterus has been prepared adequately. Oestrogen/progestogen-substitution should be started at least 1 year before assisted reproduction. To be ready for donation, the thickness of the endometrium should reach 7 mm. TS women do have an increased rate of maternal complications, in part because of their small size. Only one embryo should be transferred to avoid the additional risks of a multiple pregnancy.

Reports of fatal aortic dissection during pregnancy and the postpartum period have raised concern about the safety of pregnancy in TS. Therefore, spontaneous or assisted pregnancy in TS should be undertaken only after thorough cardiac evaluation. It is recommended to consider a history of surgically repaired cardiovascular defect, the presence of BAV, or current evidence of aortic dilatation or systemic hypertension as relative contraindications to pregnancy. The possibility of prenatal genetic testing has to be offered.

Women with TS who have spontaneous menstrual cycles and ovulate normally should not postpone the timing of pregnancies without good reason because of the increased risk of premature ovarian failure. They have to be informed about the possibility of oocyte or embryo cryopreservation [107, 108], although these techniques are far from being an established method in TS.

Other Forms of Gonadal Dysgenesis

Mixed gonadal dysgenesis (45X/46, XY), female 46/XY gonadal dysgenesis ("pure" gonadal dysgenesis "XY type", also called "XY females") and "pure" gonadal dysgenesis ("XX type" or "XX gonadal dysgenesis") are rare. They have no Turner stigmata. Complete and partial forms are observed. Pure 46/XX is at least in part due to ODGI gene mutation, inherited as an autosomal recessive, female-limited disorder [109]. SRY Mutations in XY females may lead to complete 46,XY gonadal dysgenesis or "pure" gonadal dysgenesis (also called "XY females"). These individuals suffer rapid and early degeneration of their gonads (gonadal dysgenesis), which are present in the adult as streak gonads consisting mainly of fibrous tissue and variable amounts of ovarian stroma. The external genitalia in these subjects are completely female, and Müllerian structures are normal. The frequency of SRY mutations in XY females ("pure" gonadal dysgenesis) seems to be higher than current estimates [110]. By contrast, subjects with 46,XY partial gonadal dysgenesis have ambiguous genitalia, a mix of Müllerian and Wolffian structures, and dysgenic gonads. These gonads usually consist of disorganized seminiferous tubules admixed with ovarian stroma. Again, the presence of Y chromosome material is associated with an increased risk of germ cell neoplasms so that prophylactic gonadectomy is recommended [105].

There are no practical guidelines for the clinical handling of these patients and no statistics about their later fertility available. It seems therefore logical to counsel and to treat them in analogy to the Turner Syndrome, after a full clinical and laboratory work-up including a full karyotype.

Impact on fertility There are no data pointing to the possibility of a spontaneous pregnancy. However, as long as a normal uterus is present, fertility can be reached through egg or embryo donation as clinical data confirm, describing pregnancies in pure 46/XX and pure 46/XY gonadal dysgenesis following ovum donation. Pregnancy rate per transfer was normal [111].

Noonan Syndrome

Noonan syndrome (NS) is a rare autosomal dominant disorder characterized by a phenotype [112] including short stature, facial dysmorphology and congenital heart defects.

Karyotype is normal. Noonan syndrome affects both sexes. In both sexes, there is a delay in pubertal development.

Other associated features are webbed neck, chest deformity, mild intellectual deficit, cryptorchidism, poor feeding in infancy, bleeding tendency and lymphatic dysplasias. The incidence of Noonan syndrome has been estimated to be between 1 in 1000 and 1 in 2500 live births [113]. In about 50 % of cases, NS is caused by mutations in the PTPN11 gene on chromosome 12, in a small proportion of patients by mutations in the KRAS gene. The aetiology of NS in individuals without mutations in PTPN11 or KRAS (together almost 50 % of cases) is still unknown.

NS should be considered in all foetuses with polyhydramnion, pleural effusions, oedema and increased nuchal fluid with a normal karyotype. With special care and counselling, the majority of children with NS will grow up and function normally in the adult world.

Impact on fertility Fertility appears to be normal in Noonan females but has been reported to be decreased in males, although male transmission of the disorder to the next generation is not uncommon.

Androgen Insensitivity Syndrome, Testicular Feminization ("Hairless Women")

Androgen resistance is a broad continuum reaching from male infertility to testicular feminization. Complete testicular feminization is a highly distinctive disorder where genotypic males (46/XY) are phenotypically female.

Androgen insensitivity syndrome (AIS) is a genetic condition carried on the X chromosome. Although it is inherited in an X-linked, recessive fashion in 70 %, up to 30 % of mutations are sporadic de novo mutations [114]. The estimated prevalence of AIS is between 1 in 20,000 and 1 in 99,000 genetic males. If one examines phenotypic females with inguinal hernias, the prevalence is noted to be 0.8–2.4 %.

In androgen insensitivity syndrome, there is a no activity at the androgen receptor leading to a tissue resistance to androgens. Wolffian structures are poorly (although partially) developed. Since AMH (anti-Müllerian hormone, or Müllerian inhibiting substance) is produced normally by the testes, there is a complete involution of the Müllerian ducts.

Clinical presentation [114] The typical presentation is that of primary amenorrhea in a phenotypic female adolescent. However, in an infant or child, the presentation may be of an inguinal hernia in a phenotypic female. Recent data shows a 1.1 % incidence rate of complete AIS in a child with a premenarcheal inguinal hernia, while 80–90 % of girls with complete AIS eventually develop an inguinal hernia

The external genitalia are female, breasts are developed. The "vagina" ends in a blind pouch; its average length is 2.5–3.0 cm. The testes are found in the labia majora, the inguinal canals or intra-abdominally, and should be prophylactically removed after puberty because of the risk of malignancy. Gonadectomy has to be followed by oestrogen substitution. Rates of dysgerminoma and gonadoblastoma in XY gonadal dysgenesis can rise as high as 15–30 %, but might be lower in AIS. Tumours prior to puberty are rare.

At the time of puberty (usually not delayed), testosterone levels increase in presence of abnormally high LH. Female secondary sex characteristics develop as a result of increased oestrogen levels. Sexual hair is scanty or absent because of the androgen resistance. The final diagnosis is given by the XY-karyotype.

Differential diagnosis The Mayer-Rokitansky-Küster-Hauser (MRKH) syndrome or Müllerian Agenesis is part of the differential diagnosis. MRKH is a more common cause of primary amenorrhea. Its incidence rate is 1 in 5000 [119]. MRKH, too, has a normal breast development and an underdeveloped vagina, but it has normal axillary and pubic hair and a normal female karyotype (46/XX).

Impact on fertility To enable sexual intercourse, there are different options for vaginal creation (dilatation, surgical creation). Today, there is no reasonable way to treat infertility.

Mutations in LH or FSH Receptor

Today, several different homozygous or compound heterozygous inactivating mutations of the LH receptor known. Inactivating mutations of LH receptors can be a very rare cause of delayed puberty and primary hypergonadotropic amenorrhea or premature ovarian failure [115–118]. Clinically, these patients are characterized by female external genitalia, spontaneous breast and pubic hair development at puberty, and normal or late menarche followed by oligo-amenorrhea and infertility. Oestradiol and progesterone levels are normal for the early to midfollicular phase, but do not reach ovulatory or luteal phase levels, confirming lack of ovulation. Notably, serum LH levels are high in patients with LH receptor mutations, whereas follicle-stimulating hormone levels are normal or only slightly increased. Pelvic ultrasound has demonstrated a small or normal uterus and normal or enlarged ovaries with cysts [118].

Mutations of the LH receptor gene may cause primary or secondary amenorrhea and infertility in sisters of male pseudohermaphrodites [115]. Clinically, they present a phenotype of hypergonadotropic hypogonadism ("LH resistance").

On the other hand, only few mutations of FSH receptor were discovered so far. Mutations of the FSH-receptor gene [116, 117, 120–122] cause ovarian dysgenesis leading to delayed puberty, primary or secondary hypergonadotropic amenorhea and small ovaries with variable development of female secondary sex characteristics and infertility.

Impact on fertility In the different syndromes of inactivating mutations of gonadotropin receptors, no pregnancies have been described. In contrast to the clinically similar women harbouring inactivating mutations in luteinizing hormone (LH) beta subunit that may be treated with hCG (human chorionic gonadotropin) or LH, those with mutations in LH receptor are resistant.

Galactosemia

Galactosemia is a rare inborn error of metabolism that results from impaired activity of any of the three enzymes of the Leloir pathway: galactokinase (GALK, EC 2.7.1.6), galactose-1-phosphate uridylyltransferase (GALT, EC 2.7.7.12), or UDP-galactose 4′ -epimerase (GALE, EC 5.1.3.2). Classic galactosemia (OMIM 230400), the most common clinically severe form of the disorder, results from profound impairment of GALT. Classic galactosemia impacts about 1/60,000 live births, although prevalence differs substantially among populations [123].

Sequelae include cognitive and/or behavioural impairment in close to half of all patients, speech difficulties in at least half of all patients, low bone mineral density in many patients, ataxia or tremor in some patients, absent or delayed puberty and primary or premature ovarian insufficiency (POI) in at least 80 % of all girls and women. Neonatal diagnosis with immediate dietary galactose restriction prevents or resolves the acute symptoms of classic galactosemia. However, despite presymptomatic diagnosis and strict lifelong dietary intervention, a majority of patients go on to experience a constellation of troubling long-term complications

Impact on fertility [124] In imaging studies of girls with POI examined at pubertal age or later, the ovaries are invariably abnormal and usually described as hypoplastic or "streak-like." Histological examination most often shows few if any follicles; in the cases where follicles have been observed they did not appear to have matured beyond the primordial stage. The streak-like transformation of the ovaries may be related to accumulated galactose ootoxicity over time. One study of a small cohort of galactosemic women looked at spontaneous fertility outcomes (Gubbels et al. 2008) and reported that galactosemia patients with a diagnosis of POI may be more likely to conceive than women who have POI due to other causes. In a study, [124] 22 galactosemic women were followed. Nine women have tried to conceive, of which four were successful. Three mothers were diagnosed with POF before the first pregnancy and/or in between pregnancies. In the literature, 50 pregnancy reports were found. The genotype and GALT-activity do not seem to predict the chance of becoming pregnant, whereas the occurrence of spontaneous menarche might. For those women with galactosemia who do achieve pregnancy, evidence from studies of small cohorts suggests that there are no adverse effects on the galactosemic mother or her infant.

Options to preserve endogenous fertility in galactosemia need to be explored further. For postpubertal women, freezing embryos after in vitro fertilization is an option.

11.4.3.2 Acquired Forms

Delayed Puberty and Reduced Fertility After Cancer Treatment

Childhood cancer is relatively rare, with an incidence of around 110 cases per million children per year [125, 126]. The Belgian Society of Pediatric Haematology and Oncology (unpublished date, in [108]) estimated childhood cancers are to occur in approximately 13 of 100,000 children under 15 years of age, with 45 % being cases of leukaemia and lymphoma, 20 % craniospinal tumours, 8 % neuroblastomas, 8 % soft tissue tumours, 7 % nephroblastomas, 3 % retinoblastomas and 9 % other rare tumours. The majority of children diagnosed with cancer are expected to be cured and become long-term survivors. The remarkable success in improving childhood cancer survival is exemplified by the 5-year survival rate for all leukaemias approaching 80 % (Office for National Statistics, 2004, UK) [125]. In 2010, in the USA, a total of 10,700 children and adolescents under the age of 14 were diagnosed with cancer. More than 80 % will survive the disease. For some common paediatric cancers such as Wilms' tumour, Hodgkin's disease (HD), and B-cell non-Hodgkin lymphoma (B-NHL) cure rates approach 90 % [127]. As such, it has been estimated that at the start of the twenty-first century, one in 1000 young adults in their third decade is a survivor of childhood cancer [126].

The results from the large and important *Childhood Cancer Survivor Study* (CCSS; [128]) show the natural outcome, without fertility preservation measures, of treatment for cancer diagnosed during childhood or adolescence on ovarian function and reproductive outcomes. The frequency of acute ovarian failure, premature menopause, live birth, stillbirth, spontaneous and therapeutic abortion and birth defects in the participants have been reviewed in the CCSS. Acute ovarian failure (AOF) occurred in 6.3 % of eligible survivors. Exposure of the ovaries to high-dose radiation (especially over 10 Gy), alkylating agents and procarbazine, at older ages, were significant risk factors for AOF. Premature nonsurgical menopause (PM) occurred in 8 % of participants versus 0.8 % of siblings (rate ratio = 13.21; 95 % CI, 3.26–53.51; $P = .001$). Risk factors for premature menopause included attained age, exposure to increasing doses of radiation to the ovaries, increasing alkylating agent score, and a diagnosis of Hodgkin's lymphoma. 1915 female survivors reported 4029 pregnancies. Offspring of women who received uterine radiation doses of more than 5 Gy were more likely to be small for gestational age (birth weight < 10 percentile for gestational age; 18.2% v 7.8%; odds ratio=4.0; 95% CI, 1.6–9.8; $P=.003$). The CCSS did not reveal any differences in the proportion of offspring with simple malformations, cytogenetic syndromes, or single-gene defects.

The CCSS demonstrates that women treated with pelvic irradiation and/or increasing alkylating agent doses were at risk for acute ovarian failure, premature menopause, and small-for-gestational-age offspring. There was no evidence for an increased risk of congenital malformations.

Based on these data, although problems with fertility do not become apparent until after puberty, it is clear that many treatments for childhood cancer can lead to infertility and subfertility in later life. Having survived cancer as a child, it can be very difficult for many patients to accept that they cannot produce their own children because of the treatment they received during childhood.

How can this outcome after cancer treatment be improved? Fertility preservation is becoming increasingly important to improve the quality of life in cancer survivors. Despite guidelines suggesting that discussion of fertility preservation should be done prior to starting cancer therapies, there is a lack of implementation in this area. The need for fertility preservation has to be weighed against morbidity and mortality associated with cancer. Thorough psychological counselling is required. Recommendations should be individualized and should not violate the ethical principles.

Particularly in young girls and in adolescents, there is a need for a multidisciplinary collaboration between oncologists, paediatrician and reproductive specialists to improve awareness and availability.

Effect of Chemotherapy and Radiotherapy

Children that undergo treatment for cancer are at risk of suffering from primary amenorrhea, delayed puberty, hormonal dysfunction and subfertility. Both chemotherapy and radiotherapy have a major impact on the gonadal axis and its hormonal and reproductive potential.

The oocyte has been in an arrested stage of meiosis since before birth and remains so until the onset of puberty, and this does not advance until ovulation. Chemotherapy, radiotherapy and surgery can all have adverse affects on reproduction. It is the effects on the nongrowing stockpile of primordial follicles that is of particular importance for future reproductive potential (Fig. 11.8) [129]. The mechanism by which chemotherapy causes loss of primordial follicles is, however, poorly understood. At present, it is impossible to predict the functional life span of the chemotherapeutically damaged ovary and the reproductive potential of patients with cancer.

It is important to emphasize that there is no evidence to suggest that the prepubertal female (or male) reproductive tract is protected from the adverse effects of cancer therapies. The danger of pelvic radiotherapy is significantly greater than the risk of all kinds of chemotherapy. The susceptibility of the prepubertal uterus to radiotherapy is also clearly demonstrated [108, 129].

Chemotherapy

Chemotherapeutic drugs act by interrupting vital cell processes and arresting the normal cellular proliferation cycle. They cause DNA abnormalities as well as

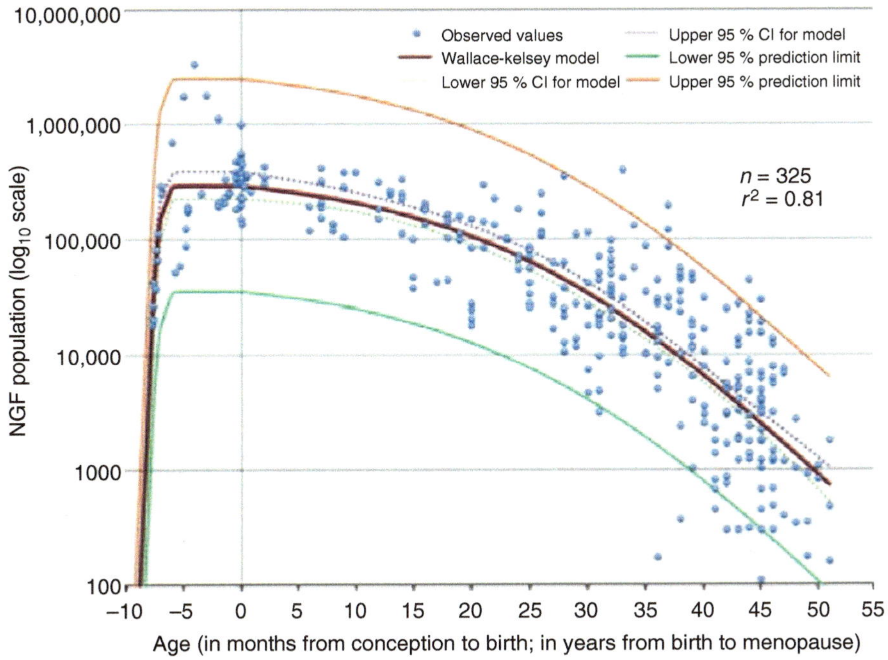

Fig. 11.8 The number of nongrowing follicles in the ovary is increasing as a function of time. Inversely, the number of potentially fertile promordial follicle available for recruitment is decreasing already before birth

oxidative damage in somatic and germ cells. Persistent unrepaired DNA double-strand breaks activate apoptotic death in oocytes. Genetic effects on the oocyte result in aneuploidy and early embryonic mortality.

In contrast to the effects on male fertility, females are, in general, less susceptible to the gonadotoxic effects of chemotherapy [130]. The clinical impact of chemotherapeutic drugs on the ovary is variable, ranging from no effect to complete ovarian atrophy. The degree of damage is dependent upon the type of the chemotherapeutic agent used, dose given, age of the patient and her baseline ovarian reserve. The prepubertal ovary is less susceptible to damage by chemotherapeutic agents. Compared to older women, early postpubertal adolescents have a higher ovarian reserve and are less susceptible to premature ovarian failure (POF). Fibrosis of stromal blood vessels adds to the ovarian damage.

Depending on the chemotherapy used, the clinical manifestation of the follicular loss ranges from a complete amenorrhea to POF and to varying degree of infertility (Table 11.9) [131]. Some paediatric chemotherapy regimens such as MOPP (mustagen, oncovin, procarbazine, and prednisone) for Hodgkin's disease, and high-dose cyclophosphamide and busulfan for bone marrow transplantation, cause sterility in a significant number of patients. Other regimens such as high dose cyclophosphamide for B-NHL and Ewing sarcoma are associated with a significant risk for fertility impairment [131]. Because no systematic comprehensive data exists on the exact rates of fertility impairment associated with current paediatric oncology therapeutic regimens, the following grading of the damaging potential is derived from adult data [125, 132]:

Alkylating agents such as cyclophosphamide and procarbazine are high risk drugs with the highest age-adjusted odds ratio of ovarian failure rates.

Platinum-based compounds such as cisplatin cause DNA damage. They carry a medium risk of amenorrhea.

Anthracycline antibiotics such as doxorubicin (DXR) induce oxidative stress. The amenorrhea and fertility risk is medium to low with this group of drugs. DXR administration in female mice caused dominant lethal mutations and aneuploidy in maturing/preovulatory oocytes.

Vinca alkaloids do not seem to increase the risk of ovarian failure though animal experiments show a high rate of oocyte aneuploidy.

Anti-metabolites like methotrexate and 5-fluorouracil do not seem to affect the ovary based on the limited current data available. Methotrexate is commonly used to treat the ectopic pregnancy without any effect on subsequent fertility.

Taxanes: The data available for taxanes are controversial. Some studies show increased risk of ovarian failure, others suggest that there is no increased risk.

Biological targeted therapies (herceptin, tamoxifen, rituximab) are designed to interfere with specific receptors or molecules expressed by tumours (herceptin or tamoxifen), or act via the immune system (rituximab). Fertility risk data for these drugs are limited. Since they target specific cells, it is believed that the risk should be low.

The risk of POF with polyagent adjuvant chemotherapy has been reported to range from 53 to 89 %. The risk of POF is related to the patient's age, treatment protocol and type of malignancy [125]. Restoration of menstruation after CRA is possible. Again this is influenced by age and duration of follow-up and has been estimated at 39–55 % in younger women (<40 years) and 0–11 % in older patients (>40 years) [133]. However, women who maintain normal menses throughout

Table 11.9 Gonadotoxic chemotherapy agents

Alkylating agents
Cyclophosphamide
Ifosfamide
Nitrosureas, e.g., carmustine and lamustine
Chlorambucil
Melphalan
Busulphan
Vinca-alkaloids
Vinblastine
Antimetabolites
Cytarabine
Others
Cisplatin
Procarbazine

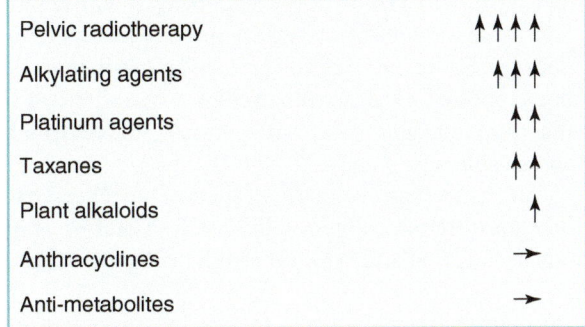

Toxicity of different oncological chemotherapies on ovarian reserve

Pelvic radiotherapy	↑↑↑↑
Alkylating agents	↑↑↑
Platinum agents	↑↑
Taxanes	↑↑
Plant alkaloids	↑
Anthracyclines	→
Anti-metabolites	→

Fig. 11.9 Comparison of the ovarian toxicity exerted by the main groups of cytotoxic drugs with the damaging effect of pelvic radiotherapy. The number of *arrows* indicates their relative potency. No particular risk is known for substances marked by a *horizontal arrow* (Modified from Meirow et al. [131])

chemotherapy remain at risk for developing POF. This is evident from the high rates of POF seen in adolescents receiving alkylating agents for cancer [134]. There are no reports of uterine damage after chemotherapy [135] (Fig. 11.9).

Effect of Radiotherapy

Unlike chemotherapy, radiotherapy affects both the ovary and the uterus [129].

Human oocyte is sensitive to radiation, with an estimated median lethal dose (LD) of <2 Gy. Damage to the ovary by radiotherapy is dependent on the age of the patient and dose of the ovarian exposure. The effective sterilizing dose (ESD) is the dose of fractionated radiotherapy (Gy) at which POF occurs immediately after treatment in 97.5 % of patients. The degree of damage depends on the radiation dose and field, fractionation schedule, and the patient's age. A radiation dose of 2 Gy is estimated to damage 50 % of ovarian follicles irreversibly; doses ranging from 5 to 20 Gy cause complete loss of ovarian function resulting in sterility [136]. The number of primordial follicles present at the time of treatment and the dose of radiation received by the ovaries determines the fertility "window." In females, it has been shown that for a given dose of radiation, the younger the patient at the time of treatment, the later the onset of premature menopause, and inversely, the higher ESD to cause permanent ovarian failure [131, 132, 136, 137]: ESD is 20.3 Gy at birth, 18.4 Gy at 10 years, 16.5 Gy at 20 years, and 14.3–16 Gy at 30 years, with only 6 Gy being required in women over 40. With total body irradiation, the location of the radiation field impacts the degree of ovarian damage (10–15.75 Gy) observed to result in ovarian failure in 90 % of patients in long-term follow-up. After abdominal radiation, ovarian failure rates may be as high as 97 %. [131].

After abdominal, pelvic, or TBI, the uterus is at risk of damage in a dose- and age-dependent manner [135]. Uterine growth and uterine blood flow start at puberty and are completed almost 7 years after menarche. Exposure to radiation leads to reduced vascularity, damage to myometrium leading to fibrosis and hormone dependent endometrial insufficiency. These uterine damages result in adverse reproductive outcomes such as increased rates of infertility, miscarriage, preterm labour, intra-uterine growth retardation and low birth weight.

Uterine function may be impaired after radiation doses of 14–30 Gy as a consequence of disruption to the uterine vasculature and musculature elasticity. In adults, an exposure to TBI of 12 Gy is associated with significant uterine damage. In childhood, radiation doses of >25 Gy directly to the uterus appears to induce irreversible damage. However, even lower dose of irradiation, as in total body irradiation, have been reported to cause impaired growth and blood flow. There is no agreement on the dose of radiation to the uterus, above which a pregnancy would not be sustainable.

Efforts to improve uterine function have been tried. However, there was no significant difference noted with regard to uterine volume, endometrial thickness, or uterine artery blood flow after high dose oestrogen replacement.

Preventive measure Ovarian transposition has been recommended to get the ovary out of the radiation field (laparoscopic "ovarian suspension" or "oophoropexy"; [132]).

Estimation of the Damage Induced by Chemotherapy and Radiotherapy by Biological Markers and By Sonography

In a prospective cohort study on girls treated for cancer, AMH, inhibin B, and FSH have been measured before, during, and after completion of treatment [138]. The aim of our study was to evaluate these biochemical measures as potential markers of early gonadotoxicity in young girls treated for cancer. As a result, AMH has been shown to be a clinically useful marker of damage to the ovarian reserve in girls receiving treatment for cancer. AMH is detectable in girls of all ages and falls rapidly during cancer treatment in both prepubertal and pubertal girls [138, 139]. Both the fall during treatment and recovery thereafter varied with risk of gonadotoxicity. In medium/low risk patients, AMH recovery is highly significant and reaches pretreatment levels [139]. The value of FSH and Inhibin B as markers of ovarian activity is limited by very low/undetectable concentrations before puberty and the need for measurement in the early follicular phase thereafter [129, 138].

The number of small antral follicles within the ovary (AFC) counted by transvaginal ultrasound, too, provide substantially more accurate indicators than FSH (or inhibin B) of what is known as the ovarian reserve. AFC allows to mean the number of primordial follicles remaining in the ovary. Both AMH and AFC show very good correlation with oocyte yield following superovulation needed for mature oocyte preservation, with a very high correlation between the two [129]. Today, this elegant method is not yet validated for abdominal transvesical ultrasound in prepubertal children.

The assessment of ovarian reserve in the prepubertal girl who has been successfully treated for cancer remains difficult. Larsen et al. evaluated ovarian function in 100 childhood cancer survivors and 21 controls of similar age [140]. Survivors with spontaneous menstrual cycles ($n=70$) were found to have smaller ovarian volume per ovary compared with controls (median, 4.8 cm^3 vs. 6.8 cm^3; $P<.001$) and a lower number of antral follicles (AFC) per ovary (median, 7.5 AFC vs. 11 AFC; $P<.001$). A regression analysis was performed to predict the total AFC number per ovary, which demonstrated a reduced number in women who were treated with ovarian irradiation (beta=−.40; $P<.001$), alkylating chemotherapy (beta=−.25; $P=.01$), older age at diagnosis (beta=−.25; $P=.01$), and longer time period off treatment (beta=−.19; $P=.044$) [140].

Fertility Preservation in Young Girls and in Adolescents

Oncological Indications

In general, fertility preservation before cancer treatment is strongly recommended if the chance of losing fertility is over 30 % with cancer therapy. In adult patients that have a partner, cryopreservation of embryos remains the most reliable method to preserve fertility in women < 35 years of age. Another efficient option is vitrification of mature unfertilized oocytes. Today, an extensive database is available for adult cancer patients [107, 141].

Children and adolescents represent a special patient group. Jadoul et al. published in 2010 an important review of ovarian cryopreservation in adults and, more specifically, in children using the PubMed databases and added their own experience with cryopreservation in children [108]. They conclude that ovarian cortex cryopreservation is feasible and as safe as comparable operative procedures in children. However, the absence of consensus on the indications for fertility preservation, as well as the optimal timing and quantity of ovarian cortex for cryopreservation, should be taken into consideration when discussing fertility issues with girls at risk of POF and their parents.

Cryopreservation of embryos and vitrification of mature unfertilized oocytes require both hormonal stimulation and delay of treatment; thus, they cannot be offered to prepubertal patients and to adolescents that must receive urgent treatment. Therefore, cryopreservation of gonadal tissue is the only option today to be offered to young prepubertal girls with malignancies that require gonadotoxic therapy [108, 129], although no births have yet resulted from freeze-thawing of prepubertal ovarian cortex.

Wallace et al. recommended the following risk assessment for fertility preservation in girls [146]:

- Intrinsic factors
  Health status of patient
  Consent (patient/parent)
  Assessment of ovarian reserve in girls/young women
- Extrinsic factors
  Nature of predicted treatment (high/medium/low/uncertain risk)
  Time available
  Expertise available

A series of women having undergone ovarian cryopreservation has shown that these patients did not necessarily need reimplantation of the ovarian tissue to get pregnant. Of the 36 women treated by cytostatic agents (20 % by cyclophosphamide because of generalized Lupus erythematodes), 11 had died at the time of last follow-up, but 5 experienced spontaneous pregnancies, with none to date having requested reimplantation of their stored ovarian tissue [142].

Is there a lower limit of age? Michaeli et al. [143] consider that ovary cryopreservation can be safely offered even to younger girls since the potential benefits are currently more evident and the risks of anaesthesia appear not to be increased, although they earlier recommended a lower limit of 3 years of age. They believe that there is an ethical obligation of clinicians to offer fertility preservation and to discuss fertility issues with cancer patients or their parents, in order to provide the opportunity for future parenthood.

Postpubertal girls from puberty to the age of 18 may be candidates for mature oocyte cryopreservation following ovarian stimulation.

The exact procedures for these modern techniques of fertility preservation including the benefits and risks of later autotransplantation of ovarian tissue as well as pregnancy outcome in high-risk survivors of cancer are summarized in specialized reviews [107, 108, 129, 132, 135, 138–140, 143].

Non-Oncological Indications

Non-oncological indications for fertility preservation procedures include haematological or autoimmune diseases, as well as certain genetic conditions such as Fragile-X and Turner syndrome, which predispose women to premature ovarian failure. In addition, repeated surgery due to ovarian cysts or ovarian torsion may result in decreased ovarian reserve [108].

Ethical Considerations

There is a need for extreme sensitivity when broaching the topic of fertility preservation. This also may be an option for adolescents who are peripubertal, but still premenarchal. In vitro maturation (IVM) and ovarian tissue conservation (OTC) can also be offered. In prepubertal girls, OTC is currently the only way to cryopreserve gametes. Careful counselling and informed consent is especially recommended. In children, OTC implies the removal of an entire ovary because of its small size. Prepubertal girls who do not have any other options have to be informed about a high risk for POF when significant loss of ovarian follicles in the remaining ovary is anticipated with cancer therapy.

Parents have to be given full information of the invasive process needing a total anaesthesia, the associated risks and the success rates. The patient and her parents should understand the still experimental nature and the potential risks of cancer cell transmission.

Wallace et al. recommend applying the Edinburgh selection criteria to young girls and adolescents. The Edinburgh selection criteria accurately identify the few girls and young women who will develop premature ovarian insufficiency. They have been validated recently for their use for selection of patients for ovarian tissue cryopreservation [144]:

- Age younger than 35 years
- No previous chemotherapy or radiotherapy if aged 15 years or older at diagnosis, but mild, non-gonadotoxic chemotherapy acceptable if younger than 15 years

- A realistic chance of surviving for 5 years
- A high risk of premature ovarian insufficiency (>50 %)
- Informed consent (from parents and, where possible, patient)
- Negative serology results for HIV, syphilis, and hepatitis B
- Not pregnant and no existing children

It has always to be kept in mind that these procedures are in part still experimental and not yet clinical routine. As Wallace and Barr stated recently, it is not likely to be feasible or indeed ethical to perform a randomized study in a well-characterized group of young women to test laparoscopic collection of ovarian cortex versus either dummy laparoscopy or indeed no intervention. In their opinion, and in mine too, it is highly unlikely that IRBs would pass such a study, or indeed that such a randomized study would be able to recruit sufficient patients [145]. Therefore, all treatments for fertility preservation in young girls and adolescents should be done in accredited centres, documented and the data pooled so that a true and accurate description of the success of ovarian cryopreservation for young women at risk of a premature menopause can be provided.

Acquired Delayed Puberty and Reduced Fertility Due to Other Causes

Ovarian Torsion and Gonadectomy

Usually, ovarian torsion and gonadectomy are listed in this category. However, unilateral loss of an ovary by torsion or gonadectomy has no impact on the age of puberty and on later fertility.

The loss of both ovaries implies a timely induction of puberty by the slowly progressive administration of oestradiol and, in a second time, oestradiol combined with a progestatif. Fertility can be reached only by egg or embryo donation if these methods are legal in the country where the patient is living.

Autoimmune Diseases

In young girls and in adolescents, endocrine and non-endocrine autoimmune diseases involving the ovary and provoking a progressive destruction of the ovarian tissue may cause exceptionally a delayed puberty. The more common physiopathology leading to a delayed puberty in presence of an autoimmune disease involves functional hypothalamic hypogonadism (see above).

However, there are reports showing an early progressive destruction of the ovarian tissue by autoimmune processes, mainly in young girls and adolescents suffering from generalized lupus erythematodes [142, 146]. Later infertility can be prevented by applying the same methods of cryopreservation of ovarian tissue recommended for young cancer patients (see above).

Endocrine Disruptors

There have been speculations about a potential responsibility of endocrine disruptors in causing delayed puberty. However, ES have been shown mostly to advance and less to delay puberty. The potential of EDs to cause precocious puberty has first been noticed in the early 1990s and has been confirmed in numerous animal studies. Subsequently, the use of some of these substances has been prohibited in products used by humans and domestic animals.

In the last years, several environmental endocrine disruptors (EDs) such as phytooestrogens, topical and natural oestrogens, pesticides, industrial chemicals and phthalates have been identified as possible agents affecting pubertal development in humans in different ways [148, 149]. EDs exert their effects through different mechanisms: by binding to the relevant hormone receptors; by direct action on cell signalling pathways or on the central nervous system and the neuroendocrine system, by suppression of hormone synthesis or through their toxic effects on the relevant organs. ES may influence puberty through their oestrogenic, antioestrogenic, androgenic, antiandrogenic effects or through their direct effects on the gonadotropin-releasing hormone (GnRH). EDs may affect puberty by inhibiting the synthesis of endogenous hormones such as testosterone, 17 beta-oestradiol and adrenal steroids via competitive inhibition of P450 steroidogenic enzymes (C17,20-lyase, aromatase). Other environmental chemicals may impair neuroendocrine functions through their effect on the central nervous system and the hypothalamic-hypophyseal-gonadal (HHG) axis. These include pesticides such as thiram, molinate, metam sodium, chlordimeform, amitraz, triazoles, dichloroacetic acid, atrazine, propazine, simazine, methanol and linuron. Depending on their mechanism of action, EDs may lead to precocious puberty, to delayed puberty, or to sexual differentiation disorders.

However, in humans, most known ES exposures lead to early pubarche and menarche in girls.

Delayed puberty has been reported by exposure to imidazole group fungicides, ketoconazole and fadrozole in the peripubertal period in animals. In a study on rats, atrazine caused delayed puberty by suppressing luteinizing hormone (LH) and prolactin levels. Another pesticide, prochloraz, suppresses oestrogen and androgen synthesis via inhibition of aromatase and 17,20-lyase [148].

In humans, Den Hond et al. [150] observed a reduction in testicular volume in boys and a delay in telarche in girls exposed to a substance with dioxin-like activity, but failed to note a change in pubertal development, or a change in the age of pubarche or menarche. Another study confirmed the relation between prenatal PCDD/F exposure and later initiation of breast development [151].

The heavy metal lead, one of the major environmental pollutants, has also been found to affect puberty [149, 152, 153]. Menarche and pubarche were delayed in girls with high serum lead levels. In addition, blood lead concentration was inversely and significantly associated with IQ. In the linear model, each increase of 10 μg per deciliter in the lifetime average blood lead concentration was associated with a 4.6-point decrease in IQ ($P = 0.004$). When estimated in a nonlinear model with the full sample, IQ declined by 7.4 points as lifetime average blood lead concentrations increased from 1 to 10 μg per deciliter [154].

In conclusion, there are several alarming reports showing that ES and the heavy metal lead influence pubertal development. The only way to stop this inacceptable poisoning of animals and of humans is the strict observance and enforcement of the already existing legal prescriptions and the targeted formulations of new laws protecting the environment against endocrine disruptors.

References

1. Marshall WA, Tanner JM (1970) Variations in the pattern of pubertal changes in boys. Arch Dis Child 45:13–23
2. Lee PA (1980) Normal ages of pubertal events among American males and females. J Adolesc Health Care 1:26–29
3. Speroff, Fritz (2005) Clinical gynecological endocrinology and infertility, 7th edn, LipinCott, Williams & Wilkins, Philadelphia
4. Largo RH, Prader A (1983) Pubertal development in Swiss girls. Helv Paediatr Acta 38(3):229–243
5. Tanner JM (1962) Growth at adolescence. Charles C Thomas, Springfield
6. Stavrou I, Zois C, Ioannidis JPA, Tsatsoulis A (2002) Association of polymorphisms of the estrogen receptor gene with the age of menarche. Hum Reprod 17:1101–1105
7. Parent A-S, Teilmann G, Juul A, Skakkebaek NE, Toppari J, Bourguignon J-P (2003) The timing of normal puberty and the age limits of sexual precocity: variations around the world, secular trends, and changes after migration. Endocr Rev 24(5):668–693
8. Kaplan SL, Grumbach MM (1990) Pathogenesis of sexual precocity. In: Grumbach MM, Sizonenko PC, Aubert ML (eds) Control of the onset of puberty. Williams and Wilkins, Baltimore, pp 620–660
9. Smail PJ, Faiman C, Hobson WC et al (1982) Further studies on adrenarche in nonhuman primates. Endocrinology 111:844–848
10. Ebling FJP, Cronin AS (2000) The neurobiology of reproductive development. Neuroreport 11:R23–R33
11. Bourguignon JP, Lebrethon MC (2000) Le primum movens du déclenchement puber-taire: signaux hypothalamiques, périphériques et environnementaux. J Gynecol Obstet Biol Reprod 29:295–297
12. Smith R, Mesiano S, Chan EC et al (1998) Corticotropin – releasing hormon directly and preferentially stimulates dehydroepiandrosterone sulfate secretion by human fetal adrenal cortical cells. J Clin Endocrinol Metab 83:2916–2920
13. Biason-Lauber A, Zachmann M, Schoenle EJ (2000) Effect of leptin on CYP17 enzymatic activities in human adrenal cells: new insight in the onset of adrenarche. Endocrinology 141:1446–1454
14. Crofton PM, Illingworth PJ, Groome NP et al (1997) Changes in dimeric inhibin A and B during normal early puberty in boys and girls. Clin Endocrinol 46(1):109–114
15. Leyendecker G, Wildt L (1996) From physiology to clinics – 29 years of experience with pulsatile GnRH. Eur J Obstet Gynecol Reprod Biol 65:S3–S12
16. Leyendecker G (1978) Die normoprolaktinämische sekundäre Ovarialinsuffizienz; Pathophysiologie, Diagnostik und Therapie. Arch Gynecol 228:503–517
17. Hadžiomerović D, Wildt L (2006) Hypothalamische Ovarialinsuffizienz. Gynäkologische Endokrinologie 4:27–32
18. Ojeda SR, Hill J, Hill DF et al (1999) The Oct-2 POU-domain gene in the neuroendocrine brain: a transcriptional regulator of mammalian puberty. Endocrinology 140:3774–3789
19. Lee BJ, Cho GJ, Norgren R et al (2001) TTF-1, a homeodomain gene required for diencephalic morphogenesis, is postnatally expressed in the neuroendocrine brain in a developmentally regulated and cell-specific fashion. Mol Cell Neurosci 17:107–126

20. Rampazzo A, Pivotto F, Occhi G et al (2000) Characterization of C14orf4, a novel intron-less human gene containing a polyglutamine repeat, mapped to the ARVD1 critical region. Biochem Biophys Res Commun 278:766–774
21. Heger S, Mastronardi C, Dissen GA et al (2007) Enhanced at puberty 1 (EAP1) is a new transcriptional regulator of the female neuroendocrine reproductive axis. J Clin Invest 117(8):2145–2154
22. Ohtaki T, Shintani Y, Honda S et al (2001) Metastasis suppressor gene KiSS-1 encodes peptides ligand of a G-protein-coupled receptor. Nature 411:613–617
23. Steeg PS, Ouatas T, Halverson D et al (2003) Metastasis suppressor genes : basic biology and potential clinical use. Clin Breast Cancer 4:51–62
24. Shahab M, Mastronardi C, Seminara SB et al (2005) Increased hypothalamic GPR-54 signaling: a potential mechanism for initiation of puberty in primates. Proc Natl Acad Sci U S A 102:2129–2134
25. Irwig MS, Fraley GS, Smith JT et al (2005) Kisspeptin activation of gonadotropine releasing hormone neurons and regulation of KiSS-1 mRNA in the male rat. Neuroendocrinology 80:264–272
26. Gottsch ML, Cunninghanam MJ, Smith JT et al (2004) A role for kisspeptins in the regulation of gonadotropine secretion in the mouse. Endocrinology 145:4073–4077
27. Muir AI, Chamberlain L, Elshourbagy NA et al (2001) AXOR12, a novel human G protein-coupled receptor, activated by the peptide KiSS-1. J Biol Chem 276:28969–28975
28. Kotani M, Detheux M, Vandenbogaerde A et al (2001) The metastasis suppressor genes KiSS-1 encodes kisspeptins, the naturals ligands of the orphan G protein-coupled receptor GPR54. J Biol Chem 276:34631–34636
29. Tena-Sempere M (2006) GPR54 and kisspeptin in reproduction. Hum Reprod Update 12:631–639
30. Navarro VM, Castellano JM, Fernandez-Fernandez R et al (2004) Advanced vaginal opening and precocious activation of the reproductive axis by KiSS-1 peptide, the endogenous ligand of GPR54. J Physiol 561:379–386
31. Han SK, Gottsch ML, Lee KJ et al (2005) Activation of gonadotropin-releasing hormone neurons by kisspeptin as a neuroendocrine switch for the onset of puberty. J Neurosci 25:11349–11356
32. Smith JT, Cunningham MJ, Rissman EF et al (2005) Regulation of Kiss1 gene expression in the brain of the female mouse. Endocrinology 146:3686–3692
33. Smith JT, Dungan HM, Stol EA et al (2005) Differential regulation of KiSS-1 mRNA expression by sex steroids in the brain of the male mouse. Endocrinology 146:2976–2984
34. Castellano JM, Navarro VM, Fernandez-Fernandez R et al (2005) Changes in hypothalamic KiSS-1 system and restoration of pubertal activation of the reproductive axis by kisspeptin in undernutrition. Endocrinology 146:3917–3925
35. Cunningham MJ, Clifton DK, Steiner RA (1999) Leptin's actions on the reproductive axis: perspectives and mechanisms. Biol Reprod 60:616–622
36. Ojeda SR, Lomniczi A, Mastronardi C (2006) Minireview: the neuroendocrine regulation of puberty: is the time ripe for a systems biology approach? Endocrinology 147: 1166–1174
37. Tena-Sempere M (2005) Hypothalamic KiSS-1: the missing link in gonadotropine feed-back control? Endocrinology 146:3683–3685
38. Clement K, Vaisse C, Lahlou N et al (1998) A mutation in the human leptin receptor gene causes obesity and pituitary dysfunction. Nature 392:398–401
39. Azziz R (1989) Reproductive endocrinologic alterations in female asymptomatic obesity. Fertil Steril 52:703–725
40. Bussen S, Sutterlin M, Steck T (1999) Endocrine abnormalities during the follicular phase in women with recurrent spontaneous abortion. Hum Reprod 14:18–20
41. Mann DR, Johnson A, Gimpel T, Castracane D (2003) Changes in circulating leptin, leptin receptor, and gonadal hormones from infancy until advanced age in humans. J Clin Endocrinol Metab 88:3339–3345

42. Grumbach MM, Styne DM (1998) Puberty: ontogeny, neuroendocrinology, physiology, and disorders. In: Wilson JD, Foster DW, Kronenberg HM, Larsen PR (eds) Williams textbook of endocrinology, 9th edn. WB Saunders Company, Philadelphia, pp 1509–1625
43. Byrd W, Bennett MJ, Carr BR, Dong Y, Wians F, Rainey W (1998) Regulation of biologically active dimeric inhibin A and B from infancy to adulthood in the male. J Clin Endocrinol Metab 83(8):2849–2854
44. Phillips DJ, de Kretser DM (1998) Follistatin: a multifunctional regulatory protein. Front Neuroendocrinol 19:287–322
45. Foster CM, Phillips DJ, Wyman T, Evans LW, Groome NP, Padmanabhan V (2000) Changes in serum inhibin, activin and follistatin concentrations during puberty in girls. Hum Reprod 15(5):1052–1057
46. Meachem SJ, Nieschlag E, Simoni M (2001) Inhibin B in male reproduction: pathophysiology and clinical relevance. Eur J Endocrinol 145:561–571
47. Horlick MB, Rosenbaum MN, Levine LS et al (2000) Effect of puberty on the relationship between circulating leptin and body composition. J Clin Endocrinol Metab 85:2509–2518
48. Ghizzoni L, Barreca A, Mastorakos G et al (2001) Leptin inhibits steroid biosynthesis by human granulosa-lutein cells. Horm Metab Res 33:323–328
49. Ibanez L, Virdis R, Potau N et al (1992) Natural history of premature pubarche : an auxological study. J Clin Endocrinol Metab 74:254–257
50. Wickman S, Saukkonen T, Dunkel L (2002) The role of sex steroids in the regulation of insulin sensitivity and serum lipid concentrations during male puberty: a prospective study with a P450-aromatase inhibitor. Eur J Endocrinol 146:339–346
51. Bottner A, Kratzsch J, Muller G, Kapellen TM, Bluher S, Keller E, Bluher M, Kiess W (2004) Gender differences of adiponectin levels develop during the progression of puberty and are related to serum androgen levels. J Clin Endocrinol Metab 89:4053–4061
52. Winter S, Ousidhoum A, McElreavey K, Raja Brauner R (2016) Constitutional delay of puberty: presentation and inheritance pattern in 48 familial cases. BMC Pediatr 16:37–44
53. Herman-Giddens ME, Slora EJ, Wasserman RC et al (1997) Secondary sexual characteristics and menses in young girls seen in office practice: a study from the pediatric research in office settings network. Pediatrics 99:505–512
54. Kaplowitz PB, Oberfield SE, Drug and Therapeutics and Executive Committees of the Lawson Wilkins Pediatric Endocrine Society (1999) Reexamination of the age limit for defining when puberty is precocious in girls in the United States: implications for evaluation and treatment. Pediatrics 104:936–941
55. Brämswig J, Dübbers A (2009) Disorders of pubertal development. Dtsch Arztebl Int 106(17):295–304
56. Kaplowitz P (2004) Clinical characteristics of 104 children referred for evaluation of precocious puberty. J Clin Endocrinol Metab 89:3644–3650
57. Kahl HSRA, Schlaud M (2007) Sexuelle Reifung von Kindern und Jugendlichen in Deutschland. Ergebnisse des Kinder- und Jugendgesundheitssurveys (KiGGS). Bundesgesundheitsbl-Gesundheitsforsch-Gesundheitsschutz 50:677–685
58. Reindollar RH, Tho SPT, McDonough PG (1989) Delayed puberty: an updated study of 326 patients. Trans Am Gynecol Obstet Soc 8:146–162
59. Harrington J, Palmert MR (2012) Distinguishing constitutional delay of growth and puberty from isolated hypogonadotropic hypogonadism: critical appraisal of available diagnostic tests. J Clin Endocrinol Metab 97:3056–3067
60. Lunsford AJ, Whelan K, McCormick K, McLaren JF (2014) Antimüllerian hormone as a measure of reproductive function in female childhood cancer survivors. Fertil Steril 101:227–231. pii: S0015-0282(13)03018-5
61. Traggiai C, Stanhope R (2003) Disorders of pubertal development. Best Pract Res Clin Obstet Gynaecol 17(1):41–56
62. Yollin E, Jonard S, Reyss A-C et al (2006) Delayed puberty with extreme uterine hypotrophy: do not conclude too early to the absence of the uterus. Gynecol Obstet Fertil 34:1029–1035

63. Stanhope R, Adams J, Jacobs HS, Brook CG (1985) Ovarian ultrasound assessment in normal children, idiopathic precocious puberty, and during low-dose pulsatile gonadotrophin-releasing hormone treatment of hypogonadotrophic hypogonadism. Arch Dis Child 60:116–119
64. Dwyer AA, Phan-Hug F, Hauschild M, Elowe-Gruau E, Pitteloud N (2015) Hypogonadism in adolescence. Eur J Endocrinol 173:R15–R24
65. Palmert MR, Dunkel L (2012) Clinical practice. Delayed puberty. N Engl J Med 366:443–453
66. Sedlmeyer IL, Palmert MR (2002) Delayed puberty: analysis of a large case series from an academic center. J Clin Endocrinol Metabol 87:1613–1620
67. Bonjour J-P (1998) Delayed puberty and peak bone mass. Eur J Endocrinol 139:257–259
68. Bertelloni S, Baroncelli GI, Ferdeghini M, Perri G, Maggese G (1998) Normal volumetric bone mineral density and bone turnover in young men with histories of constitutional delay of puberty. J Clin Endocrinol Metab 83:4280–4283
69. Gourmelen M, Pham-Huu-Trung MT, Girard F (1979) Transient partial GH deficiency in prepubertal children with delay of growth. Pediatr Res 13:221–224
70. Lanes R, Bohorquez MDSL, Leal V, Hernandez G, Borges M, Hurtado E et al (1986) Growth hormone secretion in patients with constitutional delay of growth and pubertal development. J Pediatr 109:781–783
71. Reiter EO, Lee PA (2002) Delayed puberty. Adolesc Med 13(1):101–118
72. Reiter EO, Kaplan SL, Conte FA, Grumbach MM (1975) Resposivity of pituitary gonadotropins to luteinizing hormone-releasing factor in idiopathic precocious puberty, precocious thelarche, precocious adrenarche and in patients treated with medroxyprogesterone acetate. Pediatr Res 9:111–115
73. Bierich JR (1989) Therapy with growth hormone – old and new indications. Horm Res 32:153–165
74. Loche S, Cambiaso M, Setzu S et al (1994) Final height after growth hormone therapy in non-growth-hormone-deficient children with short stature. J Pediatr 125:196–200
75. Bernasconi S, Street ME, Volta C, Mazzardo G (1997) Final height in non-growth hor-mone deficient children treated with growth hormone. The Italian multicentre study group. Clin Endocrinol 47(3):261–266
76. Quinton R, Duke VM, Robertson A et al (2001) Idiopathic gonadotrophin deficiency: genetic questions addressed through phenotypic characterization. Clin Endocrinol (Oxf) 55:163–174
77. Brioude F, Bouligand J, Trabado S et al (2010) Non- syndromic congenital hypogonadotropic hypogonadism: clinical presentation and genotype–phenotype relationships. Eur J Endocrinol 162:835–851
78. Lewkowitz-Shpuntoff HM, Hughes VA, Plummer L et al (2012) Olfactory phenotypic spectrum in idiopathic hypogonadotropic hypogonadism: pathophysiological and genetic implications. J Clin Endocrinol Metabol 97:E136–E144
79. de Morsier G (1962) Median cranioencephalic dysraphias and olfactogenital dysplasias. World Neurol 3:485–506
80. Villanueva C, Argente J (2014) Pathology or normal variant: what constitutes a delay in puberty? Horm Res Paediatr 82:213–221
81. Mitchell AL, Dwyer A, Pitteloud N, Quinton R (2011) Genetic basis and variable phenotypic expression of Kallmann syndrome: towards a unifying theory. Trends Endocrinol Metab 22:249–258
82. Raivio T, Avbelj M, McCabe MJ, Romero CJ, Dwyer AA, Tommiska J, Sykiotis GP, Gregory LC, Diaczok D, Tziaferi V et al (2012) Genetic overlap in Kallmann syndrome, combined pituitary hormone deficiency, and septo-optic dysplasia. J Clin Endocrinol Metabol 97:E694–E699
83. Jongmans MC, van Ravenswaaij-Arts CM, Pitteloud N, Ogata T, Sato N, Claahsen-van der Grinten HL, van der Donk K, Seminara S, Bergman JE, Brunner HG et al (2009) CHD7 mutations in patients initially diagnosed with Kallmann syndrome-the clinical overlap with CHARGE syndrome. Clin Genet 75:65–71

84. Thébaut A, Amouyal M, Besançon A et al (2013) Puberty, fertility and chronic diseases. Arch Pediatr 20(6):673–684
85. Codner E, Merino PM, Tena-Sempere M (2012) Female reproduction and type 1 diabetes: from mechanisms to clinical findings. Hum Reprod Update 18:568–585
86. Schweiger BM, Snell-Bergeon JK, Roman R et al (2011) Menarche delay and menstrual irregularities persist in adolescents with type 1 diabetes. Reprod Biol Endocrinol 9:61–68
87. Munoz MT, Argente J (2002) Anorexia nervosa in female adolescents: endocrine and bone mineral density disturbances. Eur J Endocrinol 147:275–286
88. Roth D, Meyer Egli C, Kriemler S, Birkhäuser M et al (2000) Female athlete triad. Schweizerische Zeitschrift für Sportmedizin und Sporttraumatologie 48(3):119–132
89. Jackman S, Diamond F (2013) Pituitary adenomas in childhood and adolescence. Pediatr Endocrinol Rev 10:450–459
90. Armstrong GT, Chow EJ, Sklar CA (2009) Alterations in pubertal timing following therapy for childhood malignancies. Endocr Dev 15:25–39
91. Muller J (2002) Disturbance of pubertal development after cancer treatment. Best practice & research. Clin Endocrinol Metab 16:91–103
92. Lenz AM, Root AW (2012) Empty sella syndrome. Pediatr Endocrinol Rev 9(4):710–715
93. Colao A, Savastano S (2011) Medical treatment of prolactinomas. Nat Rev Endocrinol 7:267–278
94. Park JK, Lee EJ, Kim SH (2012) Optimal surgical approaches for Rathke cleft cyst with consideration of endocrine function. Neurosurgery 70:250–257
95. Zada G, Laws ER (2010) Surgical management of craniopharyngiomas in the pediatric population. Horm Res Paediatr 74:62–66
96. Chandler WF, Barkan AL (2008) Treatment of pituitary tumors: a surgical perspective. Endocrinol Metab Clin North Am 37:51–66
97. Easter A, Treasure J, Micali N (2011) Fertility and prenatal attitudes towards pregnancy in women with eating disorders: results from the Avon Longitudinal Study of Parents. BJOG 118(12):1491–1498
98. Bulik CM, Sullivan PF, Fear JL et al (1999) Fertility and reproduction in women with anorexia nervosa: a controlled study. J Clin Psychiatry 60(2):130–135
99. Micali N, dos-Santos-Silva I, De Stavola B et al (2014) Fertility treatment, twin births, and unplanned pregnancies in women with eating disorders: findings from a population-based birth cohort. BJOG 121:408–416
100. Leyendecker G, Wildt L (1982) Pulsatile treatment with gonadotropin-releasing hormone (Gn-Rh). Geburtsh Frauenheilk 42:689–699
101. Birkhäuser MH (1989) Pulsatile Therapie mit LH-RH. Arch Gynecol Obstet 246(Suppl 1):38–44
102. Lunenfeld B, Insler V (1995) In: Wallach EE, Zacur HE (eds) Reproductive medicine and surgery. Mosby-Year Book, St. Louis, p 617
103. Wildt L, Leyendecker G (1987) Induction of ovulation by the chronic administration of naltrexone in hypothalamic amerorrhea. J Clin Endocrinol Metabol 64:1334–1335
104. Bondy CA, The Turner Syndrome Consensus Study Group* Clinical Practice Guideline (2007) Care of girls and women with turner syndrome: a guideline of the turner syndrome study group. J Clin Endocrinol Metab 92:10–25
105. Gibbons B, Tan SY, Yu CC-W et al (1999) Risk of gonadoblastoma in female patients with Y chromosome abnormalities and dysgenetic gonads. J Paediatr Child Health 35:210–213
106. Meyer L, Birkhäuser MH, Bühler E, Pavic N (1989) Fertilität und Turner-Mosaik-Syndrom. Geburtsh Frauenheilk 49:825–829
107. von Wolff M et al (2015) Fertility-preservation counselling and treatment for medical reasons: data from a multinational network of over 5000 women. Reprod Biomed Online 31(5):605–612
108. Jadoul P, Dolmans MM, Donnez J (2010) Fertility preservation in girls during childhood: is it feasible, efficient and safe and to whom should it be proposed? Hum Reprod Update 16:617–630

109. Aittomäki K (1994) The genetics of XX gonadal dysgenesis. Am J Hum Genet 54:844–851
110. Hawkins JR, Taylor A, Goodfellow PN et al (1992) Evidence for increased prevalence of SRY mutations in XY females with complete rather than partial gonadal dysgenesis. Am J Hum Genet 51:979–984
111. Cornet D, Alvarez S, Antoine JM et al (1990) Pregnancies following ovum donation in gonadal dysgenesis. Hum Reprod 5(3):291–293
112. Ankarberg-Lindgren C, Westphal O, Dahlgren J (2011) Testicular size development and reproductive hormones in boys and adult males with Noonan syndrome: a longitudinal study. Eur J Endocrinol 165:137–144
113. Ineke van der Burgt I (2007) Review: Noonan syndrome. Orphanet J Rare Dis:2–4. doi:10.1186/1750-1172-2-4
114. Oakes MB, Eyvazzadeh AD, Quint E, Smith YR (2008) Complete androgen insensitivity syndrome—a review. J Pediatr Adolesc Gynecol 21:305–310
115. Toledo SPA, Bruner HG, Kraaij R et al (1996) An inactivating mutation of the LH receptor causes amenorrhea in a 46, XX female. J Clin Endocrinol Metab 82:3850–3854
116. Latronico AC, Arnhold IJ (2006) Inactivating mutations of LH and FSH receptors--from genotype to phenotype. Pediatr Endocrinol Rev 4:28–31
117. Huhtaniemi IT (2002) LH and FSH receptor mutations and their effects on puberty. Horm Res 57(suppl 2):35–38
118. Arnhold IJ, Lofrano-Porto A, Latronico AC (2009) Inactivating mutations of luteinizing hormone-subunit or luteinizing hormone receptor cause oligo-amenorrhea and infertility in women. Horm Res 71:75–82
119. Raga F, Bauset C, Remohi J et al (1997) Reproductive impact of congenital Müllerian anomalies. Hum Reprod 12:2277–2281
120. Aittomäki K, Herva R, Stenman U-H et al (1996) Clincal features of primary ovarian filkaure caused by a point mutation in the FSH receptor gene. J Clin Endocrinol Metab 81:3722–3726
121. Meduri G, Touraine P, Beau I et al (2003) Delayed puberty and primary amenorrhea associated with a novel mutation of the human follicle-stimulating hormone receptor: clinical, histological, and molecular studies. J Clin Endocrinol Metab 88:3491–3498
122. Achrekar SK, Modi DN, Meherji PK et al (2010) Follicle stimulating hormone receptor gene variants in women with primary and secondary amenorrhea. J Assist Reprod Genet 27:317–326
123. Fridovich-Keil J, Gubbels CS, Spencer JB et al (2011) Ovarian function in girls and women with GALT-deficiency galactosemia. Galactosemia J Inherit Metab Dis 34:357–366
124. Gubbels GC, Land JA, Rubio-Gozalbo ME (2008) Fertility and impact of pregnancies on the mother and child in classic galactosemia. Obstet Gynecol Surv 63(5):334–343
125. Singh KL, Davies M, Chatterjee R (2005) Fertility in female cancer survivors: pathophysiology, preservation and the role of ovarian reserve testing. Hum Reprod Update 11:69–89
126. Bath LE, Wallace WH, Critchley HO (2002) Late effects of the treatment of childhood cancer on the female reproductive system and the potential for fertility preservation. Br J Obstet Gynaecol 109:107–114
127. Smith MA, Seibel NL, Altekruse SF et al (2010) Outcomes for children and adolescents with cancer: challenges for the twenty-first century. J Clin Oncol 28:2625–2634
128. Green DM, Sklar CA, Boice CD et al (2009). Ovarian failure and reproductive outcomes after childhood cancer treatment: results from the Childhood Cancer Survivor study. Clin Oncol 27:2374–2381
129. Anderson RA, Wallace WHB (2011) Fertility preservation in girls and young women. Clin Endocrinol (Oxf) 75:409–419
130. Brougham MFH, Wallace WHB (2005) Subfertility in children and young people treated for solid and haematological malignancies. Br J Haematol 131:143–155

131. Meirow D, Biedermann H, Anderson RA, Wallace WHB (2010) Toxicity of chemotherapy and radiation on female reproduction. Clin Obstet Gynecol 53:727–739
132. Irtan S, Orbach D, Helfre S, Sarnacki S (2013) Ovarian transposition in prepubescent and adolescent girls with cancer. Lancet Oncol 14:601–608
133. Bines J, Oleske DM, Cobleigh MA (1996) Ovarian function in premenopausal women treated with adjuvant chemotherapy for breast cancer. J Clin Oncol 14:1718–1729
134. Byrne J, Fears TR, Gail MH et al (1992) Early menopause in long-term survivors of cancer during adolescence. Am J Obstet Gynecol 166:788–793
135. Wallace WHB (2011) Oncofertility and preservation of reproductive capacity in children and young adults. Cancer 117(10 suppl):2301–2310
136. Wallace WH, Thomson AB, Saran F, Kelsey TW (2005) Predicting age of ovarian failure after radiation to a field that includes the ovaries. Int J Radiat Oncol Biol Phys 62: 738–744
137. Wallace WH, Thomson AB, Kelsey TW (2003) The radiosensitivity of the human oocyte. Hum Reprod 18:117–121
138. Brougham MF, Crofton PM, Johnson EJ, Evans N, Anderson RA, Wallace WH (2012) Anti-Müllerian hormone is a marker of gonadotoxicity in pre- and postpubertal girls treated for cancer: a prospective study. J Clin Endocrinol Metab 97:2059–2067
139. Wallace WHB, Anderson RA (2013) Antimüllerian hormone, the assessment of the ovarian reserve, and the reproductive outcome of the young patient with cancer. Fertil Steril 99:1469–1475
140. Larsen EC, Muller J, Schmiegelow K, Rechnitzer C, Andersen AN (2003) Reduced ovarian function in long-term survivors of radiation- and chemotherapy-treated childhood cancer. J Clin Endocrinol Metab 88:5307–5314
141. von Wolff M (ed) (2016) Perspektive Fertilität Indikation und Durchführung fertilitätsprotektiver Massnahmen bei onkologischen und nicht-onkologischen Erkrankungen. Schmidt & Klaunig, Druckerei und Verlag, Kiel, 1. Auflage. ISBN-Nr.: 978-3-88312-127-7
142. Anderson RA, Wallace WH, Baird DT (2008) Ovarian cryopreservation for fertility preservation: indications and outcomes. Reproduction 136:681–689
143. Michaeli J, Weintraub M, Gross E et al (2012) Fertility preservation in girls. Obstet Gynecol Int 2012. Article ID 139193, 10 pages
144. Wallace WHB, Grove Smith A, Kelsey TW, Edgar AE, Anderson RA (2014) Fertility preservation for girls and young women with cancer: population-based validation of criteria for ovarian tissue cryopreservation. Lancet Oncol 15:1129–1136
145. Wallace WHB, Barr RD (2010) Fertility preservation for girls and young women with cancer: what are the remaining challenges? Hum Reprod Update 16:614–616
146. Oktem O et al (2015) Ovarian function and reproductive outcomes of female patients with systemic lupus erythematodes and the strategies to preserve their fertility. Obstet Gynecol Surv 70(3):196–210
147. Wallace WHB, Critchley HOD, Anderson RA (2012) Optimizing reproductive outcome in children and young people with cancer. J Clin Oncol 30:3–5
148. Oezen S, Darcan S (2011) Effects of environmental endocrine disruptors on pubertal development. J Clin Res Pediatr Endocrinol 3(1):1–6
149. Buck Louis GM, Gray LE, Marcus M et al (2008) Environmental factors and puberty timing: expert panel research needs. Pediatrics 121(Supplement 3):S192–S207
150. Den Hond E, Roels HA, Hoppenbrouwers K et al (2002) Sexual maturation in relation to polychlorinated aromatic hydrocarbons: Sharpe and Skakkebaek's hypothesis revisited. Environ Health Perspect 110:771–776
151. Leijs MM, Koppe JG, Olie K et al (2008) Delayed initiation of breast development in girls with higher prenatal dioxin exposure; a longitudinal cohort study. Chemosphere 37(6): 999–1004

152. Wu T, Buck GM, Mendola P (2003) Blood lead levels and sexual maturation in US girls: the Third National Health and Nutrition Examination Survey, 1988–1994. Environ Health Perspect 111:737–741
153. Selevan SG, Rice DC, Hogan KA, Euling SY, Pfahles-Hutchens A, Bethel J (2003) Blood lead concentration and delayed puberty in girls. N Engl J Med 348:1527–1536
154. Canfield RL, Henderson CR, Cory-Slechta DA et al (2003) Intellectual impairment in children with blood lead concentrations below 10 μg per deciliter. N Engl J Med 348(16):1517–1526
155. Beier KM, Bosinski HA, Loewit K (2005) Sexualmedizin, 2nd edn. Urban & Fischer, München
156. Leyendecker G, Wildt L, Plotz EJ (1982) Gynäkologe 14:84

Premature Ovarian Failure in Adolescence and Young Adults: From Diagnosis to Therapy and Follow-up for Fertility Preservation

12

Andrea Giannini, Andrea R. Genazzani, and Tommaso Simoncini

Primary ovarian failure (POF) is a subclass of ovarian dysfunction in which the cause is within the ovary. POF is a primary ovarian defect characterized by absent menarche (primary amenorrhea) or premature depletion of ovarian follicles before the age of 40 years (secondary amenorrhea). It is an heterogeneous disorder affecting approximately 1 % of women <40 years, 1:10,000 women by age 20 and 1:1000 women by age 30 [1] (Table 12.1).

Various terms have been suggested to define deviation from healthy ovarian function, including premature menopause (PM) or premature ovarian insufficiency (POI). Many authors regard ovarian insufficiency as more accurate than ovarian failure, because ovarian insufficiency can be used to described a wide range of impaired ovarian function. The term also suggests that ovarian follicular activity might intermittently recover, even years after diagnosis and lead to pregnancy in about 5–10 % of these women [2].

Follicle depletion or dysfunction in adolescent or young women may be caused by many different factors. POF might also result from genetic defects, chemotherapy, radiotherapy, or surgery. A common cause of POF in adolescent is gonadal dysgenesis, with or without Turner syndrome. When ovarian failure presents as a primary amenorrhea and no associated comorbidities, approximately 50 % are found to have abnormal karyotypes. However, most causes of spontaneous POF present as secondary amenorrhea and among younger women aged 30 years or younger with secondary amenorrhea, 13 % also have been noted to have an abnormal karyotype. Thus, in most cases the diagnosis will be 46, XX spontaneous POF, meaning the karyotype is normal [2]. In 90 % of cases an unknown mechanism leads to premature exhaustion of the resting pool of primordial follicles and no etiology for spontaneous POF will be

A. Giannini (✉) • A.R. Genazzani • T. Simoncini, MD, PhD (✉)
Division of Obstetrics and Gynecology, Department of Experimental and Clinical Medicine, University of Pisa, Via Roma, 67, 56100 Pisa, Italy
e-mail: argenazzani@gmail.com; tommaso.simoncini@med.unipi.it

C. Sultan, A.R. Genazzani (eds.), *Frontiers in Gynecological Endocrinology*, ISGE Series, DOI 10.1007/978-3-319-41433-1_12

Table 12.1 Etiology of Premature Ovarian Failure (POF)

Primary POF	Genetic aberrations	X-linked (monosomy, trisomy, deletions, translocations, fragile X)
		Autosomal dominant (FSH receptor gene polymorphism, inhibin B mutation, etc.)
	Enzyme deficiency	Metabolic
	Autoimmune disease	
Secondary POF	Surgical	Bilateral oophorectomy
		Hysterectomy without oophorectomy/uterine artery embolization
	Chemotherapy or radiotherapy	
	Infections	

identified even after a thorough evaluation. Approximately 4 % of women with 46, XX spontaneous POF will have steroidogenic cell autoimmunity as the mechanism of POF [3]. Approximately 6 % of women with 46, XX spontaneous POF will have premutations in the FMR1 gene. This is the gene responsible for fragile X syndrome, the most common cause of familial mental retardation. The risk of having an FMR1 premutation is higher if there is a family history of POF, therefore, in these patients it is crucial to take a family history, and women who have relatives with spontaneous POF should be referred for genetic counseling. Moreover, approximately 6 % of women with familial POF will have a premutation in the FMR1 gene as compared with 2 % of women with isolated POF. Women found to have a premutation in the FMR1 gene are at risk of having a child with mental retardation, should they be one of the 5–10 % who conceive [4]. There are other rare genetic causes of familial POF for which routine genetic testing in sporadic cases is now not clinically indicated, such as mutations involving FSHR (FSH receptor), GALT (galactose-1-phosphate uridylyltransferase associated with galactosemia), FOXL2 (a forkhead transcription factor associated with the blepharophimosis/ptosis/epicanthus inversus syndrome), INHA (inhibin alpha gene), EIF2B (a family of genes associated with central nervous system leukodystrophy and ovarian failure), BMP15 (bone morphogenetic protein 15), and AIRE (autoimmune regulator gene associated with the autoimmune polyendocrinopathy-candidiasis-ectodermal dystrophy syndrome) [5] (Table 12.2).

POF can be explained by different autoimmune mechanisms including a general immune dysregulation such as polyglandular syndrome (i.e., hypothyroidism, adrenal insufficiency, and hypoparathyroidism 14–27 %), dry-eye syndrome, myasthenia gravis (2 %), rheumatoid arthritis, diabetes mellitus (2 %), or systemic lupus erythematosus. It might also arise from an inflammatory autoimmune process against ovarian-specific germ line antigens or regulatory factors, making the disorder more complex than initially thought. The prevalence of these diseases in women with POF is higher than in the general population, suggesting that there may be an autoimmune component in these women that is not well understood. Autoimmunity in ovarian failure can be divided into two categories: ovarian failure associated with autoimmune adrenal insufficiency and ovarian failure associated with other autoimmune

Table 12.2 Genes implicated in Premature Ovarian Failure (POF)

Categories	Chromosomes	Gene
Identified mutations	X	FMR1, 2, BMP15
	Autosomal genes	FOXL2, FSHR, LHR, FSHβ, LHβ, inhibin A, GALT, AIRE, NOGGIN, POLG
Unidentified mutations	X	AT2, c-kit, sox 3
	Autosomal genes	MIS
Candidate genes	X	DIAPH2, DFFRX, XPNPEP2, 2FX, FSHPRH1, XIST
	Autosomal genes	WT1, ATM

disease. It is only when POI is associated with adrenal autoimmunity or insufficiency that true autoimmune oophoritis can be demonstrated. Approximately 2–10% of POF is associated with adrenal failure or autoimmunity and would thus be expected to result from autoimmune oophoritis. Circulating steroidogenic cell antibodies have been recorded in these autoimmune cases, therefore, steroid cell and/or enzyme antibody markers are present in 60–87% of women with secondary amenorrhea and adrenal autoimmunity and/or Addison's disease; therefore, it has been suggested that antibodies discriminate best between autoimmune POF and POF of other etiologies. However, ovarian antibody assays have a poor specificity and testing is therefore not recommended in women with primary ovarian insufficiency [6]. Although POF can happen as a result of ovarian surgery, oophorectomy, or exposure to viral or environmental toxic agents such as smoking, the most common cause of acquired disorder is chemotherapy or radiotherapy for cancer treatment. Chemotherapy-induced ovarian damage can arise through impairment of follicular maturation or primary follicle depletion, or both. Moreover, oocytes are very sensitive to radiation and age of the patient, and extent, type, and schedule of irradiation are key prognostic factors for development of primary ovarian failure. One dose is more destructive to the oocytes than are fractionated doses, and pelvic and abdominal irradiation has the highest risk, although scatter radiation can cause substantial damage even when the ovaries are not within the radiation field [7].

In the absence of symptoms, a change in the regular menstrual bleeding pattern is the main presenting symptom with POF. The absence of the menses in a 15-year-old girl (primary amenorrhea) or the cessation of menses for 4 months or more (secondary amenorrhea) can point towards the diagnosis; however, there is no consensus on criteria to identify primary ovarian failure in adolescence and delay in diagnosis is common. Some adolescent females report hot flushes and night sweats or vaginal symptoms like dryness or dyspareunia, low libido, low energy levels, sleep disturbance, lack of concentration, stiffness, skin/hair changes, and mood swings, however the most frequent symptoms of POF is primary or secondary amenorrhea. Among patients with amenorrhea, the incidence of POF ranges from 2 to 10%. Abnormal bleeding patterns also include oligomenorrhea (bleeding that occurs less frequently than every 35 days), non-structural causes of abnormal uterine bleeding (ovulatory dysfunction, iatrogenic, or not classified), or polymenorrhea (bleeding that occurs more often than every 21 years). Because irregular menstrual cycles are both common during early adolescence and an initial symptom of early POF, diagnosis can be difficult in this population. Although less than 10 % of women presenting abnormal menses will ultimately be found to have POF, the condition has such detrimental consequences on bone health that early diagnosis of this condition is important [8]. Therefore in young female it is important to evaluate amenorrhea or change from regular to irregular menses for three or more consecutive months in the absence of hormonal preparations such as oral contraceptives (OCs). Differential diagnosis is based on the exclusion for all potential causes of primary and secondary amenorrhea including pregnancy, polycystic ovary syndrome, hypothalamic amenorrhea, thyroid abnormalities, and hyperprolactinemia. In a woman aged less than 40 years, the diagnosis of POF is usually confirmed by the combination of the triad of oligo/amenorrhea for at least 4–6 months, sex steroids deficiency, and two recording of serum concentrations of follicle-stimulating hormone (FSH) of more than 30–40 IU/L at least 1 month apart. If the result indicates that FSH is elevated, a diagnosis of POF can be established. Estradiol levels of less than 50 pg/ml indicate hypoestrogenism. However FSH is not an ideal diagnostic tool because it rises only in the later stages of follicle depletion, has marked cycle- to-cycle variability, and it is poor at predicting reproductive status. In this view, there has been interest in more direct markers of ovarian reserve such as anti-Mullerian hormone (AMH), which closely follows the reduction in follicle number over time in healthy women and falls to very low levels prior to menopause. In assessment of amenorrhea, AMH or transvaginal ultrasound scan will exclude polycystic ovarian syndrome as a cause. In POF, the antral follicle count is very low, and seeing this as a related marker of ovarian function may help to understand the diagnosis. However, even in POF, the intermittent ovarian function means that follicular activity is seen in the majority of women [9, 10].

In the absence of an obvious cause of POF (oophorectomy, chemotherapy, or pelvic radiotherapy), young women should be offered investigation in etiology, however, in the majority of cases no cause is found. Even if causation is established, the management, including fertility options, remains unchanged. E genetic etiology will be identified in approximately 5 % and autoimmune in up to 30 % [10]. Genetic counseling is nowadays recommended for several reason when a genetic form of POF is suspected or identified and a karyotype should be offered to women with POF in the onset of amenorrhea or oligomenorrhea before age 25. A karyotype is also indicated in women of any age in whom Turner's syndrome mosaicism is suspected, as well as e FMR1 (fragile x) permutation testing. Overall the permutation is found in 4–5 % of women with POF, among those with a family history of POF, 14 % have a positive result, in this view a full family history is important as many cases of spontaneous POF appear to be inherited, estimates vary from 4 to 31 %. Thirty percent of the cases of POF are estimated to be owing to autoimmunity. Presumed autoimmune etiology may be inferred from a family history of autoimmune disease or a positive anti-thyroid antibody result, which is found in approximately 24 % of women affected by POF. If a POF patient appears to be a sporadic and not hereditary case, the risk of other female relatives developing POF will probably be equal to the risk in the general population [11].

For adolescents with POF, the objective of treatment is to replace the hormones that the ovary would be producing before the age of menopause (51 years), making the treatment specifically different from hormonal therapy for menopause that focuses on the treatment of menopausal symptoms. The aims of hormonal therapy extend beyond simply symptom relief to levels that support bone, cardiovascular (CV), and sexual health. Regardless of the etiology, patients with POF are estrogen deficient. Thus, young women with POF may need higher doses of estrogen than menopausal women to ensure adequate replacement and optimal bone health. In girls with absent or incomplete breast development, estrogen therapy should be initiated and increased slowly before administration of graduated progesterone dosages until breast development is complete to prevent tubular breast formation. For those patients who have not initiated or completed pubertal growth and sexual maturity, consultation with a specialist in growth and development and hormonal therapy in children is recommended. Once pubertal development is complete, ongoing hormonal therapy will be necessary for long-term health. Hormonal support involves daily therapy with the goal of maintenance of normal ovarian functioning levels of estradiol (E2). There are no controlled studies regarding the ideal hormone replacement strategy for young women with spontaneous POF. There is room for individualization. Most women do well using a 100-μg E2 transdermal patch, which averts the first-pass effect on the liver and can be considered full-dose physiologic replacement for young women. On average this achieves a serum E2 level of 100 pg/mL, near the normal mean E2 level for normally cycling women of 104 pg/mL. Oral E2 can be given to women who prefer this route of administration, however, oral E2 increases the potential for thromboembolism relative to transdermal estradiol due to the first-pass effect on the liver. Typically, about twice as much E as is required for postmenopausal women is needed to alleviate the symptoms (100-μg E2 patch, 2 mg daily dose of oral micronized E2, or 1.25 mg of conjugated equine E). Cyclic medroxyprogesterone acetate (MPA; 10 mg/day) or oral micronized P (200 mg/day) for 12 days each month should be given to induce regular monthly withdrawal bleeding. Progestin withdrawal less frequently than each month has been associated with the development of endometrial hyperplasia in older women. A case can be made for providing a 10-mg dose of MPA or equivalent to fully induce a secretory pattern [12, 13]. Lower doses may reduce side effects but require monitoring. Still some patients may prefer a less frequent progestin withdrawal with appropriate monitoring. Oral contraceptives contain higher doses of estrogen than are necessary for hormonal therapy; therefore, they are not recommended as first-line hormonal therapy.

Estrogens are important in the process of bone remodeling. Consequently, estrogen deficiency results in an imbalance between osteoclast and osteoblast activity and a progressive loss of trabecular bone. Osteoporosis can be diagnosed by the assessment of bone density, with a reasonable ability to predict fracture risk. Decreased bone density can be noted within 6 months of the start of severe ovarian suppression by gonadotrophin-releasing hormone agonists given for steroid-dependent disease. Increased bone fragility leads to a 50 % lifetime risk of fracture and a 15 % risk of hip fracture—a major cause of disability and death—in white women with a normal age of menopause. There are no reports that suggest the chance of fracture is increased with POF; however, because these women are at increased risk for osteoporosis, they should also be advised regarding calcium intake (1200–1500 mg/dl), daily weight bearing exercise, and the need to take daily multivitamin to avoid vitamin D deficiency.

Data have documented androgen deficiency in patients affected by POF, but whether exogenous androgen is indicative is uncertain. The benefits and risks of androgen therapy have not been established and data are controversial and androgen replacement therapy has only been studied in the context of surgical menopause. On the other hand, presumably androgen replacement would be more beneficial for young women with very low levels of circulating androgen than for postmenopausal women with relative androgen deficiency. In the absence of evidence, it seems reasonable to give a trial of testosterone, in the form of patch or gel, if low libido or lack of energy persists despite adequate estrogen replacement [14].

A 5–10 % background pregnancy rate is seen in spontaneous POF. It is important to counsel patients about the small chance of spontaneous conception, and the need to use contraception if pregnancy is not desired. The COC (combined oral contraceptive) may be a good choice for these women because HRT (hormone replacement therapy) is not contraceptive. It is not possible to predict which patients will conceive, although positive prognostic factors include short duration of amenorrhea, autoimmune etiology, and ovarian activity seen on ultrasound scan. Ultrasound monitoring might benefit conception rates by improving timing of intercourse; however, monitoring has not been examined in a controlled manner. In our own experience, monitoring ovarian activity can help patients accept their diagnosis and move ahead with alternate family planning options if no follicle activity is observed or pregnancy achieved after an agreed upon timeframe [15]. Pregnancy can occur in young women despite very low AMH. Sadly, no intervention has been found to improve conception rates: ovarian stimulation, FSH suppression, and the use of steroids in autoimmune POF are all ineffective. The only treatment option is in vitro fertilization with donor oocytes. Prior to embryo transfer, the endometrium is thickened using high-dose HRT. Treatment has a high success rate (which can reach 50 % per cycle) dependent on the age of the donor. The psychological and ethical implications must be carefully considered, and counseling is mandatory for both the recipient and donor. Fertility-preservation options can be suggested to some patients with cancer and those at risk of early menopause, such as those with familial cases of POF. Early diagnosis of familial POF should provide the opportunity to predict the likelihood of early menopause, and allow other reproductive choices to be made, such as freezing embryos or having children earlier [16] (Table 12.3).

Menopause condition adversely affects cognitive function, and surgical menopause has been associated with distinct impairment of cognitive function and memory. In 100 women diagnosed with POF, substantial changes in social anxiety, depression, and self-esteem have been described. Increased risks of minor cognitive impairment or dementia, depressive and anxiety symptoms, parkinsonism, and increased mortality from neurological and mental diseases have been noted in a cohort of over 2000 women who had had unilateral or bilateral oophorectomy, in

Table 12.3 Diagnosis, initial evaluation, and management of Premature Ovarian Failure (POF)

Definition
At least 3–4 months of amenorrhea in association with menopausal levels of serum FSH concentration on two occasions
Initial assessment and investigations
Good history, including family history
Tests
Serum FSH, LH, prolactin, TSH, estradiol; if FSH in menopausal range, repeat. AMH? Inhibin B?
Further investigations
Chromosomal and genetic studies: karyotype, FMR1 gene mutation if family history of POF, fragile X syndrome or mental retardation
Autoantibodies: autoimmune screen for polyendocrinopathy, thyroid antibodies, anti-adrenal antibodies? ovarian antibodies
DEXA: estimation of bone mineral density
Pelvic ultrasonography
Management
Provide counseling, information and emotional support
Provide HRT/COC up to age 50 years and then yearly review as required
Provide calcium and vitamin supplements and encourage weight-bearing exercise
Provide contraception if required and advice on fertility issues

FSH follicle-stimulating hormone, *LH* luteinizing hormone, *TSH* thyroid-stimulating hormone, *AMH* anti-Mullerian hormone, *FMR1* gene responsible for fragile X syndrome, *DEXA* dual-energy X-ray absorptiometry, *HRT* hormone replacement therapy, *COC* combined oral contraceptive

this view it is crucial to treat adolescent and young women affected by POF in order to prevent long-term risk of cognitive impairment [17].

When POF is diagnosed in the adolescent female, the patient and her family are often unprepared for such news with its implications for compromised fertility and impaired self-image and the need for long-term hormonal therapy. It is best to inform the patient and family by having a direct conversation. Adolescents may demonstrate myriad emotions ranging from apathy or denial to remorse or sadness, and these emotions may be different from those of their parents or guardians. Psychological counseling also should be offered because impaired self-esteem and emotional distress have been reported after diagnosis of primary ovarian insufficiency. Because many patients will use the Internet to learn more about their diagnoses, referral to appropriate sources for support is an efficient means to enhance patient care. A greater understanding of female reproductive biology and the physiologic effect of POF enables health care providers to offer counseling for these young women. Once POF is diagnosed, patients should be evaluated at least annually. Physicians should address the special needs of this population and counsel family members and patients on the risk of comorbidities associated with primary ovarian insufficiency and the condition's potential for genetic inheritance [18].

Concluding, as POF has cumulative negative effects over time, it is important for clinicians to make a timely diagnosis and bring appropriate strategies for symptoms management, emotional support, and risk reduction. Therapies in patients affected by POF need to be individualized and depend on the endpoints of treatment in different moments of women's life. The approach to POF patients should be multidisciplinary and the management of these patients includes counseling and emotional support, planning fertility and a hormonal replacement strategy up to at least age of natural menopause, therefore, long-term deprivation of estrogen has serious implications for female health for bone density, cardiovascular and neurological systems, wellbeing, and sexual health in particular.

References

1. Santoro N (2003) Mechanisms of premature ovarian failure. Ann Endocrinol (Paris) 64:87–92
2. Nelson L, Covington S, Rebar R (2005) An update: spontaneous premature ovarian failure is not an early menopause. Fertil Steril 83:1327–1332
3. Bakalov VK, Vanderhoof VH, Bondy CA et al (2002) Adrenal antibodies detect asymptomatic auto-immune adrenal insufficiency in young women with spontaneous premature ovarian failure. Hum Reprod 17:2096–2100
4. Marozzi A, Vegetti W, Manfredini E et al (2000) Association between idiopathic premature ovarian failure and fragile X premutation. Hum Reprod 15:197–202
5. Broekmans F, Soules M, Fauser B (2009) Ovarian aging: mechanisms and clinical consequences. Endocr Rev 30:465–493
6. LaBarbera AR, Miller MM, Ober C et al (1988) Autoimmune etiology in premature ovarian failure. Am J Reprod Immunol Microbiol 16:115–122
7. Sonmezer M, Oktay K (2004) Fertility preservation in female patients. Hum Reprod Update 10:251–266
8. Nelson LM (2009) Clinical practice. Primary ovarian insufficiency. N Engl J Med 360:606–614
9. Broer SL, Eijkemans MJ, Scheffer GJ et al (2011) Anti-mullerian hormone predicts menopause: a long-term follow-up study in normo-ovulatory women. JCEM 96:2532–2539
10. Conway GS, Kaltsas G, Patel A et al (1996) Characterization of idiopathic premature ovarian failure. Fertil Steril 65:337–341
11. van Kasteren YM, Hundscheid RD, Smits AP et al (1999) Familial idiopathic premature ovarian failure: an overrated and underestimated genetic disease? Hum Reprod 14:2455–2459
12. Chetkowski RJ, Meldrum DR, Steingold KA et al (1986) Biologic effects of transdermal estradiol. N Engl J Med 314:1615–1620
13. Rebar R (2007) Premature ovarian failure. In: Lobo RA (ed) Treatment of the postmenopausal woman: basic and clinical aspects, 3rd edn. Academic Press, Oxford, pp 99–109
14. Rebar RW (2009) Premature ovarian failure. Obstet Gynecol 113:1355–1363
15. Bidet M, Bachelot A, Touraine P (2008) Premature ovarian failure: predictability of intermittent ovarian function and response to ovulation induction agents. Curr Opin Obstet Gynecol 20:416–420
16. American College of Obstetrics and Gynecology (2006) Ovarian tissue and oocyte cryopreservation. Fertil Steril 86:S142–S147
17. Rocca W, Grossardt B, Geda Y et al (2008) Long-term risk of depressive and anxiety symptoms after early bilateral oophorectomy. Menopause 15:1050–1059
18. Groff AA, Covington SN, Halverson LR et al (2005) Assessing the emotional needs of women with spontaneous premature ovarian failure. Fertil Steril 83:1734–1741

Emergency Contraception 13

Sharon Cameron

Abbreviations

EC	Emergency contraception
IUD	Copper bearing intrauterine device
LH	Luteinising hormone
LNG	Levonorgestrel
PK	Pharmacokinetic
POP	Progestogen only pill
PRM	Progesterone receptor modulator
UPA	Ulipristal acetate

13.1 Introduction

Emergency contraception (EC) is defined as any drug or device that is used after sexual intercourse to prevent unwanted pregnancy. Abortion is defined as termination of an established pregnancy, i.e., of an embryo that has already implanted in the uterus. The World Health Organization (WHO) recently published a report on sexual health, human rights and the law, that specified that the evidence shows that for adolescents increased access to EC protects from negative health outcomes, and does not increase the risk of unwanted pregnancies, or sexually transmitted infections [1]. The WHO list of essential medicines includes EC and also includes the medical abortion drugs mifepristone and misoprostol [2].

The methods of EC that are in current use include the copper bearing intrauterine device (IUD), and the oral methods of levonorgestrel (LNG) and ulipristal acetate

S. Cameron, MD, MFSRH, FRCOG
Chalmers Centre, NHS Lothian and University of Edinburgh,
2 a Chalmers Street, Edinburgh EH3 9ES, UK
e-mail: Sharon.cameron@ed.ac.uk

C. Sultan, A.R. Genazzani (eds.), *Frontiers in Gynecological Endocrinology*,
ISGE Series, DOI 10.1007/978-3-319-41433-1_13

(UPA). Mifepristone is also used for oral EC, but it is only available in China, Russia, Armenia, Ukraine and Vietnam [3].

13.2 Efficacy Assumptions

There has never been a randomized placebo-controlled trial of EC. The efficacy of EC in clinical trials is therefore calculated from the number of observed pregnancies compared to the number of expected pregnancies (in the absence of EC), based on the conception probability at the time in the menstrual cycle when intercourse occurred [4]. In most clinical trials, the expected pregnancy rates in the absence of EC have been low, in the region of 5 %. In the clinical trials of oral LNG compared to UPA for EC, the observed pregnancy rate was 1–2 % [5]. On this basis, we might conclude that oral EC prevents one half to two thirds of pregnancies that might otherwise have occurred. However, these calculations are based on a number of assumptions. Firstly, we assume that we can accurately determine the phase in the menstrual cycle when intercourse took place. In clinical studies, as many as 30 % of women who stated that were sure of the date of their last menstrual period and believed that they were in the first half of the cycle when they took EC, had actually already ovulated (based upon subsequent urine or serum hormone analyses) [6, 7]. In addition, we know that many women have had more than one episode of unprotected sexual intercourse when they request EC [6]. Efficacy calculations also assume that sperm have entered the reproductive tract. However, in a study of women presenting for EC that assessed the presence of sperm on vaginal smears, there was no sperm present in one third of cases [8]. We do know however, that oral EC methods can delay or inhibit ovulation, so on this basis alone they have to be better than nothing [9].

13.3 Effectiveness, Acceptability and Availability

The IUD is by far the most effective method of EC. In a systematic review of more than 40 studies involving over 7000 women, the observed pregnancy rate was one in 1000 [10]. The IUD can also be used over a wider time period than oral EC. It can be inserted up to 5 days after the earliest estimated date of ovulation. It also can be retained as an ongoing method of highly effective, long acting reversible contraception. But the IUD is not popular. In the UK, where women can access the IUD for EC at no financial cost to themselves, only 2–5 % of women seeking EC choose the IUD [11, 12].

There have been two comparative randomised controlled trials (RCTs) conducted to date of UPA versus LNG, with over 3400 women treated [5, 13]. In the meta-analysis of these trials, use of UPA was associated with almost halving of the risk of pregnancy for women treated within 120 h of unprotected sex. For women who were treated within 24 h of intercourse, the difference was more marked, with women receiving UPA having approximately one third the risk of pregnancy, compared to women receiving LNG [5]. Both LNG and UPA are well tolerated and associated with a similar side effect profile [5]. The European Medicines Authority (EMA) recently reviewed the safety and efficacy data pertaining to UPA and recommended that UPA should be available throughout Europe without the need for a prescription [14]. The EMA's decision on UPA also resulted in LNG becoming available without prescription in many of those countries (e.g., Italy, Germany), where LNG had formerly required a prescription.

13.4 Mechanism of Action and Effect on Pregnancy

The IUD has both pre- and post-fertilization effects. Copper ions are toxic to sperm and oocytes. The IUD also induces a local inflammatory reaction in the endometrium that may prevent implantation [15]. It should not be inserted for EC beyond 5 days after the earliest date of ovulation as this could potentially disrupt an early pregnancy. Generally, the IUD should be removed if possible, in women who become pregnant with an IUD in situ, given the higher risk of adverse outcome such as septic abortion [16].

It is generally accepted that both LNG and UPA exert their contraceptive effect as EC through their ability to delay ovulation by up to 5 days (presumed lifespan of sperm in the reproductive tract). However, once the Luteinising Hormone (LH) surge (ovulatory trigger) has started, then LNG is no longer able to delay ovulation, although UPA still remains able to delay ovulation until the LH peak [9]. There is good evidence that LNG does not prevent implantation and is not abortifacient. Bio medical studies have demonstrated that the EC dose of LNG when given after ovulation, does not affect the development of a secretory endometrium at either histological level, molecular level nor at electron microscopic level [17]. Furthermore, an in vitro model of blastocyst implantation showed that the addition of LNG was unable to prevent implantation [18]. LNG use is not associated with a higher risk of miscarriage, ectopic or pregnancy complications and there is no adverse effect on children conceived after exposure to LNG for EC [19, 20].

There is also evidence that the EC dose of UPA does not exert significant effects on the endometrium [21]. Although immediate post-ovulatory administration of the EC dose of UPA has been associated with a reduction in endometrial thickness, the thickness remains within the normal range and histological assessment showed that secretory development was unaffected [21]. Furthermore, serum progesterone levels remained in the normal range for the luteal phase, suggesting that there would be sufficient luteal support for an implanting embryo. In vitro studies have also shown that UPA does not prevent implantation of blastocysts [22]. Safety data regarding the effects of UPA on pregnancy are inevitably limited since use of UPA for EC has been limited. Also, pregnancy rates after use are low, most women chose to terminate an unintended pregnancy after UPA, and the outcome of pregnancies that continue to birth are unlikely to be reported unless there is a complication. However, the available data from over one million women who used UPA in the clinical trials and post marketing surveillance have been consistent with no increased risk of miscarriage or ectopic or congenital abnormality in babies after exposure to UPA [23].

Table 13.1 Risk factors for failure of EC (LNG or UPA) from Glasier et al. [24]

	Odds ratio [95 % CI]	*P* value
Cycle day of intercourse[a]	4.4 [2.3–8.2]	$P<0.0001$
Further UPI[a]	4.6 [2.2–9.0]	$P<0.0002$
BMI Obese vs. normal	3.6 [1.96–6.53]	$P<0.0001$

[a]No treatment group effect

Table 13.2 Risk of pregnancy in women with obese BMI vs. normal BMI and EC treatment (LNG or UPA) from Glasier et al. [24]

BMI group	LNG OR (95 % CI)	UPA OR (95 % CI)
Obese vs. normal	4.41 (2.05–9.44)[a]	2.62 (0.89–7.00)

[a]$P=0.0002$

13.5 Factors Predictive of Failure of EC

In a secondary analysis of the meta-analysis of the RCTs of UPA and LNG, three factors were significant for failure of EC: (i) cycle day that intercourse occurred, (ii) further episodes of sex in the same cycle after EC and (ii) obesity [24] (Table 13.1).

Cycle day when sex occurs and further sex after EC have previously been established as risk factors [25], however, obesity (Body mass index ≥30 kg/m^2) as a risk for failure was a new finding.

Further statistical analysis of this dataset showed that there was a treatment effect with women with a BMI ≥30 kg/m^2 having an almost fourfold increased risk of EC failure compared to women of normal BMI receiving LNG [24]. In contrast, women with a BMI ≥30 kg/m^2 who received UPA had a doubling risk of pregnancy compared to women of normal BMI receiving UPA compared to women of normal BMI receiving LNG (Table 13.2).

Additional analysis showed that the limit of efficacy (when the observed pregnancy rate is no less than the expected rate in the absence of EC) was reached with LNG at a BMI of 26 kg/m^2, yet this limit of efficacy was not reached with UPA until n a BMI of 35 kg/m^2. Similar analyses were conducted for weight alone, and showed that the limit of efficacy with LNG and UPA was reached at weights of 70 and 88 kg respectively. However, the findings came from secondary analysis of studies that were not designed to address the issue of BMI and efficacy of EC. In addition, as for most clinical trials that have strict inclusion/exclusion criteria, the numbers of women with BMI ≥30 kg/m^2 were low as were the number of pregnancies in this group. Also, in a substantial proportion of all participants, the height and weight had been self-reported, which introduces inaccuracies in BMI determination [5, 13].

Previous studies of LNG for EC conducted by the WHO had failed to show an impact of BMI upon pregnancy rate [26]. The EMA reviewed the data from the clinical trials, together with data from unpublished studies of LNG for EC and concluded that the data were not sufficiently robust to conclude that obesity was associated with a decrease in efficacy of EC, and recommended that women with obesity could continue to use either UPA or LNG [27]. Nevertheless, the uncertainty remains. Also, there is some pharmacokinetic (PK) data that might some support the notion that efficacy of LNG for EC may be adversely impacted upon by obesity. Specifically a PK study of low dose combined contraceptive pill containing LNG showed that in women with obesity, LNG takes a longer time to achieve steady state levels than in women of normal BMI [28]. Whilst it is very unlikely that there will be a definitive RCT of women with/without obesity with efficacy of EC as an end-point, ongoing studies examining the PK of UPA in women with/without obesity will provide useful information to inform this debate.

13.6 Can EC Prevent Abortion?

The evidence from both population studies and clinical trials of advance provision of EC (supply to keep at home in case of need) would indicate that use of EC does not reduce unintended pregnancy rates or abortion rates at population level. Indeed, a Cochrane review of six RCTs of over 6300 women (with one or more supplies of EC at home) compared to standard access, failed to demonstrate any reduction in pregnancy rates at 3, 6 or 12 months [29].

In Norway, availability of LNG for EC from the pharmacy without prescription was associated with 30-fold increase in sales over 10 years, but the abortion rate remained unchanged over this time [30]. Similarly, in Great Britain, abortion rates continued to increase up to 2008, some 7 years after availability of LNG for EC from the pharmacy [31]. However, abortion rates are influenced by many factors and demographic changes in society with earlier age of coitarche, later age at first birth, relationship break ups and divorce may mean that women now spend a greater proportion of their reproductive lives at risk of unintended pregnancy. Also, we know from the clinical trials of advance provision of EC that women do not use EC for every episode of unprotected sex [29].

Studies conducted in UK, France and Denmark amongst women requesting abortion have shown that 12 % of women have used EC in the conception cycle to try to prevent the pregnancy [32–34]. Furthermore, a survey of women requesting abortion in the UK showed that although availability of LNG EC at 'no cost' from the pharmacy did not affect this percentage, in spite of most respondents being aware that EC was free at the pharmacy [32].

Research has also shown that women often fail to recognize that they are at risk of pregnancy, neglect the risk or are deterred from using EC due to stigma, or misconceptions about the method [33, 34]. It has also been suggested that the increase in EC use may be amongst women who are least at risk of an unintended pregnancy, but are anxious about that risk [30]. In addition, we do know that many women may have more episode(s) of sex in the same cycle after using EC, and that further sex increases the risk of pregnancy [25].

13.7 Establishing Effective Contraception After EC

Given the higher risk of pregnancy if further sex occurs in the same cycle after EC, it is important that women start an effective method of ongoing contraception as soon as possible. The term 'quick start' is used to denote starting a method of contraception at any point in the menstrual cycle, without waiting for the next menses. If women attend a family planning (FP) service for EC, then they can be provided with ongoing contraception at this same visit. A study from the UK suggested that 23 % of women attending a FP service for EC chose to start effective contraception, usually the combined oral contraceptive pill [11]. Of course, women are increasingly choosing to access EC from the pharmacy (in countries where this is available without prescription), and most pharmacists cannot provide hormonal contraception without a prescription. A pilot study from the UK examined two pharmacy -based interventions designed to facilitate access to effective contraception after EC [35]. It randomised 12 pharmacies to provide women with either (i) standard care, i.e., pharmacist provides EC as usual (LNG), or (ii) pharmacist supplied a 1 month supply of the progestogen only pill (POP) with EC – so that women could start the POP immediately and have up to 1 month to arrange an appointment with their usual care provider for effective ongoing contraception or (iii) women had a rapid access pathway to the local FP for contraception upon presentation of their empty EC box. Women in this study consented to be contacted by the researcher 8 weeks later to determine what method of contraception they were using. Although, it was a small study with just under 60 participants in each of the arms of the study, there was a significantly higher proportion of women in the POP (52 %) and rapid access arm (52 %) using effective contraception than in the standard care arm alone (16 %). This suggests that provision of a POP or rapid access to a FP could prove to be an effective measure to increase the uptake of effective contraception after EC from the pharmacy. In addition, the POP is a very safe method of contraception and could be provided more easily than a combined oral contraceptive pill. Larger robust studies in this area are therefore needed.

13.8 Contraception After Ulipristal Acetate for Contraception

UPA is a progesterone receptor modulator (PRM), and PRMs may interfere with the action of progestogen containing contraception. There is concern therefore that UPA may affect the efficacy of UPA or vice versa. Guidelines from the Faculty of Sexual and Reproductive Healthcare UK advise that women can commence hormonal contraception after UPA, but should rely on additional barrier contraception or abstain for 14 days if the method is a COC [36]. This is based upon an estimated 7 days to clear UPA (based upon its half life of 32 h) plus a further 'theoretical' 7 days to induce ovarian quiescence with a COC.

A recent placebo-controlled RCT that examined the effects of quick starting a COC after UPA in healthy volunteers with a follicle of at least 13 mm in size (equivalent to mid follicular phase), showed that there was no difference between UPA and placebo in either the proportion of women who achieved ovarian quiescence on

Table 13.3 Strategies to improve effectiveness of EC

Increase use of IUD for EC
No further sex in same cycle after oral EC
Commence effective ongoing contraception
Develop a more effective oral EC

a COC nor the number of days to achieve quiescence [37]. This study design was such that it could not determine whether the COC might impact upon the ability of UPA to delay ovulation. A further RCT study has examined the effects of starting a progestogen only pill (POP) containing desogestrel, the day after the UPA or placebo [38]. This study demonstrated that although UPA did not affect the contraceptive actions of this POP (ovarian suppression and cervical mucus), that the POP did affect the ability of UPA to delay ovulation [38]. In view of this, guidelines advise that women should not start a hormonal method of contraception for at least five days after using UPA for EC [39].

13.9 A More Effective Oral EC

Prostaglandins play a critical role at the time of follicle rupture and the cyclo- oxygenase- 2 inhibitor meloxicam inhibits prostaglandin synthesis. A pilot RCT comparing the effect of the EC dose of LNG plus meloxicam versus LNG and placebo on follicle rupture when administered to healthy female volunteers in the preovulatory phase of the cycle demonstrated that there was no ovulation at 5 days (i.e., lifespan of spermatozoa in the female reproductive tract) in 39 % of participants receiving LNG and meloxicam vs. 16 % of those receiving LNG and placebo [40]. This suggests that perhaps a combination of meloxicam and LNG might increase the efficacy of LNG for EC. It is also possible that meloxicam combined with UPA might increase the efficacy of UPA further. Large robust trials are now required.

A Cochrane review demonstrated that mid doses of mifepristone (25–50 mg) are more effective than LNG [25]. Studies have also shown that higher doses of mifepristone (200 mg) have profound effects on endometrial secretory development that may prevent implantation [41, 42]. Further research into the development of more effective oral ECs is therefore warranted.

Conclusion

So what strategies can we adopt in order to maximize the chances that EC can prevent unintended pregnancy? (Table 13.3). Given the fact that the IUD is the most effective method of EC it seems only logical to promote increased use of the IUD for EC. With increasing proportions of women choosing to access EC from the pharmacy, developing close links between IUD providers (FP clinics/ Gynaecology) and pharmacies will therefore be required.

However, if an IUD for EC is not acceptable to a woman or available, then UPA is more effective than LNG. In addition, there should be no further episodes of unprotected sex after oral EC and women should establish an effective ongoing method of contraception as soon as possible.

More research is required to explore the efficacy of the approach of providing a temporary supply of the POP with oral EC from the pharmacy.

We also need more research into the possible impact of obesity on efficacy of oral EC and we need to have a more effective oral EC; that also prevents implantation.

References

1. World Health Organization. Sexual health, human rights and the law. Human reproduction program. June 2015. http://www.who.int/reproductivehealth/publications/sexual_health/sexual-health-human-rights-law/en/. Access 13 Jul 2015
2. WHO model list of essential medicines Apr 2015. http://www.who.int/medicines/publications/essentialmedicines/en/. Access date 13 Jul 2015
3. International Consortium for Emergency Contraception. In depth country information. http://www.cecinfo.org/country-by-country-information/in-depth/. Access date 13 Jul 2015
4. Trussell J, Ellertson C, von Hertzen H, Bigrigg A, Webb A, Evans M, Ferden S, Leadbetter C (2003) Estimating the effectiveness of emergency contraceptive pills. Contraception 67(4):259–65
5. Glasier A, Cameron ST, Logan S, Fine P et al (2010) Ulipristal acetate versus levonorgestrel for emergency contraception: a randomised non-inferiority trial and meta-analysis of ulipristal acetate versus levonorgestrel. Lancet 375(9714):555–62
6. Stirling A, Glasier A (2002) Estimating the efficacy of emergency contraception – how reliable are the data? Contraception 66(1):19–22
7. Novikova N, Weisberg E, Stanczyk FZ, Croxatto HB, Fraser IS (2007) Effectiveness of levonorgestrel emergency contraception given before or after ovulation – a pilot study. Contraception 75(2):112–8
8. Espinós-Gómez JJ, Senosiain R, Mata A, Vanrell C, Bassas L, Calaf J (2007) What is the seminal exposition among women requiring emergency contraception? A prospective, observational comparative study. Eur J Obstet Gynecol Reprod Biol 131(1):57–60
9. Brache V, Cochon L, Deniaud M, Croxatto HB (2013) Ulipristal acetate prevents ovulation more effectively than levonorgestrel: analysis of pooled data from three randomized trials of emergency contraception regimens. Contraception 88(5):611–8
10. Cleland K, Zhu H, Goldstuck N, Cheng L, Trussell J (2012) The efficacy of intrauterine devices for emergency contraception: a systematic review of 35 years of experience. Hum Reprod 27(7):1994–2000
11. Cameron ST, Glasier A, Johnstone A, Rae L (2011) Ongoing contraception after use of emergency contraception from a specialist contraceptive service. Contraception 84(4):368–371
12. Baird AS (2013) Use of ulipristal acetate, levonorgestrel and the copper-intrauterine device for emergency contraception following the introduction of new FSRH guidelines. J Fam Plann Reprod Health Care 39(4):264–9
13. Creinin MD, Schlaff W, Archer DF, Wan L, Frezieres R, Thomas M, Rosenberg M, Higgins J (2006) Progesterone receptor modulator for emergency contraception: a randomized controlled trial. Obstet Gynecol 108(5):1089–97
14. European Consortium for emergency contraception. Emergency contraception availability in Europe. http://www.ec-ec.org/emergency-contraception-in-europe/emergency-contraception-availability-in-europe/. Access date 13 Jul 2015
15. Ortiz ME, Croxatto HB (2007) Copper-T intrauterine device and levonorgestrel intrauterine system: biological bases of their mechanism of action. Contraception 75(6 Suppl):S16–30, Review

16. Brahmi D, Steenland MW, Renner RM et al (2012) Pregnancy outcomes with an IUD in situ: a systematic review. Contraception 85:131–139
17. Gemzell-Danielsson K, Berger C, Lalitkumar PG (2014) Mechanisms of action of oral emergency contraception. Gynecol Endocrinol 30(10):685–7
18. Lalitkumar PG, Lalitkumar S, Meng CX, Stavreus-Evers A, Hambiliki F, Bentin-Ley U, Gemzell-Danielsson K (2007) Mifepristone, but not levonorgestrel, inhibits human blastocyst attachment to an in vitro endometrial three-dimensional cell culture model. Hum Reprod 22(11):3031–7
19. Cleland K, Raymond E, Trussell J, Cheng L, Zhu H (2010) Ectopic pregnancy and emergency contraceptive pills: a systematic review. Obstet Gynecol 115(6):1263–6
20. Zhang L, Ye W, Yu W, Cheng L, Shen L, Yang Z (2014) Physical and mental development of children after levonorgestrel emergency contraception exposure: a follow-up prospective cohort study. Biol Reprod 91(1):27
21. Stratton P, Levens ED, Hartog B, Piquion J, Wei Q, Merino M, Nieman LK (2010) Endometrial effects of a single early luteal dose of the selective progesterone receptor modulator CDB-2914. Fertil Steril 93(6):2035–41
22. Berger C, Boggavarapu NR, Menezes J, Lalitkumar PG, Gemzell-Danielsson K (2015) Effects of ulipristal acetate on human embryo attachment and endometrial cell gene expression in an in vitro co-culture system. Hum Reprod 30(4):800–11
23. Levy DP, Jager M, Kapp N, Abitbol JL (2014) Ulipristal acetate for emergency contraception: postmarketing experience after use by more than 1 million women. Contraception 89(5):431–3
24. Glasier A, Cameron ST, Blithe D, Scherrer B, Mathe H, Levy D, Gainer E, Ulmann A (2011) Can we identify women at risk of pregnancy despite using emergency contraception? Data from randomized trials of ulipristal acetate and levonorgestrel. Contraception 84(4): 363–367
25. Cheng L, Che Y, Gülmezoglu AM (2012) Interventions for emergency contraception. Cochrane Database Syst Rev (8):CD001324. DOI: 10.1002/14651858.CD001324.pub4. Access date 13 Jul 2015
26. Von Hertzen H, Piaggio G, Peregoudov A, Ding J, Chen J, Song S, Ba'rtfai G, Ng E, Gemzell-Danielsson K, Oyunbileg A, WHO Research Group on Post-ovulatory Methods of Fertility Regulation et al (2002) Low dose mifepristone and two regimens of levonorgestrel for emergency contraception: a WHO multicentre randomised trial. Lancet 360:1803–1810
27. European Medicines Agency, assessment report for emergency contraceptive medicinal products containing levonorgestrel or ulipristal. http://www.ema.europa.eu/docs/en_GB/document_library/EPAR_-_Assessment_Report_-_Variation/human/001027/WC500176357.pdf. Access date 13 Jul 2015
28. Edelman AB, Carlson NE, Cherala G, Munar MY, Stouffer RL, Cameron JL, Stanczyk FZ, Jensen JT (2009) Impact of obesity on oral contraceptive pharmacokinetics and hypothalamic-pituitary-ovarian activity. Contraception 80(2):119–27
29. Polis CB, Schaffer K, Blanchard K, Glasier A, Harper CC, Grimes DA (2007b) Advance provision of emergency contraception for pregnancy prevention (full review). Cochrane Database Syst Rev (2):CD005497
30. Pedersen W (2008) Emergency contraception: why the absent effect on abortion rates? Acta Obstet Gynecol Scand 87(2):132–3
31. Department of Health. Abortion statistics, England and Wales: 2014. https://www.gov.uk/government/uploads/system/uploads/attachment_data/file/319460/Abortion_Statistics__England_and_Wales_2014.pdf. Access date 13 Jul 2015
32. Cameron ST, Gordon R, Glasier A (2012) The effect on use of making emergency contraception available free of charge. Contraception 86(4):366–9
33. Sørensen M, Pedersen B, Nyrnberg L (2000) Differences between users and non-users of emergency contraception after a recognized unprotected intercourse. Contraception 62:1–3

34. Moreau C, Bouyer J, Goulard H, Bajos N (2005) The remaining barriers to the use of emergency contraception: perception of pregnancy risk by women undergoing induced abortions. Contraception 71:202–207
35. Michie L, Cameron ST, Glasier A, Larke N, Muir A, Lorimer A (2014) Pharmacy-based interventions for initiating effective contraception following the use of emergency contraception: a pilot study. Contraception 90:447–453
36. Faculty of sexual and reproductive healthcare. Quick start guidance. Sept 2010 www.fsrh.org.uk. Access date 13 Jul 2015
37. Cameron ST, Berger C, Michie L, Klipping C, Gemzell-Danielsson K (2015) The effects on ovarian activity of ulipristal acetate when 'quickstarting' a combined oral contraceptive pill: a prospective, randomized, double-blind parallel-arm, placebo-controlled study. Hum Reprod 30(7):1566–72
38. Brache V, Cochon L, Duijkers IJM, et al. (2015). A prospective, randomized, pharmacodynamic study of quick-starting a desogestrel progestin-only pill following ulipristal acetate for emergency contraception. Hum Reprod;30:2785–93
39. Faculty of Sexual and Reproductive Healthcare statement on quickstarting after upa/www.fsrh.org/documents (access date 1 September 2016)
40. Massai MR, Forcelledo ML, Brache V, Tejada AS, Salvatierra AM, Reyes MV, Alvarez F, Fau'ndes A, Croxatto HB (2007) Does meloxicam increase the incidence of anovulation induced by single administration of levonorgestrel in emergency contraception? A pilot study. Hum Reprod 22:434–439
41. Cameron ST, Critchley HOD, Buckley CH, Kelly RW, Baird DT (1997) Effect of two antiprogestins (mifepristone and onapristone) on endometrial factors of potential importance for implantation. Fertil Steril 67:1046–1053
42. Gemzell-Danielsson K, Svalander P, Swahn ML, Johannisson E, Bygdeman M (1994) Effects of a single post-ovulatory dose of RU486 on endometrial maturation in the implantation phase. Hum Reprod 9(12):2398–404

Adolescent Pregnancy and Contraception

14

Matan Elami-Suzin and Joseph G. Schenker

Key Points

- There is much difference in the incidence of adolescent pregnancy between various nations, but in recent years, the overall incidence has decreased.
- Adolescent pregnancy is a medical and social problem.
- Adolescents vary in their ability to implement various types of contraception.
- Sexually active adolescents are more likely to seek contraception if they perceive pregnancy as a negative outcome, have long-term educational goals, are older, experience a pregnancy scare or actual pregnancy, or have family, friends, and/or a clinician who encourage the use of contraception.
- Barriers that may impede adolescent access to contraceptive services include lack of access to confidential services and concerns about side effects such as weight gain, loss of bone density, and increased risk of thromboembolism or pelvic inflammatory disease.
- Before initiating contraception, it is important to review the adolescent's history for absolute or relative contraindications, discuss the risks and benefits, and obtain consent.
- Contraception counseling should include education about the anticipated adverse effects, the need to use condoms to protect against sexually transmitted infections, the availability of and indications for emergency contraception, and strategies to increase adherence.

M. Elami-Suzin, MD • J.G. Schenker, MD, FRCOG, FACOG (✉)
Department of Obstetrics and Gynecology, Hebrew University – Hadassah Medical Centre, Jerusalem, Israel
e-mail: joseph.schenker@mail.huji.ac.il

C. Sultan, A.R. Genazzani (eds.), *Frontiers in Gynecological Endocrinology*,
ISGE Series, DOI 10.1007/978-3-319-41433-1_14

14.1 Adolescent Pregnancy [1–3]

Adolescent pregnancy is defined as a pregnancy in an adolescent girl, usually within the ages of 13–19.

About 16 million girls aged 15–19 and some one million girls under 15 give birth every year. Ninety-five per cent of these births occur in low- and middle-income countries. The proportion of births that take place during adolescence is about 2 % in China, 18 % in Latin America and the Caribbean and more than 50 % in sub-Saharan Africa. In low- and middle-income countries, almost 10 % of girls become mothers by age 16 years, with the highest rates in sub-Saharan Africa and south-central and south-eastern Asia.

In South Asia, the Middle East and North Africa, age at marriage has traditionally been low in kinship-based societies. In such cases, most girls married soon after menarche, fertility is high, and consequently many children were born from adolescent mothers.

In developing countries, declining age at menarche and increased schooling have prolonged the period of adolescence. Together with a growing independence from parents and families, this has led to premarital sexual relations and increasing numbers of adolescent pregnancies

Children age 12–14 years old are more likely than other adolescents to have unplanned sexual intercourse.

The risk factors for adolescent pregnancy are: school drop-out, absence of future plans, low self-esteem, alcohol and drug abuse, lack of knowledge as to sexuality, and inappropriate use of contraceptive methods.

In sub-Saharan Africa, South Asia and Latin America, unsafe abortion is a frequent phenomenon and a cause of illness and even death, especially among young girls. In the USA, Europe and sub-Saharan Africa, high frequencies of physical abuse are reported in pregnant adolescents. In a number of African countries, female genital mutilation in young girls is a traditional practice, with possible consequences for the course of labor.

14.1.1 Complications During Pregnancy

Complications during pregnancy and childbirth are the second cause of death for 15–19-year-old girls globally.

In Latin America, the risk of maternal death is four times higher among adolescents younger than 16 years than among women in their twenties. Although some of this risk can be attributed to factors other than young age – e.g., giving birth for the first time, lack of access to care, or socioeconomic status – there appears to be an independent effect of young maternal age on pregnancy risk to the mother. Prenatal care tends to be inadequate among adolescent mothers which shows the importance of prenatal visits to decrease complications of pregnancy in this age group.

Young adolescents may still grow during pregnancy. Comparison of measurements of maternal height in adolescents and older mothers indicate that the mean height of the adolescents was significantly smaller than the height of older pregnant women.

Anemia frequently occurs in pregnant women. In a number of studies, anemia appears to be higher in pregnant adolescents than in older pregnant women. The cause is often nutritional deficiency and this can be treated adequately during antenatal care, if such care is available.

Infectious diseases like malaria, hookworm and HIV infection play an important role. In developing countries, malaria parasitemia occurs frequently during pregnancy, especially in primigravida. Adolescents are at increased risk of contracting HIV infection. Modern antiretroviral combination therapy during pregnancy considerably reduces mother-to-child transmission.

Reviewing the literature, there is no evidence that the incidence of hypertensive disease in adolescent pregnancies is higher than the incidence in adult women of the same parity; and there is also no indication of a difference between countries.

Rates of ectopic pregnancy, pre-eclampsia, eclampsia, preterm labor, premature rupture of membrane and cesarean section were significantly higher among adolescents <15 years of age; the risk then decreased steadily with age and became comparable with the control group after 16 years of age.

Labor As a result of insufficient prenatal care, the global incidence of premature births and low birth weight is higher among teenage mothers. Risks for medical complications are greater for girls 14 years of age and younger. An underdeveloped pelvis can lead to difficulties in childbirth. Young women under 20 face a higher risk of obstructed labor, which if cesarean section is not available can cause an obstetric fistula, a tear in the birth canal that creates leakage of urine and/or feces. At least two million of the world's poorest women live with fistulas. Higher incidence of postpartum hemorrhage and mental disorders, such as depression, were observed in adolescent pregnancy.

14.1.2 Adolescent Pregnancy—Effect on Newborn

Stillbirths and death in the first week of life are 50 % higher among newborn to mothers younger than 20 years than among babies born to mothers 20–29 years old. Deaths during the first month of life are 50–100 % more frequent if the mother is an adolescent versus older, and the younger the mother, the higher the risk.

The rates of preterm birth, low birth weight and asphyxia are higher among the children of adolescents, all of which increase the chance of death and of future health problems for the baby. Approximately 14 % of infants born to adolescents 17 years or younger are preterm versus 6 % for women 25–29 years of age. Young adolescent mothers (14 years and younger) are more likely than other age groups to give birth to underweight infants, and this is more pronounced in black adolescents.

Pregnant adolescents are more likely to smoke and use alcohol than are older women, which can cause many problems for the child after birth.

14.1.3 Social Aspects

Teenage mothers are at risk for long-term problems in many major areas of life, including school failure, poverty, and physical or mental illness. Teenage pregnancy is usually a crisis for the pregnant girl and her family. Common reactions include anger, guilt, and denial. If the father is young and involved, similar reactions can occur in his family.

Pregnant teenagers require special understanding, medical care, and education, particularly about nutrition, infections, substance abuse, and complications of pregnancy. Pregnant teens can have many different emotional reactions: some may not want their babies, others may view the creation of a child as an achievement and not recognize the serious responsibilities. Depression is common among pregnant teens, some teenage become overwhelmed by guilt, anxiety, and fears about the future.

Rates of ectopic pregnancy, pre-eclampsia, eclampsia, preterm labor, premature rupture of membrane and cesarean section were significantly higher among adolescents <15 years of age; the risk then decreased steadily with age and became comparable with the control group after 16 years of age.

Rates of adolescent childbearing have dropped significantly in most countries and regions in the past two decade.

Teenage girls account for 14 % of the estimated 20 million unsafe abortions performed each year, which result in some 68,000 deaths.

14.2 Adolescent Contraception

As a means of preventing teenage pregnancy and reducing the amount of induced abortions, adolescents may be offered a variety of contraceptive methods. Choosing a contraceptive method in adolescents may not be an easy task. The features of an ideal contraceptive method would be that it is: cheap; highly effective; have no side effects; independent of intercourse; does not require a regular action on the part of the user; is acceptable to all cultures and religions, and; is easily distributed and administered by non-healthcare personnel.

There is no one method that fits all of these criteria, and one must choose from a variety of available methods – each with its own advantages and disadvantages.

Adolescents may vary in their ability to initiate, and continue using, various types of contraception. Thus, prescribing "The Pill" for an adolescent patient – a contraceptive method that requires planning and forethought to prevent possible pregnancy – may not necessarily be the best option for them.

The intention of the present chapter is to demonstrate on ways of initiating the use of contraceptives by adolescents, overcoming barriers and solving problems regarding its use.

The female adolescent is more likely to seek contraception if she [4] perceives pregnancy as a negative outcome, is older, has future educational goals, is afraid of becoming pregnant, and has family, friends or physician who encourage the use of contraception.

14.3 Barriers for Contraception Use

As clinicians treating adolescents, we should strive to identify and overcome various barriers that prevent use of contraceptives. Female teens perceive cost, lack of information, and lack of access to confidential healthcare services, as significant barriers. Other barriers include concerns regarding potential pelvic examination and fear from side effects.

A prospective cohort study, which included 1404 urban female teens, has shown that removal of major barriers appears to be associated with use of more effective methods of contraception and decreased rates of pregnancy [5]. About 50 % of participants had experienced a past pregnancy; minors had parental consent to participate. Participants were educated about reversible contraception, with an emphasis on the benefits of long-acting reversible contraception. They were provided with their choice of reversible contraception at no cost, and followed for 2–3 years. Nearly 75 % chose an intrauterine device (IUD) or implant. Younger adolescents tended to choose the implant and older ones the IUD. Compared with sexually active United States teenagers in 2008, study participants had lower rates of pregnancy (34.0 versus 158.5 per 1000), birth (19.4 versus 94.0 per 1000), and abortion (9.7 versus 41.5 per 1000).

Confidentiality The adolescent's need for privacy should be recognized and respected. Health providers are required to develop and maintain a stable relationship with the adolescent, independently from the relationship with her parents. She should be given the chance to ask questions and tell her concerns freely, and to obtain gynecologic and sexual information directly from the clinician. The adolescent's age is a factor in whether she will choose an option of total confidentiality. A young teenager may ask her mother to stay with her through the entire office visit, especially if her mother is aware of her sexual behavior and is the one who desires the teenager to use a contraceptive method. Nevertheless, encouraging some independent time with the adolescent is important to obtain a more detailed history about other possible high-risk behaviors.

Pelvic Examination Many teenagers are afraid to consult healthcare providers, fearing that pelvic examination would have to be carried in order for them to receive contraception [6]. The physical exam of a female adolescent who seek contraception should perform general physical examination, including inspection of the external genitalia, but internal pelvic examination is only needed for insertion of an intrauterine device [7]. No specific findings on pelvic examination would be a contraindication for the initiation or restitution of oral contraceptives (OCs), contraceptive patch, vaginal ring, and progesterone implant or progesterone injections. Speculum and bimanual examination may be necessary to test for sexually transmitted infections (STI) if urine or vaginal swab tests are not available.

Legal Issues A minor's right to access contraceptive services in a health care setting without parental involvement varies among different countries, and the clinicians treating adolescents should be familiar with local law, protocols, and regulations.

Concerns Regarding Side Effects Adolescents have specific fears and concerns regarding use of contraception.

- Weight Gain – Many teenagers fear of gaining weight with the use of hormonal contraception. However, they should be reassured that available evidence does not support this regarding OCs. In the case of depot medroxyprogesterone acetate (DMPA), weight gain might be a concomitant event, but no causal relationship has been established. Factors other than DMPA may contribute to weight gain.
- Bone Density – Ultra-low dose estrogen (20 mcg) OCs and DMPA might interfere with achieving peak bone mass in teenagers and young adults. Rare cases of osteoporosis, including fractures, have been reported in patients taking DMPA, and the prescribing information for DMPA includes a boxed warning that DMPA should be used as a long-term birth control method (e.g., longer than 2 years) only if other birth control methods are inadequate [8]. It is vital to share information with the adolescent regarding the potential effects of DMPA on bone density. There is a general convention that DMPA should be avoided early puberty, but there is lack of evidence to limit its use in older adolescents. In fact, some experts argue that for adolescents in whom DMPA is the only acceptable contraceptive option, the benefit of pregnancy prevention outweighs the potential risk to bone health.
- The Society for Adolescent Health and Medicine has published a position paper regarding the boxed warning for DMPA [9]. This paper suggest that:
  - With adequate explanation of benefits and potential risks, *DMPA may continue to be prescribed to adolescent girls* who need contraception.
  - Decisions regarding bone density monitoring of adolescents using DMPA for contraception should be individualized; the decisions should be made by the clinician in concert with the adolescent, and potentially the adolescent's guardian.
  - *Duration of use of DMPA need not be restricted to 2 years.*
  - *Adolescents using DMPA should be encouraged to take 1300 mg of elemental calcium and 400 international units vitamin D and to exercise each day.*
  - *Estrogen supplementation should be considered* for girls who are doing well on DMPA and have osteopenia or are at risk for osteopenia and who have no contraindications to estrogen.
- Thromboembolism – Probably one of the most feared negative consequence of combined estrogen-progestin hormonal contraception is venous thromboembolism (VTE). Use of combined OCs increases VTE risk by two to fourfold compared to non-users. *However, this should be put readily in perspective, because the absolute risk is still very low* (increases from 2–3:10,000 non-users to 8–12:10,000 current users) *and much lower than the VTE risk during pregnancy and postpartum period* (60–80:10,000). It is, indeed, safer to prevent an unwanted pregnancy than terminating or continuing carrying it !

  Although reducing the estrogen dose had improved the safety and side-effects profile of OCs, it did not eliminate completely the increased risk of VTE [10–12]. There are several factors which influence the risk:

Table 14.1 Options for emergency contraception with reported efficacies

Method	Dose	Timing of use after unprotected intercourse (better to use as soon as possible)	Reported efficacy
Levonorgestrel	0.75 mg given twice, 12 h apart *or* 1.5 mg given as a single dose	Up to 3 days (72 h)	59–94 % of pregnancies prevented
Estrogen plus progesterone (Yuzpe regimen)	100–120 micrograms ethinyl estradiol plus 500–600 mcg levonorgestrel in each dose, given twice, 12 h apart	Up to 5 days (120 h)	47–89 % of pregnancies prevented
Mifepristone	Single 600 mg dose	Up to 5 days (120 h)	99–100 %
Copper intrauterine device	Inserted within 120 h after intercourse	Up to 5 days (120 h)	At least 99 %
Ulipristal	Single oral dose of 30 mg	Up to 5 days (120 h)	98–99 %

Experts recommend that ulipristal acetate be avoided in women using enzyme-inducing drugs or who have taken them within the last 28 days. Patients should also be advised to avoid ulipristal if they are currently taking drugs that increase gastric pH (e.g., antacids, histamine H2 antagonists, and proton pump inhibitors).

14.4.3 Contraindications

Although the Centers for Disease Control and Prevention (CDC) and the World Health Organization's (WHO) Medical Eligibility Criteria for Contraceptive Use applies contraindications to daily use of hormonal contraceptives in some women based on their medical history, these contraindications do *not* apply to adolescents and women seeking emergency contraception. In particular, cardiovascular disease, thrombophilic disorders, migraine, liver disease, and breastfeeding are considered conditions where the advantages of using the method generally outweigh the theoretical or proven risks [36].

The medical eligibility guidelines do not include information about ulipristal. Contraindications to its use are available in the package insert and include suspected pregnancy, poorly controlled asthma, and hepatic dysfunction.

Contraindications to copper IUD use include severe uterine distortion, active pelvic infection, copper allergy, and suspected pregnancy.

14.4.4 Efficacy of EC in Overweight and Obese Adolescents

Some data suggest levonorgestrel and ulipristal emergency contraception may be less effective in overweight or obese women. A 2015 study reported that levonorgestrel emergency contraception was less effective at preventing pregnancy as weight and body mass index increased [37]. The women in the 80 kg group had a pregnancy risk of 6 %, which was similar to the pregnancy risk as if no contraceptive had been used. At least one pharmaceutical package insert for levonorgestrel emergency contraception warns of reduced contraceptive efficacy in women weighing ≥75 kg. However, the European Medicines Association concluded that the available data were too limited and not robust enough to be certain the contraceptive efficacy of levonorgestrel or ulipristal emergency contraception is reduced with increased bodyweight and that the benefits of taking these medications outweigh any risks [38].

We counsel overweight and obese adolescents of potentially reduced or absent efficacy of levonorgestrel emergency contraception as BMI increases above 30 kg/m^2 or at weight ≥75 kg, and offer them a copper-releasing IUD as first-line therapy to prevent pregnancy. There is no evidence of impaired contraceptive efficacy for obese women who rely on the copper IUD for contraception. If the IUD is not an option, ulipristal is more likely to be effective than levonorgestrel.

14.4.5 Resuming or Initiating Hormonal Contraception

The duration of effectiveness of emergency contraception has not been determined. Thus it is not clear when regular contraception should be resumed or initiated within the menstrual cycle of emergency contraceptive use [39]. The safest approach is to advise adolescents using emergency contraception pills that a risk of pregnancy still exists if they have unprotected sexual intercourse after the emergency contraceptive pills have been taken; therefore, they should immediately initiate an effective contraceptive method.

For those taking levonorgestrel or combined estrogen-progestin emergency contraception, any regular contraceptive method can be started immediately after the use of the emergency contraceptive [36]. Backup methods of contraception (e.g., condom or diaphragm) or abstinence are required during the first 7 days of use. Although efficacy is not compromised by immediate initiation, it is prudent to avoid starting longer-acting hormonal methods (e.g., depot-medroxyprogesterone acetate, etonogestrel implant, levonorgestrel-releasing intrauterine devices) until it is certain that pregnancy has not occurred. However, this concern should be balanced against risk of unintended pregnancy if initiation of one of these methods is delayed.

For those taking ulipristal for emergency contraception, there is theoretical concern that starting a hormonal method after taking ulipristal could make either the ulipristal or the hormonal method less effective by competitive binding to the progestin receptors. In 2015, the US Food and Drug Administration amended the package insert and stated that progesterone-containing contraceptives should not be used with ulipristal or for 5 days following ulipristal use [40]. The ulipristal package insert recommends using a barrier method for the remainder of the cycle to avoid any potential drug interactions with a hormonal contraceptive. Some experts advise waiting 7 days after ulipristal to start a hormonal method. A guideline from the United Kingdom recommends that additional precautions be taken for 14 days after taking ulipristal (9 days if using or starting the progestogen-only pill, 16 days for estradiol valerate/dienogest pill) [41].

14.4.6 Repeated Emergency Contraception

There is no contraindication to giving a second dose of hormonal emergency contraception if a second episode of unprotected intercourse occurs any time after the first dose was administered. In contrast, there is no support for use of ulipristal more than once per cycle or if there has been another episode of unprotected sexual intercourse outside the treatment window (>120 h) [36].

14.4.7 Adolescents Who Are Using EC as a Primary Method

This is also commonly encountered situation. Hormonal emergency contraception is less effective, contains higher hormone levels per dose, and causes more menstrual irregularities than ongoing use of combined or progestin-only oral contraceptives [36]. The key to proper use of EC is education by the healthcare provider.

14.5 "Getting Started" with Contraception

When discussing contraceptive use with the adolescent, several points must be stressed:

1. The selection of the contraceptive method is based on effectiveness, frequency of use, and personal convenience (Fig. 14.1). Recently, the long-acting reversible contraceptives (LARC), including the etonogestrel implant and intrauterine devices (copper and levonorgestrel) have been recommended by both the American College of Obstetricians and Gynecologists (ACOG) and the American Academy of Pediatrics (AAP), as the most effective means for prevention of an unintended pregnancy [42].
2. Adverse effects
3. Tips on increasing adherence and to promote use
4. Protection against STIs (i.e., use of condoms)
5. Availability and indications for emergency contraception

There are many sexually active teenagers who are worried about becoming pregnant, but also not sure if to start using contraception, and what kind of. The encounter with the teen should be focused on her thoughts and concerns, reviewing stories and beliefs about contraceptives that she heard from friends or family members, and stressing the importance of dual protection (i.e., both against pregnancy and STIs). Teens that are not sexually active yet should be educated about the use of condoms and emergency contraception, in case their status changes.

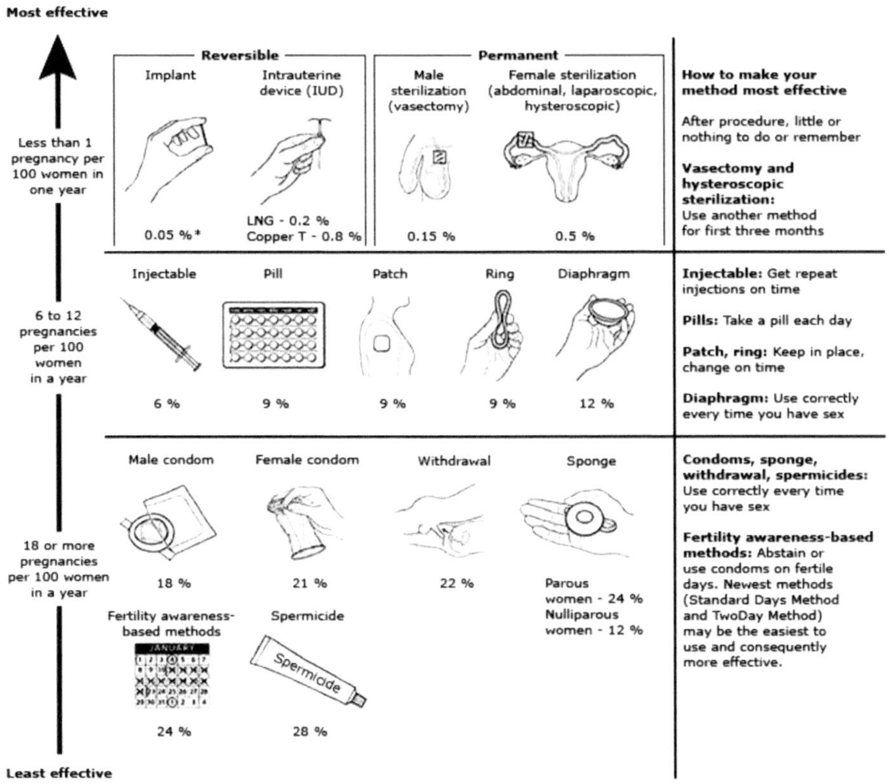

Fig. 14.1 Comparing effectiveness of contraceptive methods. Condoms should always be used to reduce the risk of sexually transmitted infections. Other methods of contraception:
Lactational amenorrhea method - LAM is a highly effective, temporary method of contraception
Emergency contraception - Emergency contraceptive pills or a copper IUD after unprotected intercourse substantially reduces risk of pregnancy
LNG levonorgestrel. * The percentages indicate the number out of every 100 women who experienced an unintended pregnancy within the first year of typical use of each contraceptive method. World Health Organization (WHO) et al. [76], Trussell [77] (Reproduced from: U.S. Selected Practice Recommendations for Contraceptive Use, 2013: Adapted from the World Health Organization Selected Practice Recommendations for Contraceptive Use, 2nd Edition. MMWR Morb Mortal Wkly Rep 2013; 62:1.)

The healthcare provider must also discuss with the adolescent potential advantages and adverse effects:

- *Benefits* – Advantages of combined estrogen-progestin hormonal contraception include improved bone density and protection against ovarian cancer, endometrial cancer, salpingitis, ectopic pregnancy, benign breast disease, dysmenorrhea, acne, and iron deficiency [43]. The same benefits, with the exception of improved bone density, are provided by DMPA. The adolescent may also view the change in menstruation pattern (i.e., fewer periods or amenorrhea), as a potential advantage.

Neither the progestin implant nor the IUDs has been associated with decreased bone density, which might also be regarded as a potential advantage.
- *Adverse effects* – The combined estrogen-progestin hormonal contraception (OCs, transdermal patch and vaginal ring), as well as DMPA, etonorgestrel implant and intra-uterine progestin systems, can cause breakthrough bleeding and/or amenorrhea. These can frighten or upset the adolescent, and she would likely discontinue the use of the method, unless she was educated in advance about these potential problems and their treatment [44].

  The transdermal patch might cause local contact dermatitis (mild or severe). Also, partial or complete detachment of the patch from the skin was reported more commonly in adolescents (up to 35 %) [45, 46] than in adults (<5 %) [47, 48]. No detachments were reported when the patch was worn on the arm. The likely explanation may be inadequate care in application and increased activity among teenagers compared with adults.

Although it is not necessary to obtain written informed consent before the initiation of hormonal contraception in adolescents, the use of a structured informed consent form can ensure that the risks and benefits are adequately discussed.

14.6 Long Acting Reversible Contraception (LARC)

14.6.1 The Intra-uterine Device (IUD)

Usually, most physicians are reluctant to insert an IUD to an adolescent, and even to nulliparous adult patient. This reluctancy stems from several reasons, including: [49] history of negative publicity; disinformation about the risk of ectopic pregnancy, infection and infertility; misconceptions about the mechanism of action of the IUD; lack of provider training; and fears of litigation.

In the 1970s, the IUD was used by 10 % of women in the United States using contraception. When the Dalkon Shield (a common IUD used in that era) was linked to pelvic inflammatory disease, utilization of all IUDs fell and litigation rose.

One probable explanation for the increased infectious morbidity in the 1970s is the construction of the IUD tail, which were multifilament and braided and acted like "ropes" that allowed bacteria to ascend upward from the lower genital tract. Coupled with the fact that no test had yet been developed to detect asymptomatic Chlamydia infection, many women developed severe pelvic infections.

Current IUDs, which have monofilament tail strings, have not been associated with an elevated infection risk, beyond the first 2–3 weeks after insertion. In 2005, the US Food and Drug Administration (FDA) approved liberalized package labeling for the copper T380A (Paragard), removing any proscription against its use in nulliparous women or in those with more than one sexual partner. Initial studies with the newest levonorgestrel releasing IUD (LNg14 IUD; Jaydess*, Skyla*) include nulliparous women. Based on the results of these trials, the product label contains no recommendation against use in nulliparous women. Although the LNg20 IUD

(Mirena*) package label contains a recommendation for its use in parous women, the LNg20 has been studied in nulliparous women and found to be safe. The American College of Obstetrics and Gynecologists (ACOG) states that IUDs are safe and appropriate for most women, including nulliparous women and adolescents, and that use of IUDs should be encouraged as a first-line approach to pregnancy prevention [42, 50]. The IUD is an attractive option for adolescents and adolescent mothers who desire long-term, uninterrupted contraception. It lasts 3–10 years depending on the type of device. Parous adolescents may be better candidates for the IUD than nulliparous adolescents because higher expulsion rates have been reported in nulliparous adolescents. However the 3- and 5-year devices have been successfully used in nulliparous adolescents. This has been shown in a large study based on medical records of 1177 female teenagers age 13–24 years [51]. In this study the first-attempt success rate was 95.8 % for nulliparous women and 96.7 % for parous women. The first-attempt success rate was 95.5 % (n = 169) for women aged 13–17 years compared with 96.3 % (n = 963) for women aged 18–24 years.

The World Health Organization suggests: [52]

- The IUD is an unacceptable risk in a woman with pelvic inflammatory disease (PID) or purulent cervicitis currently or in the past 3 months.
- The risks outweigh the advantages of inserting an IUD in a woman with multiple partners or a partner with multiple partners.
- There is no restriction on IUD placement when there is a past history of PID and no current sexually transmitted infection.

14.6.1.1 Mechanisms of Action

There are several possible mechanisms of action for IUD [53, 54], including changes in cervical mucus that inhibit sperm transport (e.g., increased copper concentration, thickening, glandular atrophy or decidualization); chronic inflammatory changes of the endometrium and fallopian tubes, which have spermicidal effects and inhibit fertilization and implantation; thinning and glandular atrophy of the endometrium, which inhibits implantation; and direct toxic effects on the oocyte. It is important to stress that *the IUD is not an abortifacient* (defined as interruption of an implanted pregnancy) [53].

14.6.1.2 Absolute and Relative Contraindications

- Absolute contraindications for any IUD placement include: possible or confirmed pregnancy; severe distortion of the uterine cavity (such as by fibroids or anatomic anomalies) that precludes IUD insertion; acute, recent (within 3 months) or recurrent uterine infection (includes sexually transmitted, postpartum and post-abortion infections); untreated cervicitis; active genital actinomycoses.
- Absolute contraindications for copper IU include Wilson's disease and known copper allergy.
- Absolute contraindications for levonorgestrel IUD include: known allergy to levonorgestrel; acute liver disease or liver tumor; and known or suspected carcinoma of the breast.

- Relative contraindications for any IUD placement include: patients at high risk for STIs (multiple sexual partners, past infections); previous IUD problem (perforation, significant cramps); unresolved abnormal uterine bleeding; known severe vasovagal reactions.
- Relative contraindications for copper IUD include current anemia or menorrhagia-associated anemia.
- Relative contraindications for levonorgestrel IUD include past intolerance to progestin and patient unwilling to accept a change in menstrual pattern (hypomenorrhea or amenorrhea).

The risks and benefits of IUD for an adolescent must be determined on a case-by-case basis.

14.6.1.3 Quick Guide for IUD Insertion

- Screen every adolescent for chlamydia and gonorrhea before insertion. If not screened and proven negative we usually give 1 g azithromycin orally at the day of insertion.
- The IUD may be inserted at any time during the cycle if pregnancy can be excluded. A pregnancy test should be obtained if pregnancy cannot be excluded clinically, and a negative result documented before insertion.
- As NSAIDs or topical anesthetics have not been found helpful to ease insertion pain, we do not use them. We also do not routinely use paracervical block, as the procedure itself is painful. Paracervical block is an option for patients at risk of *greater than average* insertional pain, such as those requiring cervical dilation or with a history of prior painful IUD insertion, and it can also be useful for patients at risk for a vasovagal reaction.
- Each IUD type has a unique insertion procedure. The provider should be familiar with device instructions and never use force when measuring the uterine cavity or passing the IUD through the cervical canal, as this increases the risk of perforation.
- We use misoprostol 400 mcg vaginally or sublingually before IUD insertion to *nulliparous* adolescents or adolescents with *previous failed insertion*.
- Although not necessary, we find it more relaxing to insert the IUD under abdominal ultrasound guidance. If the insertion was not performed under ultrasound guidance we confirm proper placement with ultrasound immediately after insertion.
- One can insert the IUD immediately after abortion or at 4–6 weeks post-partum. The copper IUD may be placed immediately following a vaginal or cesarean delivery.
- Back-up contraception is not needed after insertion of a CuT380A, but should be provided for 7 days if a levonorgestrel IUD is inserted more than 7 days from the start of menstrual bleeding.

14.6.1.4 Complications

- *Uterine perforation* – This occurs in about 1:1000 interval IUD insertions. The risk factors include cervical stenosis, inexperienced provider, postpartum period, breastfeeding and fixed or retroverted uterus. If perforation by the sound or the

IUD is suspected, the adolescent must be monitored for tachycardia, hypotension, syncope, or an acute abdomen. Even though these rarely occur after perforation, they warrant a transfer to hospital for further management. If perforation is suspected in a stable patient (which usually is the case), IUD removal can be attempted by placing gentle traction on the string. If the string is not visible, the location of the IUD can usually be determined by ultrasound examination. Depending on the location, the IUD can then be retrieved using a hysteroscope or laparoscope. Removing the IUD under direct vision helps to prevent injury to pelvic organs that could be snagged by the device. Laparotomy is required if laparoscopic or hysteroscopic removal is difficult, if perforation of intraabdominal organs is suspected or with ongoing intraperitoneal hemorrhage. Immediate intervention is not essential if the patient is stable. A uterine perforation caused by a sound or an IUD is not a contraindication for future vaginal delivery.

- *Vasovagal response* – Sometimes, the IUD insertion causes transient syncope or presyncope, hypotension, bradycardia, and/or nausea. These typically resolve by stopping the procedure, placing the adolescent in a recumbent position, and giving supportive care.
- *Postinsertion patient counseling*

We teach the adolescent to feel the IUD strings and to verify periodically and especially after the menses that the IUD is retained. We guide her, that if she doesn't feel the strings, she should schedule an appointment and use a back-up contraceptive method until her healthcare provider confirms whether or not the IUD is in place. Even with absent problems we schedule a follow-up visit in 1–3 months, because it was shown to increase continuation of the method.

14.7 Contraceptive Progestin Implant

These were also suggested (together with the IUD) as a first-line contraceptive method in adolescents [42, 43]. The contraceptive implant is potentially an attractive option for adolescents and adolescent mothers who desire long-term contraception. It provides pregnancy protection within 24 h of insertion, and fertility returns quickly after its removal. Unexpected and prolonged bleeding can be a problem and can trigger request for premature removal. One should reliably exclude pregnancy before implant insertion. Therefore the "Quick-Start" method is *not recommended* for the implant.

14.8 Depo Medroxy Progesterone Acetate (DMPA) Injections

Typically, the first injection is given during the menstrual period to ensure absence of pregnancy. Alternatively, it can be given using the Quick-Start method (Fig. 14.2) [55]. If DMPA is initiated more than 7 days after the first day of the menstrual period and she has had unprotected intercourse during the cycle, clinicians and patients must recognize that there is a small chance of preimplantation or early pregnancy despite a negative pregnancy test prior to the injection. We suggest that

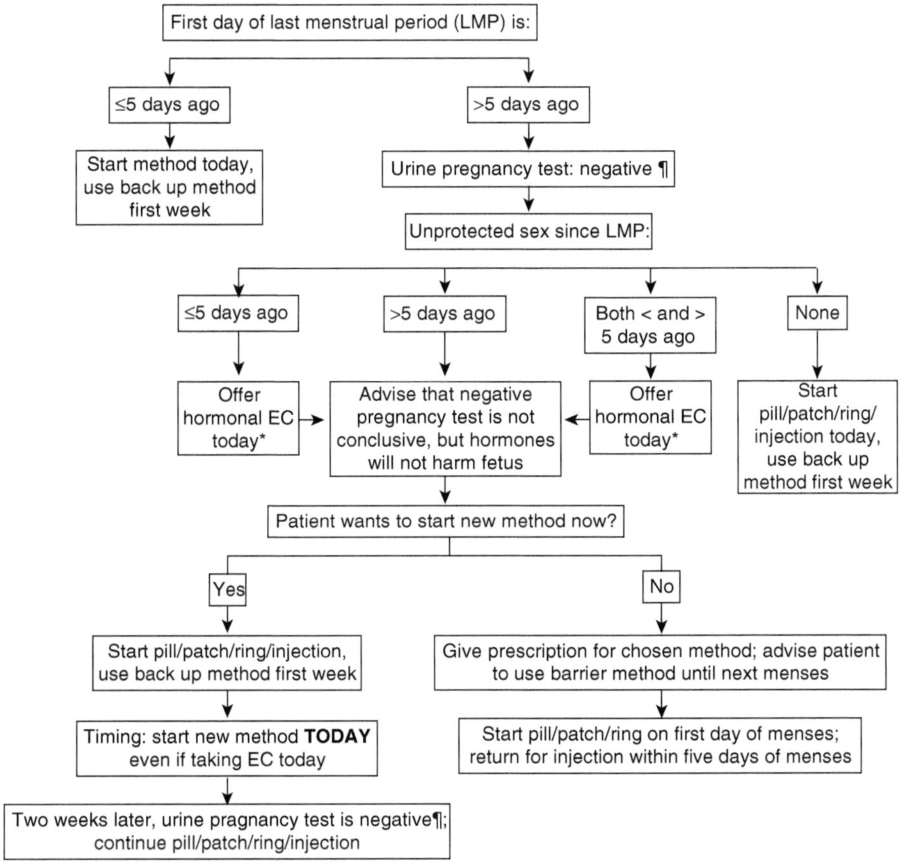

Fig. 14.2 The "Quick-Start" algorithm for initiation of short acting reversible contraception (pill, patch, vaginal ring and DMPA injection). EC emergency contraception. * Because hormonal EC is not 100 % effective, check urine pregnancy test 2 weeks after EC use. If pregnancy test is positive, provide options counseling (Reproduced with permission from: RHEDI/The Center for Reproductive Health Education In Family Medicine, Montefiore Medical Center, New York City. Copyright © 2007 RHEDI)

in these cases to receive emergency contraception if intercourse occurred within the previous 120 h, and we advise to use back-up contraception for 7 days after DMPA injection since ovulation may occur within 24 h of the initial injection, and we counsel them to repeat the pregnancy test in 2–3 weeks.

14.8.1 Switching from Another Contraceptive Method to DMPA

A common scenario is an adolescent girl not happy from one contraceptive method and asking another one. Many mistakes can be made during this changing period, both by the patients and by the providers. Table 14.2 is designed to provide short and clear guidelines regarding safe switch between various methods.

Table 14.2 Switching between various contraceptive methods

	Pill	Patch	Ring	DMPA injection	Implant	Hormonal IUD	Copper IUD
Pill	*No gap:* take first pill of new pack the day after taking any pill in old pack	Start patch *1 day before* stopping pill	*No gap:* insert ring the day after taking any pill in pack	First shot *7 days before* stopping pill	Insert implant *4 days before* stopping pill	Insert hormone IUD *7 days before* stopping pill	Can insert copper IUD up *to 5 days after stopping* the pill
Patch	Start pill *1 day before stopping* patch		*No gap:* insert ring and remove patch on the same day	First shot *7 days before* stopping patch	Insert implant *4 days before* stopping patch	Insert hormone IUD *7 days before* stopping patch	Can insert copper IUD up *to 5 days after stopping* patch
Ring	Start pill *1 day before stopping* ring	Start patch *2 days before* stopping ring		First shot *7 days before* stopping ring	Insert implant *4 days before* stopping ring	Insert hormone IUD *7 days before* stopping ring	Can insert copper IUD up *to 5 days after stopping* ring
DMPA injection	Can take first pill *up to 15 weeks after* the last shot	Can start patch *up to 15 weeks after* the last shot	Can insert ring *up to 15 weeks after* the last shot		Can insert implant *up to 15 weeks after* the last shot	Can insert hormone IUD up *to 15 weeks after the* last shot	Can insert copper IUD *up to 16 weeks after the* last shot
Implant	Start pill *7 days before implant* is remove	Start patch *7 days before* implant is removed	Start ring *7 days before* implant is removed	First shot *7 days before* implant is removed		Insert hormone IUD *7 days before* implant is removed	Can insert copper IUD up *to 5 days after implant* is removed
Hormonal IUD	Start pill *7 days before* IUD is removed	Start patch *7 days before* IUD is removed	Start ring *7 days before* IUD is removed	First shot *7 days before* IUD is removed	Insert implant *4 days before* IUD is removed		Can insert copper IUD *right after* hormone IUD is removed
Copper IUD	Start pill *7 days before* IUD is removed	Start patch *7 days before* IUD is removed	Start ring *7 days before* IUD is removed	First shot *7 days before* IUD is removed	Insert implant *4 days before* IUD is removed	Insert hormone IUD *right after* copper IUD is removed and use back-up method for *7 days*	

14.8.1.1 What to Do if She's Late for Injection?

Adolescents who are late for injection shouldn't be turned away solely because of that. After a 150 mg injection, ovulation does not occur for at least 14 weeks. Therefore, a 2-week "grace period" (repeat injection without pregnancy testing) is appropriate for adolescent women receiving injections every 3 months (13 weeks). For adolescents more than 2 weeks late for their injection (>15 weeks from the last injection), we suggest a pregnancy test before administering DMPA and back-up contraception (or abstinence) for 7 days.

As a result of a study showing that contraceptive efficacy is maintained with a "grace period" as long as 4 weeks [56], the World Health Organization (WHO) adopted a longer grace period in its updated guidelines. A limitation of these data is that more than one third of the women in the study were lactating, placing them at low baseline risk for conception. Therefore, in high-resource countries, we continue to encourage women to return on time and allow a 2-week grace period, and require documentation of a negative pregnancy test in women who present more than 2 weeks (>15 weeks from their last injection).

14.8.2 Pros and Cons of DMPA Injections

- *Advantages* of DMPA injections include: reversibility, privacy, lasts 12 weeks, effective in obese adolescents, reduces risk of ectopic pregnancy, menses decreases or ceases, reduces dysmenorrhea and other menstrual symptoms, few drug interactions, less seizures in epileptics, less pain crises in adolescents with sickle cell anemia, reduction in endometriosis related pelvic pain, reduction in abnormal uterine bleeding associated with leiomyomas, possible reduction in the incidence of PID.
- *Disadvantages* of DMPA injections include: increase in unscheduled bleeding, possible increase in weight gain, possible induction of depression, a decrease in bone density that is *usually reversible*, small risk of severe allergic reaction, a delay in return to fertility, repeated injection is needed every 12 weeks.

A thorough proactive counseling about possible side effects of DMPA, and especially menstrual irregularities and the need for repeat injections is vital for adolescents choosing this method. It was shown that women who are well informed are much more likely to become satisfied users with high continuation rates [44, 57–61].

14.9 Vaginal Contraceptive Ring

For some adolescents this is a very attractive option because it needs to be changed only every 3 weeks. However, some adolescents do not feel comfortable in insertion of things into their vaginas. Those who use tampons might be better candidates for this method. The vaginal ring can be initiated according to the Quick Start method (Fig. 14.2).

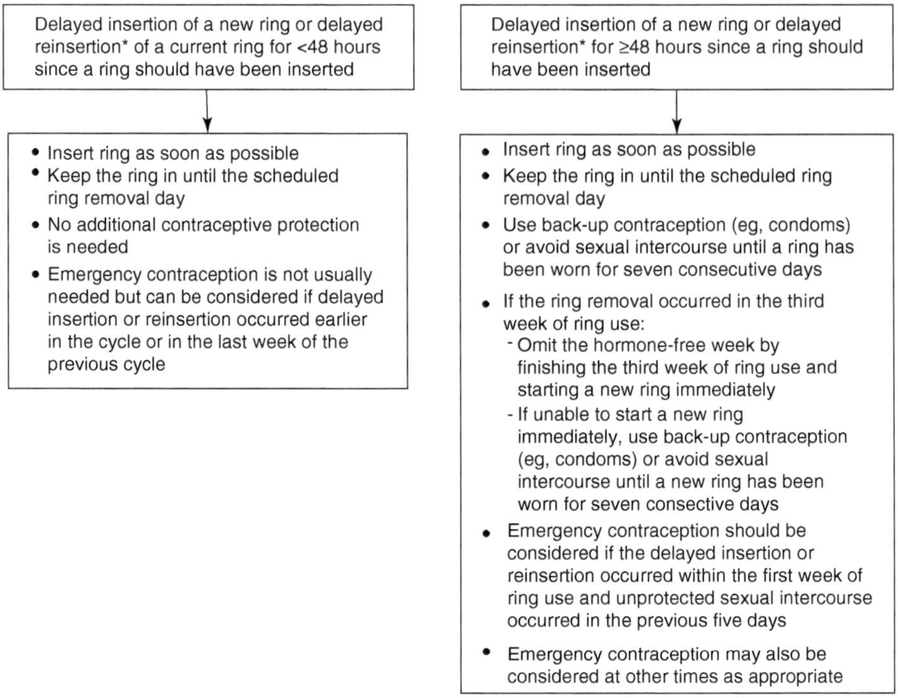

Delayed insertion of a new ring or delayed reinsertion* of a current ring for <48 hours since a ring should have been inserted
• Insert ring as soon as possible
• Keep the ring in until the scheduled ring removal day
• No additional contraceptive protection is needed
• Emergency contraception is not usually needed but can be considered if delayed insertion or reinsertion occurred earlier in the cycle or in the last week of the previous cycle
Delayed insertion of a new ring or delayed reinsertion* for ≥48 hours since a ring should have been inserted
• Insert ring as soon as possible
• Keep the ring in until the scheduled ring removal day
• Use back-up contraception (eg, condoms) or avoid sexual intercourse until a ring has been worn for seven consecutive days
• If the ring removal occurred in the third week of ring use:
- Omit the hormone-free week by finishing the third week of ring use and starting a new ring immediately
- If unable to start a new ring immediately, use back-up contraception (eg, condoms) or avoid sexual intercourse until a new ring has been worn for seven consective days
• Emergency contraception should be considered if the delayed insertion or reinsertion occurred within the first week of ring use and unprotected sexual intercourse occurred in the previous five days
• Emergency contraception may also be considered at other times as appropriate

Fig. 14.3 Management of delayed insertion or reinsertion of the contraceptive vaginal ring. * If removal takes place but the woman is unsure of how long the ring has been removed, consider the ring to have been removed for ≥48 h since a ring should have been inserted or reinserted (Reproduced from: US Selected Practice Recommendations for Contraceptive Use, 2013: Adapted from the World Health Organization Selected Practice Recommendations for Contraceptive Use, 2nd Ed. MMWR Morb Mortal Wkly Rep 2013; 62:1)

If the ring remains in place more than 3 but ≤5 weeks, it is removed and a new one is inserted after a 1-week ring-free interval; if the ring is left in place for >5 weeks, back-up contraception is recommended until a new ring has been in place for 7 days. The ring remains effective when left in place for up to 5 weeks, as the ring contains sufficient steroids to maintain stable blood concentrations for this period of time [62]. Thus, inhibition of ovulation is sufficiently maintained if an adolescent forgets to remove the ring after the usual 3-week use period. In 2013, the US Selected Practice Recommendations for Contraceptive Use published an algorithm for counseling patients who delay insertion or reinsertion of the ring (Fig. 14.3) [63].

Adolescents who desire fewer days of withdrawal bleeding and are willing to tolerate some spotting can safely use an extended ring regimen whereby the ring is changed every 3 weeks, omitting the hormone-free week for up to 1 year [64–68]. Extended use is effective and does not worsen bothersome side effects, except for unscheduled bleeding.

Unplanned removal or expulsion of the contraceptive ring can occur. The ring should not be removed during intercourse. If it accidentally falls out, it may be rinsed with cool or warm (not hot) water and reinserted into the vagina within 3 h. From our own experience, many teenagers do not feel "clean" with the vaginal ring and have a need to wash it frequently. Frequent washing decreases effectiveness and may cause intermittent bleeding or spotting.

If the ring is out of the vagina for more than 3 consecutive hours, subsequent steps depend on the week of the cycle that the ring is out:

- During the first 2 weeks of the cycle, the ring is reinserted as soon as possible. Pregnancy may not be prevented if the ring is out for more than 3 h during this time, so an additional form of contraception, such as condoms with spermicide, is used until the reinserted ring has been in place for 7 continuous days. The ring should subsequently be removed according to the original schedule, after which the adolescent can expect to have her normal period.
- During week three of the cycle, the adolescent discards the ring. She then chooses one of two different restart options:
  - Option one – Insert a new ring and begin a new 3-week cycle. Back-up contraception or abstinence is recommended until the new ring has been used continuously for 7 days. The adolescent may not have a regular period until she reaches her next ring-free week, but she may have vaginal spotting or bleeding prior to that point.
  - Option two – Insert a new ring and begin a new 3-week cycle. Back-up contraception or abstinence is recommended until the new ring has been used continuously for 7 days. The adolescent may not have a regular period until she reaches her next ring-free week, but she may have vaginal spotting or bleeding prior to that point.

These steps are consistent with recommendations from the manufacturer. In contrast, the CDC recommendations are more liberal and state that back-up contraception is not needed if reinsertion of the current ring occurs in less than 48 h (see Fig. 14.3).

14.10 Transdermal Patch

The fact that the transdermal patch does not require daily attention makes it an attractive option for adolescents. However, the need for weekly change also may promote decreased adherence. The transdermal patch can be initiated according to the Quick Start method (see Figure 14.2).

The patch is applied to the buttock, abdomen, upper arm, or upper torso (but not the breast, as it might cause breast tenderness due to high local estrogen concentration). A different site is used each time a new patch is applied. The patch is changed once a week for 3 weeks (21 total days), followed by 1 week that is patch-free. It should always be changed/applied on the same day of the week. Reminder systems are useful to ensure appropriate weekly changes. The consequences of failing to change the transdermal contraceptive patch at the appropriate time should be addressed with the adolescent.

- *Delay in beginning the first patch in a cycle* — When a new patch cycle is delayed beyond the scheduled start day, users are instructed to apply a patch as soon as they remember and use back-up contraception (or avoid sex) for at least 1 week. The day they apply the new patch becomes the new patch change day.

  Delay in beginning the second or third patch in a cycle — There is a 2-day (48 h) period of continued release of adequate contraceptive steroid levels when the patch is left on for two extra days. If users change the patch within this window, the patch change day remains the same and there is no need for back-up contraception.

  After this 2-day (48 h) time period, failure to replace the second or third patch in a cycle increases the risk for contraceptive failure. Therefore, users will need to use back-up contraception (or avoid sex) for 7 days and, in some instances, use emergency contraception, if this occurs. The day the patient remembers to apply the patch becomes the new change day.
- *Delay in removing the third patch in a cycle* — Forgetting to remove the third patch on time carries less risk than forgetting to remove the first or second patch. The user is instructed to remove the patch when she remembers; the patch change day is not altered.

These recommendations are similar to those of the 2013 US Selected Practice Recommendations for Contraceptive Use, which included the following algorithm for counseling patients who delay application of the patch (Fig. 14.4) [63]. Strategies to promote weekly changes should be reviewed with adolescents using the transdermal patch. These include using a wall, computer, or cell phone calendar; a cell phone weekly alarm; or a sticker designating the change day on the bathroom mirror.

If a patch becomes partially or completely detached for less than 24 h, it should be reapplied at the same location (if it has not lost its stickiness: ancillary adhesives or tape should *not* be used), or replaced with a new patch immediately. If detachment lasts longer than 24 h, a new patch should be applied, and this day of the week becomes the new patch change day. An additional method of contraception (e.g., condoms, spermicides) should be used for the first 7 days of this cycle or the patient should avoid sex.

In various trials, 1.8 % of transdermal patches required replacement for complete detachment and 2.9 % became partially detached [47]. Living in a warm, humid climate did not increase the risk of detachment. The quality of adherence was illustrated in a study in which 30 women were subjected to various conditions over several 7-day time periods during transdermal patch use [47]. The conditions included normal activity, use of a sauna, immersion in a whirlpool bath, use of a treadmill followed by showering, cool water immersion, and a combination of these activities. Only one patch became detached during the 87 cycles that were evaluated, suggesting that skin adherence is not adversely affected by a vigorous, athletic lifestyle.

14.11 Oral Contraceptives (OCs)

Especially in the adolescent age group there are various adherence problems with OCs:

1. Not refilling the prescription
2. Forgetting to take the pill
3. Starting next pack late
4. Using pills inconsistently and sporadically
5. Not using a back-up method when needed

One study has shown that up to 33 % of adolescents missed a pill in the previous 3 months [29]. Therefore, the adolescent should be provided clear verbal and written instructions. The clinician should ascertain that she has sufficient reading skills to interpret labels and instructions.

To optimize the adolescent's adherence to OCs, we suggest giving her only three things to remember:

1. When to start the pill
2. Take the pill every day at the same time, especially when doing something else regularly, like teeth brushing
3. Call the clinic if there are any questions

OCs can be started at any time. In adolescents, they are typically started on the first day of the next menstrual period or the Sunday after the onset of the menstrual period ("Sunday start method"). The rationale for this delayed start date is to make sure that the adolescent is not pregnant. However, as many as 25 % of adolescents who seek OCs from family planning clinics never take the first pill [69, 70].

To address this issue, a "same day" or "Quick Start" method is now the preferred approach. The Quick Start method requires increased attention to the adolescent's self-report of sexual activity since her last menstrual period, the accuracy of the pregnancy test in the context of her sexual history, and the use of emergency contraception when applicable (see Fig. 14.2). It's also, in our opinion, important to give teenage girls the regiments with less hormone free interval (i.e., 24/4 preparations instead of 21/7) because these preparations allow the adolescent to simply take a pill every day and to start the next pack immediately after finishing the previous one. This makes things easy on her and she will be less likely to forget.

14.11.1 Extended-Cycle or Continuous Pill Use

The desire to avoid monthly periods may be related to participation in athletic events or summer camps, or to the general discomfort and "hassle" of monthly periods. A schedule that involves continuous pill use for 84 days followed by a week of

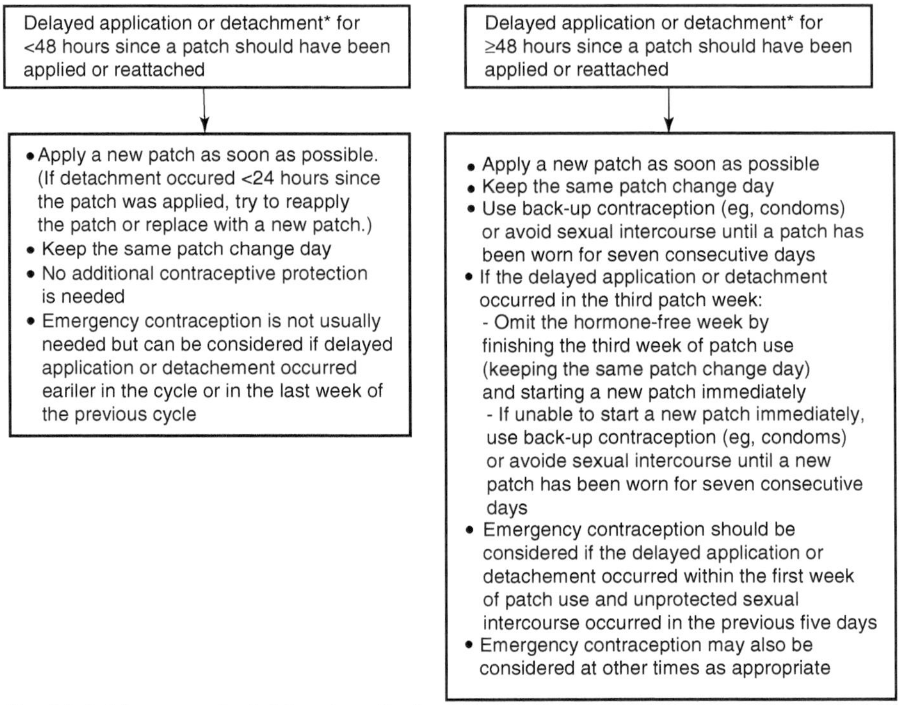
Delayed application or detachment* for <48 hours since a patch should have been applied or reattached
• Apply a new patch as soon as possible. (If detachment occured <24 hours since the patch was applied, try to reapply the patch or replace with a new patch.)
• Keep the same patch change day
• No additional contraceptive protection is needed
• Emergency contraception is not usually needed but can be considered if delayed application or detachement occurred eariler in the cycle or in the last week of the previous cycle
Delayed application or detachment* for ≥48 hours since a patch should have been applied or reattached
• Apply a new patch as soon as possible
• Keep the same patch change day
• Use back-up contraception (eg, condoms) or avoid sexual intercourse until a patch has been worn for seven consecutive days
• If the delayed application or detachment occurred in the third patch week:
- Omit the hormone-free week by finishing the third week of patch use (keeping the same patch change day) and starting a new patch immediately
- If unable to start a new patch immediately, use back-up contraception (eg, condoms) or avoide sexual intercourse until a new patch has been worn for seven consecutive days
• Emergency contraception should be considered if the delayed application or detachement occurred within the first week of patch use and unprotected sexual intercourse occurred in the previous five days
• Emergency contraception may also be considered at other times as appropriate

Fig. 14.4 Management of delayed application or detachment of the contraceptive patch. * If detachment takes place but the woman is unsure when the detachment occurred, consider the patch to have been detached for ≥48 h since a patch should have been applied or reattached (Reproduced from: US Selected Practice Recommendations for Contraceptive Use, 2013: Adapted from the World Health Organization Selected Practice Recommendations for Contraceptive Use, 2nd Ed. MMWR Morb Mortal Wkly Rep 2013; 62:1)

pill-free days may help to increase adherence in adolescents who wish to avoid a monthly period. In addition, an oral contraceptive that provides continuous, year-round contraception has been approved by the FDA. It contains levonorgestrel 90 mcg and ethinyl estradiol 20 mcg.

Until studies are conducted in adolescents, information on extended-cycle and continuous, year-round pills must be drawn from studies and clinical experience in adults. One-half to two-thirds of adult women report a decrease in breakthrough spotting or bleeding (BTB) in the second half compared with the first half of the extended or year-long regimen. To manage BTB, a 3-day, hormone-free interval was more beneficial than continuous pills [71].

A systematic review of continuous use of oral contraceptives in adult women found that other menstrual symptoms, including headaches, genital irritation, tiredness, bloating, and dysmenorrhea also improved with extended-cycle pill use [72].

14.12 Condoms

We always stress the benefit of dual-protection against both pregnancy and STIs. Girls planning to use condoms should receive them before leaving the office or clinic, if possible, to ensure availability and promote adherence.

14.13 Continuation Rate of Various Contraceptive Methods Among Adolescents

A systematic review of hormonal and intrauterine methods of contraception in young women found limited data about continuation rates [73]. Nevertheless, "zooming in" on the CHOICE project, the 12-month continuation rates among 1099 urban adolescents (age 14–19 years of age) who were provided with contraception at no cost were as follows: [74]

- Levonorgestrel intrauterine system ($n=330$) – 81 %
- Copper intrauterine device ($n=55$) – 76 %
- Etonogestrel implant ($n=378$) – 82 %
- Depot medroxyprogesterone acetate ($n=112$) – 47 %
- Oral contraceptives ($n=146$) – 47 %
- Contraceptive patch ($n=21$) – 41 %
- Vaginal ring ($n=57$) – 31 %

Continuation rates were greater among adolescents who used long-acting reversible contraception (i.e., levonorgestrel intrauterine system, copper intrauterine device, or etonogestrel implant) than other methods (84.7 versus 44 %). This study strengthens further, that *LARC should be first line contraception methods in this age group if we truly want to prevent unintended pregnancy.*

14.14 Providing Contraception to Adolescents with Chronic Illness

Hormonal contraception for the chronically ill adolescent can be a challenge. Estrogen-based hormonal contraceptives, as an example, should not be offered to an adolescent with significant valvular disease who is not being treated with an anticoagulant. Although DMPA is useful in such cases, its effect on fluid retention should be evaluated and monitored.

Similarly, estrogen-based hormonal contraceptives should not be offered to an adolescent with antiphospholipid antibody abnormalities, uncontrollable hypertension, and vascular involvement. DMPA is useful in such cases; there have been no reports of systemic lupus erythematosus flares with long-term DMPA use.

In addition, multiphasic or ultra-low dose oral estrogen-progestin contraceptives are not recommended in adolescents taking many anticonvulsants because anticonvulsants other than valproic acid increase the clearance of sex steroids. DMPA is a good alternative because progesterone levels are high enough to be unaffected by increased P-450 activity.

Other medications that alter the effectiveness of estrogen-based hormonal contraceptives by increasing clearance of sex steroids include rifampin, griseofulvin, and certain antiretroviral agents. Herbal medication such as St. John's Wort also can increase clearance of sex steroids. There are inadequate data to support any significant drug interaction between common antibiotics and estrogen-based hormonal contraceptives.

It is important to review the choice of hormonal contraceptives in the context of the chronic illness, potential increase in estrogen-related complications, and drug interactions during the counseling process. The risk of pregnancy needs to be weighed against the risk of a medical complication from hormonal contraception. In addition, emergency contraception should be discussed with adolescents whose current treatment may be teratogenic to the fetus or in whom pregnancy would severely compromise health [75].

Detailed guidelines for contraceptive methods in patients with medical issues were recently updated but the World Health Organization and are available online at http://www.who.int/reproductivehealth/publications/family_planning/MEC-5/en/

Bibliography

1. WHO publication, Adolescent pregnancy. 2012
2. Chibber R, Fouda M, Al-Hijji J et al (2014) Adverse pregnancy outcome among teenagers: a reality? J Obstetr Gynaecol J Inst Obstetr Gynaecol 34(4):297–300
3. WHO Publication, adolescent pregnancy, Fact sheet N°364. Sept 2014
4. Nelson AI, Neinstein LS (2009) Contraception. In: Neinstein LS, Gordon CM, Katzman DK (eds) Handbook of adolescent health care. Lippincott Williams & Wilkins, Philadelphia, p 389
5. Secura GM, Madden T, McNicholas C et al (2014) Provision of no-cost, long-acting contraception and teenage pregnancy. N Engl J Med 371(14):1316–1323
6. Sanfilippo JS (1991) Adolescents and oral contraceptives. Int J Fertil 36(Suppl 2):65–77; discussion 77–69
7. Braverman PK, Breech L, Committee on Adolescence, American Academy of Pediatrics (2010) Clinical report – gynecologic examination for adolescents in the pediatric office setting. Pediatrics 126(3):583–590
8. (2005) 'Black box' warning added to contraceptive injection. FDA Consum. 39(2):3
9. Cromer BA, Scholes D, Berenson A et al (2006) Depot medroxyprogesterone acetate and bone mineral density in adolescents –the black box warning: a position paper of the society for adolescent medicine. J Adolesc Health 39(2):296–301
10. Vandenbroucke JP, Rosing J, Bloemenkamp KW et al (2001) Oral contraceptives and the risk of venous thrombosis. N Engl J Med 344(20):1527–1535
11. Douketis JD, Ginsberg JS, Holbrook A, Crowther M, Duku EK, Burrows RF (1997) A reevaluation of the risk for venous thromboembolism with the use of oral contraceptives and hormone replacement therapy. Arch Intern Med 157(14):1522–1530

12. Bloemenkamp KW, Rosendaal FR, Buller HR, Helmerhorst FM, Colly LP, Vandenbroucke JP (1999) Risk of venous thrombosis with use of current low-dose oral contraceptives is not explained by diagnostic suspicion and referral bias. Arch Intern Med 159(1):65–70
13. PhVWP Monthly report on safety concerns, guidelines and general matters. European Medicines Agency; Jan 2012
14. Rosing J, Tans G, Nicolaes GA et al (1997) Oral contraceptives and venous thrombosis: different sensitivities to activated protein C in women using second- and third-generation oral contraceptives. Br J Haematol 97(1):233–238
15. Rosing J, Middeldorp S, Curvers J et al (1999) Low-dose oral contraceptives and acquired resistance to activated protein C: a randomised cross-over study. Lancet 354(9195): 2036–2040
16. Middeldorp S, Meijers JC, van den Ende AE et al (2000) Effects on coagulation of levonorgestrel- and desogestrel-containing low dose oral contraceptives: a cross-over study. Thromb Haemost 84(1):4–8
17. Kemmeren JM, Algra A, Meijers JC, Bouma BN, Grobbee DE (2002) Effects of second and third generation oral contraceptives and their respective progestagens on the coagulation system in the absence or presence of the factor V Leiden mutation. Thromb Haemost 87(2): 199–205
18. Kemmeren JM, Algra A, Meijers JC et al (2004) Effect of second- and third-generation oral contraceptives on the protein C system in the absence or presence of the factor VLeiden mutation: a randomized trial. Blood 103(3):927–933
19. Sidney S, Petitti DB, Soff GA, Cundiff DL, Tolan KK, Quesenberry CP Jr (2004) Venous thromboembolic disease in users of low-estrogen combined estrogen-progestin oral contraceptives. Contraception 70(1):3–10
20. Pomp ER, le Cessie S, Rosendaal FR, Doggen CJ (2007) Risk of venous thrombosis: obesity and its joint effect with oral contraceptive use and prothrombotic mutations. Br J Haematol 139(2):289–296
21. Abdollahi M, Cushman M, Rosendaal FR (2003) Obesity: risk of venous thrombosis and the interaction with coagulation factor levels and oral contraceptive use. Thromb Haemost 89(3):493–498
22. Nightingale AL, Lawrenson RA, Simpson EL, Williams TJ, MacRae KD, Farmer RD (2000) The effects of age, body mass index, smoking and general health on the risk of venous thromboembolism in users of combined oral contraceptives. Eur J Contracept Reprod Health Care 5(4):265–274
23. Louv WC, Austin H, Perlman J, Alexander WJ (1989) Oral contraceptive use and the risk of chlamydial and gonococcal infections. Am J Obstet Gynecol 160(2):396–402
24. Rubin GL, Ory HW, Layde PM (1982) Oral contraceptives and pelvic inflammatory disease. Am J Obstet Gynecol 144(6):630–635
25. Ness RB, Keder LM, Soper DE et al (1997) Oral contraception and the recognition of endometritis. Am J Obstet Gynecol 176(3):580–585
26. Wolner-Hanssen P, Svensson L, Mardh PA, Westrom L (1985) Laparoscopic findings and contraceptive use in women with signs and symptoms suggestive of acute salpingitis. Obstet Gynecol 66(2):233–238
27. Ness RB, Soper DE, Holley RL et al (2001) Hormonal and barrier contraception and risk of upper genital tract disease in the PID Evaluation and Clinical Health (PEACH) study. Am J Obstet Gynecol 185(1):121–127
28. Godfrey EM (2015) Helping clinicians prevent pregnancy among sexually active adolescents: U.S. medical eligibility criteria for contraceptive use and U.S. selected practice recommendations for contraceptive use. J Pediatr Adolesc Gynecol 28(4):209–214
29. Emans SJ, Grace E, Woods ER, Smith DE, Klein K, Merola J (1987) Adolescents' compliance with the use of oral contraceptives. JAMA 257(24):3377–3381
30. Bagwell MA, Thompson SJ, Addy CL, Coker AL, Baker ER (1995) Primary infertility and oral contraceptive steroid use. Fertil Steril 63(6):1161–1166

31. Trussell J, Guthrie KA (2007) Talking straight about emergency contraception. J Fam Plann Reprod Health Care 33(3):139–142
32. Gemzell-Danielsson K (2010) Mechanism of action of emergency contraception. Contraception 82(5):404–409
33. Gemzell-Danielsson K, Berger C (2013) P GLL. Emergency contraception – mechanisms of action. Contraception 87(3):300–308
34. Cheng L, Che Y, Gulmezoglu AM (2012) Interventions for emergency contraception. Cochrane Database Syst Rev 8, CD001324
35. Emergency contraception. Faculty of sexual and reproductive healthcare clinical guidance. Jan 2012
36. (2015) Practice Bulletin No. 152: emergency contraception. Obstet Gynecol. 126(3):e1–e11
37. Kapp N, Abitbol JL, Mathe H et al (2015) Effect of body weight and BMI on the efficacy of levonorgestrel emergency contraception. Contraception 91(2):97–104
38. Levonorgestrel and ulipristal remain suitable emergency contraceptives for all women, regardless of bodyweight. European Medicines Agency. Press release 24/7/2014. http://www.ema.europa.eu/ema/index.jsp?curl=pages/news_and_events/news/2014/07/news_detail_002145.jsp&mid=WC0b01ac058004d5c1ht
39. Salcedo J, Rodriguez MI, Curtis KM, Kapp N (2013) When can a woman resume or initiate contraception after taking emergency contraceptive pills? A systematic review. Contraception 87(5):602–604
40. Ulipristal acetate. US FDA approved product information. National Library of Medicine
41. Clinical Effectiveness Unit (2011) Combined hormonal contraception. Faculty of Sexual and Reproductive Healthcare, London
42. Committee on Adolescent Health Care Long-Acting Reversible Contraception Working Group, TACoO, Gynecologists (2012) Committee opinion no. 539: adolescents and long-acting reversible contraception: implants and intrauterine devices. Obstet Gynecol 120(4):983–988
43. Ott MA, Sucato GS, Committee on Adolescents (2014) Contraception for adolescents. Pediatrics 134(4):e1257–e1281
44. Hubacher D, Goco N, Gonzalez B, Taylor D (1999) Factors affecting continuation rates of DMPA. Contraception 60(6):345–351
45. Logsdon S, Richards J, Omar HA (2004) Long-term evaluation of the use of the transdermal contraceptive patch in adolescents. ScientificWorldJournal 4:512–516
46. Rubinstein ML, Halpern-Felsher BL, Irwin CE Jr (2004) An evaluation of the use of the transdermal contraceptive patch in adolescents. J Adolesc Health 34(5):395–401
47. Zacur HA, Hedon B, Mansour D, Shangold GA, Fisher AC, Creasy GW (2002) Integrated summary of ortho Evra/Evra contraceptive patch adhesion in varied climates and conditions. Fertil Steril 77(2 Suppl 2):S32–S35
48. Creasy GW, Abrams LS, Fisher AC (2001) Transdermal contraception. Semin Reprod Med 19(4):373–380
49. Stanwood NL, Garrett JM, Konrad TR (2002) Obstetrician-gynecologists and the intrauterine device: a survey of attitudes and practice. Obstet Gynecol 99(2):275–280
50. American College of Obstetricians, Gynecologists Committee on Gynecologic Practice, Long-Acting Reversible Contraception Working Group (2009) ACOG Committee Opinion no. 450: increasing use of contraceptive implants and intrauterine devices to reduce unintended pregnancy. Obstet Gynecol 114(6):1434–1438
51. Teal SB, Romer SE, Goldthwaite LM, Peters MG, Kaplan DW, Sheeder J (2015) Insertion characteristics of intrauterine devices in adolescents and young women: success, ancillary measures, and complications. Am J Obstet Gynecol 213:515.e1–515.e5
52. World Health Organization, Reproductive Health and Research (2010) Medical eligibility criteria for contraceptive use: a WHO family planning cornerstone, 4th edn. World Health Organization/Reproductive Health and Research, Geneva
53. Stanford JB, Mikolajczyk RT (2002) Mechanisms of action of intrauterine devices: update and estimation of postfertilization effects. Am J Obstet Gynecol 187(6):1699–1708
54. Rozin S, Schwartz A, Schenker JG (1969) The mode of action of an intrauterine contraceptive device. Int J Fertil 14(2):174–179

55. Rickert VI, Tiezzi L, Lipshutz J, Leon J, Vaughan RD, Westhoff C (2007) Depo now: preventing unintended pregnancies among adolescents and young adults. J Adolesc Health 40(1): 22–28
56. Steiner MJ, Kwok C, Stanback J et al (2008) Injectable contraception: what should the longest interval be for reinjections? Contraception 77(6):410–414
57. Nelson AL, Katz T (2007) Initiation and continuation rates seen in 2-year experience with same day injections of DMPA. Contraception 75(2):84–87
58. Lei ZW, Wu SC, Garceau RJ et al (1996) Effect of pretreatment counseling on discontinuation rates in Chinese women given depo-medroxyprogesterone acetate for contraception. Contraception 53(6):357–361
59. Canto De Cetina TE, Canto P, Ordonez Luna M (2001) Effect of counseling to improve compliance in Mexican women receiving depot-medroxyprogesterone acetate. Contraception 63(3):143–146
60. Westfall JM, Main DS, Barnard L (1996) Continuation rates among injectable contraceptive users. Fam Plann Perspect 28(6):275–277
61. Polaneczky M, Guarnaccia M, Alon J, Wiley J (1996) Early experience with the contraceptive use of depot medroxyprogesterone acetate in an inner-city clinic population. Fam Plann Perspect 28(4):174–178
62. Mulders TM, Dieben TO (2001) Use of the novel combined contraceptive vaginal ring NuvaRing for ovulation inhibition. Fertil Steril 75(5):865–870
63. U.S. Selected Practice Recommendations for Contraceptive Use (2013): Adapted from the World Health Organization Selected Practice Recommendations for Contraceptive Use, 2nd Edition. Recommendations and Reports 62(RR05):1–46
64. Barreiros FA, Guazzelli CA, Barbosa R, de Assis F, de Araujo FF (2010) Extended regimens of the contraceptive vaginal ring: evaluation of clinical aspects. Contraception 81(3):223–225
65. Miller L, Verhoeven CH, Hout J (2005) Extended regimens of the contraceptive vaginal ring: a randomized trial. Obstet Gynecol 106(3):473–482
66. Barreiros FA, Guazzelli CA, de Araujo FF, Barbosa R (2007) Bleeding patterns of women using extended regimens of the contraceptive vaginal ring. Contraception 75(3):204–208
67. Guazzelli CA, Barreiros FA, Barbosa R, de Araujo FF, Moron AF (2009) Extended regimens of the vaginal contraceptive ring: cycle control. Contraception 80(5):430–435
68. Barreiros FA, Guazzelli CA, Barbosa R, Torloni MR, Barbieri M, Araujo FF (2011) Extended regimens of the combined contraceptive vaginal ring containing etonogestrel and ethinyl estradiol: effects on lipid metabolism. Contraception 84(2):155–159
69. Polaneczky M, Slap G, Forke C, Rappaport A, Sondheimer S (1994) The use of levonorgestrel implants (Norplant) for contraception in adolescent mothers. N Engl J Med 331(18): 1201–1206
70. Lara-Torre E (2004) "Quick Start", an innovative approach to the combination oral contraceptive pill in adolescents. Is it time to make the switch? J Pediatr Adolesc Gynecol 17(1):65–67
71. Coffee AL, Sulak PJ, Kuehl TJ (2007) Long-term assessment of symptomatology and satisfaction of an extended oral contraceptive regimen. Contraception 75(6):444–449
72. Edelman A, Gallo MF, Nichols MD, Jensen JT, Schulz KF, Grimes DA (2006) Continuous versus cyclic use of combined oral contraceptives for contraception: systematic Cochrane review of randomized controlled trials. Hum Reprod 21(3):573–578
73. Krashin J, Tang JH, Mody S, Lopez LM (2015) Hormonal and intrauterine methods for contraception for women aged 25 years and younger. Cochrane Database Syst Rev. (8):CD009805
74. Rosenstock JR, Peipert JF, Madden T, Zhao Q, Secura GM (2012) Continuation of reversible contraception in teenagers and young women. Obstet Gynecol 120(6):1298–1305
75. Gold MA, Sucato GS, Conard LA, Hillard PJ, Society for Adolescent Medicine (2004) Provision of emergency contraception to adolescents. J Adolesc Health 35(1):67–70
76. World Health Organization (WHO), Department of Reproductive Health and Research, Johns Hopkins Bloomberg School of Public Health/Center for Communication Programs (CCP) (2011) Knowledge for health project. Family planning: a global handbook for providers (2011 update). CPP and WHO, Baltimore, Geneva
77. Trussell J (2011) Contraceptive failure in the United States. Contraception 83:397

Index

C. Sultan, A.R. Genazzani (eds.), *Frontiers in Gynecological Endocrinology*, ISGE Series, DOI 10.1007/978-3-319-41433-1